Equine Anesthesia and Pain Management

Equine Anesthesia and Pain Management: A Color Handbook brings together key information for clinicians in an easy-to-use, problem-orientated format. It disseminates a wealth of knowledge about horse, donkey and mule anesthesia and pain management in a quick reference style, with a focus on clinical practice. Fifteen chapters by expert contributors cover everything from anesthetic equipment, premedication and physical restraint, to total intravenous anesthesia, inhalant anesthesia and partial intravenous anesthesia, recovery, complications and euthanasia. Over 250 superb color photographs and diagrams bring the material to life.

This book will be invaluable to all those who need practical information easily to hand, whether equine practitioner, veterinary technician or nurse, or veterinary student.

Veterinary Color Handbook Series

PUBLISHED TITLES

A Colour Handbook of Skin Diseases of the Dog and Cat UK Version, Second Edition,
by Patrick J. McKeever, Tim Nuttall and Richard G. Harvey

Urinary Stones in Small Animal Medicine: A Colour Handbook,
by Albrecht Hesse and Reto Neiger

Small Animal Dental, Oral and Maxillofacial Disease: A Colour Handbook,
by Brook A. Niemiec

Small Animal Emergency and Critical Care Medicine: A Color Handbook,
by Elizabeth A. Rozanski and John E. Rush

Small Animal Anesthesia and Pain Management: A Color Handbook,
by Jeff Ko

Small Animal Fluid Therapy, Acid-base and Electrolyte Disorders: A Color Handbook,
by Elisa M. Mazzaferro

Skin Diseases of the Dog and Cat, Third Edition,
by Tim Nuttall, Melissa Eisenschenk, Nicole A. Heinrich and Richard G. Harvey

Small Animal Anesthesia and Pain Management: A Color Handbook, Second Edition,
edited by Jeff Ko

Infectious Diseases of the Dog and Cat: A Colour Handbook,
edited by Scott Weese and Michelle Evason

Equine Anesthesia and Pain Management: A Color Handbook,
edited by Michele Barletta, Jane Quandt and Rachel Reed

For more information about this series, please visit:
www.crcpress.com/Veterinary-Color-Handbook-Series/book-series/CRCVETCOLHAN

Equine Anesthesia and Pain Management

A Color Handbook

Edited by

MICHELE BARLETTA
JANE QUANDT
RACHEL REED

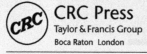

CRC Press
Taylor & Francis Group
Boca Raton London

CRC Press is an imprint of the
Taylor & Francis Group, an **informa** business

First edition published 2023
by CRC Press
6000 Broken Sound Parkway NW, Suite 300, Boca Raton, FL 33487–2742

and by CRC Press
4 Park Square, Milton Park, Abingdon, Oxon, OX14 4RN

CRC Press is an imprint of Taylor & Francis Group, LLC

© 2023 Taylor & Francis Group, LLC

ISBN: 978-1-032-30962-0 (hbk)
ISBN: 978-1-498-74958-9 (pbk)
ISBN: 978-0-429-19094-0 (ebk)

DOI: 10.1201/9780429190940

Typeset in Janson
by Apex CoVantage, LLC

CONTENTS

PREFACE

The purpose of this book is to provide a centralized resource of basic and advanced information regarding anesthesia of equine patients. Within these chapters, the reader can find the basic knowledge required to anesthetize horses and prevent and manage common complications that may develop during sedation, anesthesia and recovery. Our target audience is veterinary students, practitioners and technicians who are learning the basics of equine anesthesia as well as practitioners and technicians with more advanced skills in this field. At the end of each chapter, we reference other books and manuscripts where the reader can find more information about the topic. Several chapters also include case examples, which are meant to provide a practical scenario, including sedation and anesthetic drugs, doses and tips for the overall management of the anesthetic event.

The editors sought out authors who are leaders in their field and highly qualified to write about the topic. Our authors worked to create chapters that cover the necessary information for safe equine sedation and anesthesia.

This book is meant to be used as a practical reference for practitioners in the operating room and in the field. We chose a bullet-point format which allows the reader to quickly find the information needed.

Pictures and illustrations are included in each chapter to help explain concepts and techniques described in the text. Several tables are also provided to summarize information for the reader. Editing this book was an exciting journey for us, and we believe that the result of our efforts is a comprehensive resource on anesthesia for the equine anesthetist.

Michele Barletta, DVM, MS, PhD, ACVAA, graduated from the University of Turin, Italy, in 2002 and obtained his PhD in 2006. After completion of his degrees, he moved to the United States, where he completed a rotating internship in small animal medicine and surgery at Purdue University in 2007. After his internship he stayed at Purdue University for his anesthesiology residency and masters degree. He worked at the University of Minnesota for three years as assistant clinical professor in anesthesiology. In 2013, Dr. Barletta joined the University of Georgia, where he is currently working as associate professor. In addition to being a Diplomate of the American College of Veterinary Anesthesia and Analgesia, he has published several journal articles and book chapters and has presented at many national and international conferences on topics related to anesthesia and analgesia in both small and large animal species. His research and clinical interests include acute and chronic pain, anesthetic management of the critical patient and equine anesthesia.

Jane Quandt, DVM, MS, DACVAA, DACVECC, graduated from Iowa State University College of Veterinary Medicine in 1987. After working in small animal practice for one year, she decided to pursue an anesthesia residency. She completed the residency and masters in anesthesia at the University of Minnesota and became boarded in anesthesia in 1993. In order to improve her ability to manage critical cases she did a second residency and became boarded in small animal emergency and critical care in 2007. She was on faculty at the College of Veterinary Medicine at the University of Minnesota for ten years. She joined the faculty at the University of Georgia College of Veterinary Medicine in 2011 and is currently a tenured full professor in comparative anesthesia. She has published several journal articles and book chapters and has presented at national and international conferences on topics related to anesthesia and analgesia in both small and large animal species. Dr. Quandt has had the privilege of being awarded the Carl Norden-Pfizer Distinguished Veterinary Teacher Award and the Zoetis Distinguished Veterinary Teacher Award.

Rachel Reed, DVM, DACVAA, graduated from North Carolina State University College of Veterinary Medicine in 2011. Following graduation, Dr. Reed spent two years in mixed animal private practice before pursuing a residency in veterinary anesthesia and analgesia at the University of Tennessee in Knoxville. Following residency and board certification in the American College of Veterinary Anesthesia and Analgesia, Dr. Reed joined the anesthesia service at the University of Georgia College of Veterinary Medicine, where she is currently working as a clinical associate professor. Dr. Reed has published several journal articles and book chapters in addition to presenting at national and international conferences. Her interest is in equine analgesia and the use of opioids for management of acute pain in horses.

ACKNOWLEDGEMENT

The editors would like to thank Bonnie Lockridge BASc, RVT, VTS (Anesthesia & Analgesia) for providing several pictures included in this book.

CHAPTER 1

ANESTHESIA EQUIPMENT

Rachel Reed, Stephanie Kleine and Michele Barletta

1

1.1 INTRODUCTION

Anesthetic procedures lasting longer than one hour are best managed anesthetically with the use of equipment providing a means of oxygen delivery and positive pressure ventilation. This also allows for the use of inhalants if an anesthetic machine with a vaporizer is employed.

The equipment necessary for equine anesthesia depends on the procedure, the location and environment, and the anesthetic plan.

1.2 MEDICAL GASES

- The purity of medical gases is enforced by the Food and Drug Administration.
- Oxygen is the primary carrier gas utilized in equine anesthesia, and it is available in three forms:
  1) Compressed gas cylinders
     - The requirements for manufacturing, labeling, filling, transportation, storage, handling, maintenance, and disposition are published by the Department of Transportation.
     - Cylinders are available in various sizes classified by letters A through H, A being the smallest. Size E (**Figure 1.1**) is commonly used for situations where oxygen must be transported to or with the patient. Cylinders can be mounted to small-animal anesthesia machines to use for foals and donkeys (up to 120–150 kg body weight). Size H (**Figure 1.2**) is commonly used in veterinary hospitals

as the primary oxygen source and can be used as individual cylinders to operate large-animal anesthesia machines or connected together to form an oxygen bank. When the latter system is used, the oxygen is delivered to the desired location in the hospital via a pipeline system (**Table 1.1**).

- The body of most cylinders is composed of steel or steel carbon fiber.
- MRI-safe cylinders made of aluminum are available.
- Medical gas cylinders are color-coded. Oxygen is green in the U.S. (white internationally). Medical-grade air is yellow.
- Compressed gas cylinders are an ideal source of oxygen for ambulatory procedures and low-volume surgical clinics.
- Cylinders should be carefully stored, preferably indoors at room temperature and out of direct exposure to sunlight which could result in overheating of the cylinder. Exposure to temperatures colder than 20°F or warmer than 130°F should be strictly prohibited.
- Only personnel with cylinder safety training should transport or use the cylinder. Care should be taken to constantly support the cylinder and not allow the cylinder to fall or strike any other object with appreciable force. Damaged cylinders can become

DOI: 10.1201/9780429190940-1

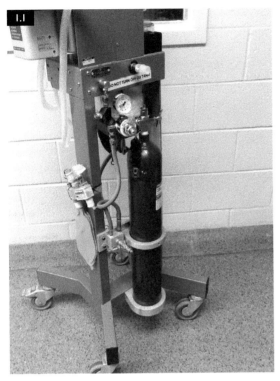

Figure 1.1 **E cylinder**

projectiles that can cause damage to property and life-threatening injury to personnel.

2) Liquid oxygen
   - Liquid oxygen units (**Figure 1.3**) are available as stationary units maintained at the location of oxygen use. They are refilled by a gas supplier as needed.
   - The liquid oxygen is stored at -148°C in an insulated container.
   - Oxygen is supplied to the hospital in gaseous form from the liquid gas source via a pipeline system.
   - It is ideal for hospitals with a high surgical case load where the financial investment in liquid oxygen is justified.

3) Oxygen concentrators
   - These units employ a molecular sieve to absorb nitrogen, carbon dioxide, carbon monoxide, and water vapor from ambient air, allowing for oxygen

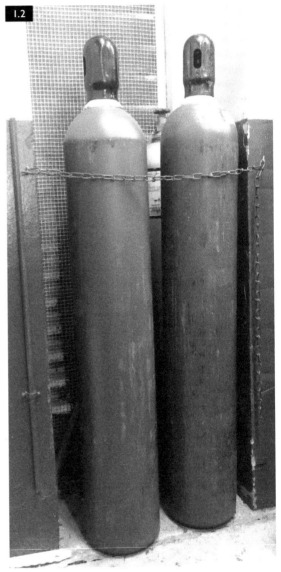

Figure 1.2 **H cylinders**

Table 1.1 **Oxygen cylinders**

SIZE	WEIGHT (LBS)	VOLUME (L)	PRESSURE (PSI)
E	14	660	1,900
H	119	6900	2,200

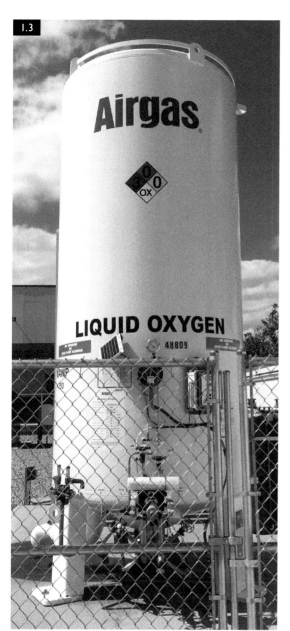

Figure 1.3 Liquid oxygen

and argon to pass through. They also filter out most airborne contaminants and are fairly reliable machines.
- The resulting gas is 90–96% oxygen, although the oxygen output might be lower (as low as 73%).

- These units can be cheaper than liquid oxygen; however, they require some maintenance, and the oxygen output should be checked periodically using an oxygen analyzer.

1.3   THE ANESTHESIA MACHINE

It is generally divided into three regions: high-, intermediate-, and low-pressure systems.

1) High-pressure system
   - Pressures in this area can be as high as 2,200 psi, depending on the existing pressure of the gas cylinder.
   - Includes cylinders, hanger yokes, yoke blocks, high pressure hoses, pressure gauges, and the pressure reducing valve.
   - Size E cylinders are commonly attached to portable anesthesia machines (used for foals and donkeys) via the yoke. The yoke serves to position and support the cylinder, provide a tight gas seal, and provide unidirectional gas flow.
   - The yoke (**Figure 1.4**) has several components. The body of the yoke is the framework of the unit. The retaining screw is used to attach the cylinder to the yoke. The nipple is the port through which gas travels to enter the machine. The index pins are a safety system ensuring that the correct gas is used in the system. The washer is used to form a seal preventing leakage of gas from the cylinder. A check valve is in place to prevent bidirectional gas flow.
   - Pressure gauges receive high-pressure gas from the cylinder, and the pressure is indicated on the gauge in either kPa or psi (**Figure 1.5**).
   - Pressure-reducing valves (regulator valves) serve to reduce the pressure in the high-pressure system to a more constant pressure of 40–55 psi and to prevent

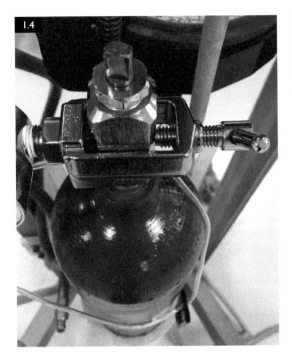

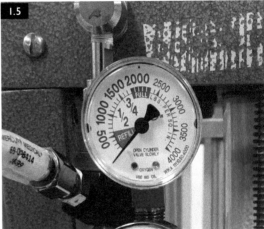

Figure 1.5 Pressure gauge

Figure 1.4 Hanger yoke

fluctuations in pressure as the cylinder empties.

2) Intermediate-pressure system
   • The intermediate-pressure system receives gas from the pressure regulator at 40–55 psi and carries it to the flush valve, demand valve, or flowmeter of the low-pressure system.
   • Intermediate-pressure hoses are color coded based on gas content in the same fashion as the cylinders.
   • Hospital pipeline systems can incorporate one of two different safety systems to ensure connection of the correct hose to the house main oxygen supply. The first is a diameter index safety system (**Figure 1.6**) in which the threads of the intermediate pressure hose of a specific gas will only fit the threads of its gas inlet. The second is a keyed quick-connect system (**Figure 1.7**) in which the position of pins in the connection device prevents connection of the hose to the wrong gas source.

   • The flush valve (**Figure 1.8**) provides a large volume of gas to the anesthetic circuit rapidly. This gas bypasses the vaporizer, therefore it does not contain inhalant anesthetic. Gas flowing through the flush valve is delivered at 35–75 l/min.
   • Demand valves (**Figure 1.9**) are used to provide positive pressure ventilation to large animals. Demand valves are triggered by two different mechanisms: 1) manually by pushing the button on the top of the valve or 2) the development of negative pressure at the valve outlet when the animal takes a breath.
     • The valve outlet is designed to fit into the opening of various endotracheal tube styles via the use of different adaptors. When attached to an

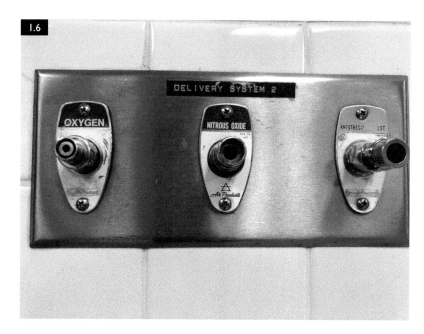

Figure 1.6 Diameter index safety system

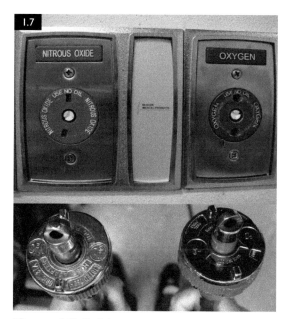

Figure 1.7 Quick-connect system

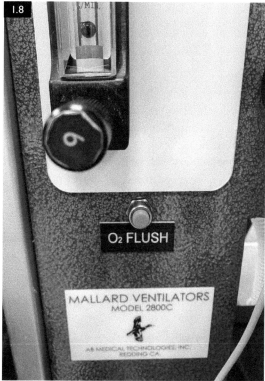

Figure 1.8 Flush valve

endotracheal tube, the demand valve will fire when the patient generates enough negative airway pressure to trigger the valve.

- If the demand valve is left in place during expiration, there is greater

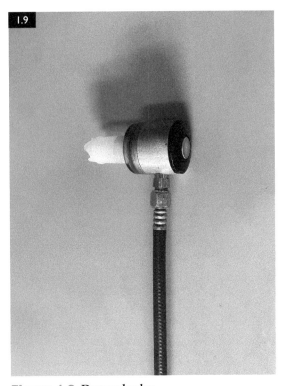

Figure 1.9 **Demand valve**

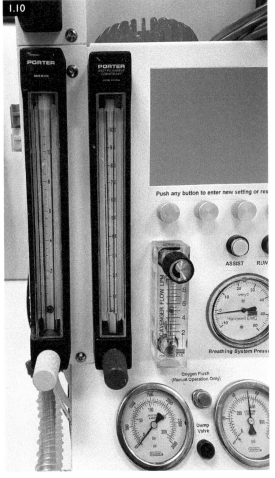

Figure 1.10 **Flowmeters**

resistance to expiration than if the demand valve is removed during this time.
- Demand valves are used extensively in equine anesthesia to deliver positive pressure ventilation in patients under anesthesia for short periods of time or to support ventilation in patients just taken off a ventilator until the patient starts to breathe spontaneously.
- They can deliver 160–200 l/min of oxygen at 50 psi.

3) Low-pressure system
- The low-pressure system of the anesthetic machine receives gas from the intermediate-pressure system at the flowmeter and includes flowmeter, vaporizer, conduit from the vaporizer to the circuit, breathing circuit, adjustable pressure limiting valve, CO_2 absorbent, and rebreathing bag.

- Flowmeters (**Figure 1.10**)
  - At this stage, the pressure of the gas is reduced from 40–50 psi down to just above ambient pressure.
  - Flowmeters control the rate of delivery of gas to the anesthetic circuit. These units generally incorporate a tapered glass tube and float.
  - Turning a knob at the bottom of the flowmeter adjusts flow through the flowmeter. As gas flow through the tube increases, the float moves higher up the tube, allowing more gas to pass

around it. The tube is labeled with the associated flow rates of various float positions.

- Several float types exist; ball type floats should be read at the middle of the ball, while other float types should be read at the top of the float.
- Flowmeters are calibrated as a unit at 760 mmHg and 20°C. If any component of the flowmeter fails, the entire unit should be replaced.
- Modern precision flowmeters have an accuracy of ± 2.5%.
- Use of a flowmeter at high altitude results in a higher flow through the flowmeter than indicated on the tube.

- Vaporizers
  - They are used to administer inhalant anesthetic agents such as sevoflurane and isoflurane. Vaporizers receive oxygen from the flowmeter, incorporate inhalant anesthetic into the carrier gas, and the mixture of oxygen and inhalant anesthetic is then directed through the common gas outlet.
  - Modern vaporizers are concentration-calibrated, agent-specific, and designed to be used outside and upstream of the breathing circuit. They are categorized based on how the inhalant enters the carrier gas into flow-over type and injection type vaporizers.
  - Flow-over type vaporizers include vaporizers designed for isoflurane, sevoflurane (**Figure 1.11**), and halothane. They incorporate a variable bypass system in which the oxygen supplied to the vaporizer is split into carrier gas, which is directed to the vaporizing chamber, and bypass gas, which goes into the bypass channel, based on the position of the concentration control dial.

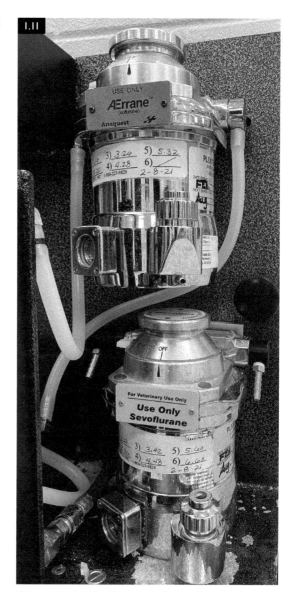

Figure 1.11 Isoflurane and sevoflurane vaporizers

As the dial is adjusted to a higher percentage, more gas passes through the vaporization chamber, picking up inhalant anesthetic before joining the bypass gas and exiting the vaporizer. This "splitting ratio" determines the partial pressure of inhalant anesthetic leaving the vaporizer. When these vaporizers are used at high altitudes, the same partial pressure of inhalant anesthetic leaves the vaporizer as would be expected at sea level. Although this partial pressure represents a greater percent concentration of ambient pressure than indicated on the vaporizer control dial, it is the partial pressure which determines the patient's anesthetic depth, and therefore the vaporizer can continue to be used in the same way.

- Injection type vaporizers are used for desflurane (**Figure 1.12**). Due to the high vapor pressure of desflurane, it is impossible to use the traditional flow-over type vaporizer and achieve precise concentrations of desflurane. The injection type vaporizers used for desflurane are electronic, requiring a source of electricity. The liquid anesthetic is heated and pressurized before being injected into the carrier gas in accordance with the vaporizer dial setting and the flow of oxygen through the machine. Injection vaporizers will continue to deliver the same percent concentration when used at high altitudes. This percent concentration now represents a smaller partial pressure due to lower ambient pressure at altitude. Therefore, use of a desflurane vaporizer at altitude may require a higher dial setting to maintain anesthesia than would be required at sea level.

1.4   THE BREATHING CIRCUIT

- The breathing circuit serves to carry gas from the common gas outlet to the patient and to remove exhaled gases from the patient.
- Breathings circuits are broadly classified into rebreathing and non-rebreathing circuits.
- Rebreathing circuits (**Figure 1.13**) incorporate a mechanism for CO_2 absorption, and gases are recycled around the circuit during the anesthetic period.
  - The most common type of rebreathing system is the circle system. In this system, gas in the breathing circuit is propelled around the circle via the inspiration and expiration of the patient, with the expiratory and inspiratory one-way valves ensuring unidirectional flow. Proper function of the inspiratory and expiratory one-way valves is critical to proper function of a circle rebreathing system.

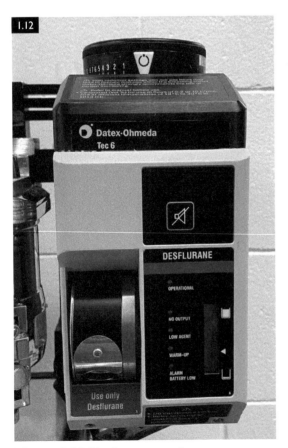

Figure 1.12 **Desflurane vaporizer**

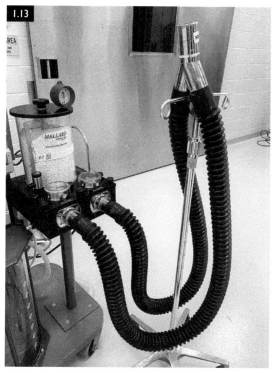

Figure 1.13 **Rebreathing circuit**

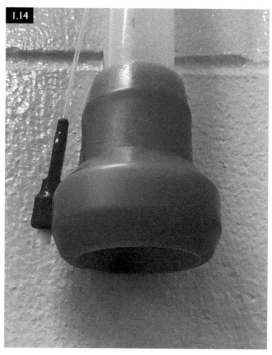

Figure 1.14 **Rubber bell**

- Another, less commonly used rebreathing circuit design is the to-and-fro circuit in which gas is expelled from the patient, through the CO_2 absorbent into a reservoir bag, and then inspired from the reservoir bag back through the CO_2 absorbent and into the patient.
- Both can be used as a closed or semi-closed system, depending on the oxygen flow. In a closed system the oxygen provided only meets the metabolic demand of the patient, while in a semi-closed system more oxygen is delivered (usually 10–20 ml/kg/min).
- Non-rebreathing circuits provide the patient's inspired tidal volume with gas directly from the common gas outlet. No rebreathing occurs thanks to the high fresh gas flow, and there is no need for CO_2 absorption. These circuits are not used in large animal patients due to the high flow rates necessary to prevent rebreathing.
- Hoses used for breathing circuits in equine anesthesia usually have an internal diameter of 50 mm. Y-pieces used on these hoses connect to endotracheal tube openings via rubber bell (**Figure 1.14**) connections or Bivona (**Figure 1.15**) insert connections.
- Hoses used in small animal anesthesia, with an internal diameter of 22 mm, can be used for smaller patients (foals and donkeys).

1.4.1 Carbon Dioxide Absorbent

- Absorption of CO_2 occurs at the carbon dioxide absorption canister. The canister is filled with commercial CO_2 absorbent granules which remove CO_2 from the airway gas via a chemical reaction.
- Canisters come in different sizes, and large canisters are mounted on the large-animal anesthesia machine. Although there is not

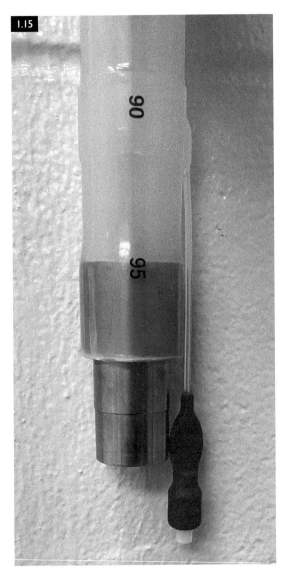

Figure 1.15   Bivona insert

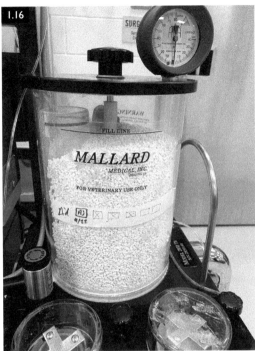

Figure 1.16 CO_2 absorbent canister

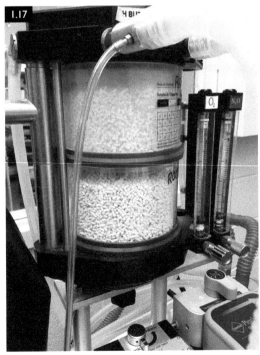

Figure 1.17   Anesthesia machine with double canister (CO_2 absorbent)

compelling evidence on the exact size, most recommend that the canister should be twice the tidal volume of the patient (in most cases this is not true for large-animal anesthesia machines) (**Figure 1.16**).

- When smaller patients (foals and donkeys) are anesthetized a small-animal anesthesia machine can be used. In this case it is recommended to use a machine with a double canister (**Figure 1.17**).

- The CO_2 absorbent granules contain a high level of calcium hydroxide, a strong base which reacts with CO_2 and water to produce carbonates.
- The CO_2 absorbent becomes exhausted as the base in the granules is depleted. There are several ways to ensure that the absorbent is changed before it has become completely exhausted.
  - To maximize its use, the CO_2 absorbent can be changed when the end tidal gas analyzer begins to indicate that the patient is rebreathing CO_2. Thus, CO_2 has made it through the absorbent canister without being removed from the circuit, which indicates absorbent exhaustion. This may be problematic if this occurs at the beginning of the anesthesia, and the CO_2 absorbent will need to be changed during the procedure.
  - A second method is to use the indicator dye that is incorporated into the absorbent. This indicator dye changes color as the pH of the absorbent begins to fall. Depending on the indicator dye in the CO_2 absorbent, the granules will begin to change color (i.e. change from white to purple with ethyl violet indicator) (**Figure 1.18**). It is recommended that when two-thirds of the granules have changed color, the canister should be refreshed. The caveat to this method is that when the machine is not in use, most granule types will return to the original color and may not be noticed by the next user until the rebreathing circuit is once again in use. Some types of CO_2 absorbent can maintain the color after the reaction, but they are more expensive.
  - Another, less precise but very safe method is to maintain a schedule in which the canisters are routinely changed after a set period of time, unless either of the above circumstances (rebreathing CO_2 or color change) are

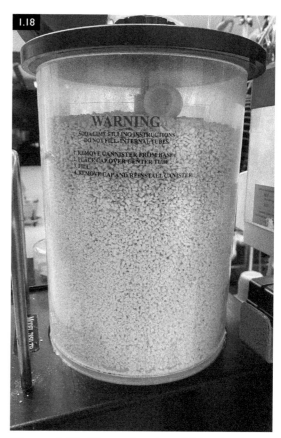

Figure 1.18 Change in color of CO_2 absorbent

met before the scheduled change occurs. This method has the added advantage of preventing use of CO_2 absorbent that has become desiccated due to prolonged disuse of an anesthesia machine resulting in drying of the absorbent granules.
- Before each use, it is recommended to crumble some granules from the canister between the fingers. If the granules break down easily, the CO_2 absorbent is still fresh; if they are hard, then it is probable that they are desiccated and ready to be changed.

1.4.2 The Reservoir Bag

- The reservoir bag serves many purposes, including providing a reserve of gas to buffer changes in circuit volume during the

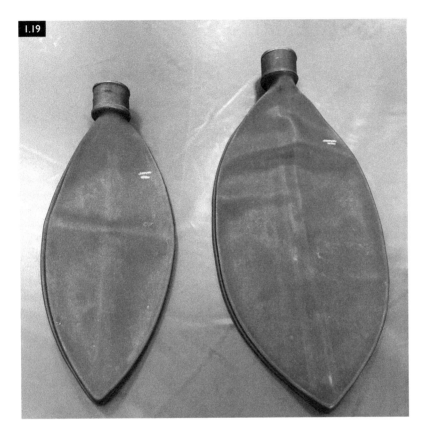

Figure 1.19 15-l and 30-l rebreathing bags

respiratory cycle, a means for administration of positive pressure ventilation, a visual aid in assessing the patient's respiratory rate and tidal volume, and direct feedback on the patient's lung compliance.

- Typically, the volume of the rebreathing bag used for a patient is calculated as five to ten times the tidal volume of the patient. Tidal volume is generally estimated to be 10–20 ml/kg. Fifteen- and 30-l rebreathing bags (**Figure 1.19**) are available for use in horses. A 5-l bag can be used for animals up to 200 kg of body weight.

1.4.3 The Adjustable Pressure Limiting Valve (APL Valve)

- The APL valve is also commonly referred to as the pop-off, the overflow, or the pressure relief valve (**Figure 1.20**).

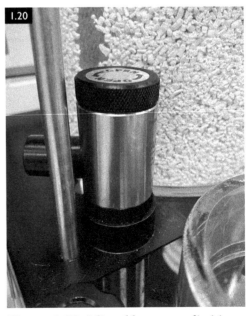

Figure 1.20 Adjustable pressure limiting (APL) valve

- This valve allows gas to escape from the circuit into the scavenge system. When completely open, APL valves are usually set to allow gas to exit the circuit when pressure within the system exceeds 1–3 cmH$_2$O.

1.5 ANESTHETIC GAS SCAVENGER

- Excess gas from the anesthetic circuit passes into the scavenge system. The scavenge system includes the APL valve, a conduit from the APL valve to the interface, a conduit from the interface to the elimination system, and the elimination system. The scavenge system can be either active or passive.
- Active scavenge systems (**Figure 1.21**) employ a suction to remove gas as it comes through the APL valve. It then passes through the interface. The interface is composed of three parts: the positive pressure relief valve, the negative pressure relief valve, and the reservoir bag. These components

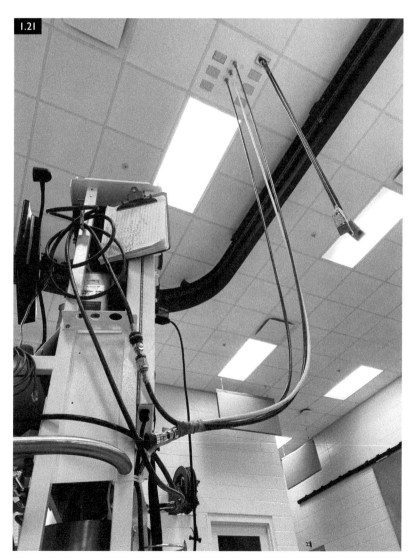

Figure 1.21 Active scavenge system

prevent adverse pressure effects on the breathing system and provide a place for gas to accumulate when not connected to suction. The waste gas is then carried to the elimination system, which can be either venting to outside air or absorption in activated charcoal.

- Passive systems (**Figure 1.22**) are much simpler. They incorporate a conduit from the APL valve either to an activated charcoal absorption canister or vented straight to the outside atmosphere.

- Scavenge systems are important to use and maintain in working order to prevent exposure of personnel to waste anesthetic gases. According to the Occupational Safety and Health Administration, scavenging systems are considered the preferred method to protect personnel from anesthetic gas exposure.

- Other measures that can be taken to limit exposure include careful filling of vaporizers in well-ventilated rooms and with minimal personnel involved

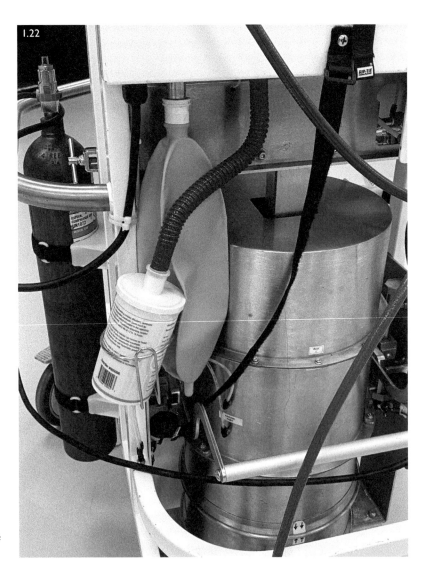

Figure 1.22 Passive scavenge system

(i.e. at the end of the day), ensuring that the anesthetic circuit is free of leaks, appropriate inflation of the endotracheal tube cuff, leaving the animal connected to the breathing circuit at the end of the procedure as long as possible, and avoidance of the patient's head and expired breath in the recovery period.

1.6   PRE-ANESTHETIC MACHINE CHECK

- Prior to use of any anesthesia machine, the machine should be evaluated to ensure proper function and to identify any leaks.
- An initial evaluation of the machine components is made, ensuring that all connections are in place and all components are properly functioning.
- The anesthetist should check to ensure that the gas source is present and with adequate oxygen supply. This involves checking the pressure of an oxygen cylinder, ensuring that the oxygen concentrator is functioning properly, or that the main oxygen supply is working appropriately.
- The machine should be leak-tested. Once all the components are in place, the APL valve is closed and the Y-piece is occluded. The circuit is then pressurized to 30 cmH$_2$O. If there is a leak greater than 250 ml/min, then the anesthetist should troubleshoot the machine to identify the leak.
- Lastly, the anesthetist should ensure that the ventilator is powered and working appropriately and that the scavenge is properly connected to the machine.

1.7   ENDOTRACHEAL TUBES

- Endotracheal intubation is used to maintain a patent airway, protect the airway from fluid or debris that may enter the oral cavity, provide a means for oxygen supplementation, allow for use of inhalant anesthetics, and allow for intermittent positive pressure ventilation.
- Although rarely contraindicated, endotracheal intubation should be mandatory in procedures where the surgeon plans to work in the oral cavity, procedures lasting longer than one hour when oxygen supplementation and positive pressure ventilation are indicated, anesthetic protocols using inhalant anesthetics, and procedures where airway patency may be compromised (i.e. myelogram).
- Endotracheal tubes used in horses are generally polyvinyl chloride, silicone, or rubber. Silicone endotracheal tubes (**Figure 1.23**) are most commonly used due to the desirable qualities of being non-reactive and capable of being heat-sterilized.
- The endotracheal tube cuff is used to eliminate any leaks around the endotracheal tube. Cuffs can be of two types: high-volume low-pressure (HVLP) or low-volume high-pressure (LVHP). HVLP cuffs have the advantage of covering a larger surface area and exerting less pressure on the tracheal mucosa. LVHP cuffs have the advantage of conforming to the shape of the tube when completely deflated and exerting pressure on a smaller surface area of tracheal mucosa than the HVLP type cuff. LVHP cuffs are commonly used in equine anesthesia.
- Murphy type endotracheal tubes present a "murphy eye" at the patient end of the tube. The purpose of this hole is to provide an alternate path for airway gas to take should the patient end of the endotracheal tube become occluded.
- The connection to the breathing circuit can be the rubber bell design (**Figure 1.14**) or the metal connector designed for the Bivona insert (**Figure 1.15**).
- Endotracheal tubes should have several markings, including the internal diameter in millimeters, length markings in centimeters

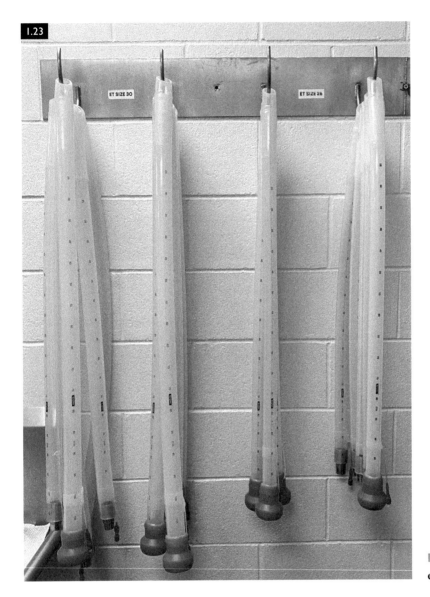

Figure 1.23 Silicone endotracheal tubes

from the patient end of the tube, and possibly markings indicating it has been tested for tissue toxicity (i.e., Z-79, F-29).

- Most average-size horses weighing 500 kg can accommodate a 26-mm internal diameter endotracheal tube. Larger horses and drafts, especially, may accommodate a 30-mm internal diameter endotracheal tube. Smaller tubes should be available at the time of intubation in case of difficulty in intubation (**Table 1.2**).

- Horses are generally intubated blindly either in sternal or lateral recumbency. A mouth speculum should be used to prevent damage to the endotracheal tube.

- A mouth speculum can be made by using a small piece of PVC pipe with a large enough bore to accommodate the endotracheal tube. The pipe is placed between the incisors, and the tube is advanced through the pipe segment (**Figure 1.24**).

Table 1.2 **Endotracheal tube (ETT) size (ID = internal diameter) appropriate for different size horses**

BODY WEIGHT	70–150 KG (150–350 LB)	150–250 KG (350–550 LB)	250–350 KG (550–750 LB)	350–450 KG (750–1000 LB)	450–550 KG (1000–1200 LB)
ETT size (ID in mm)	14–18	18–22	22–24	24–26	26–30

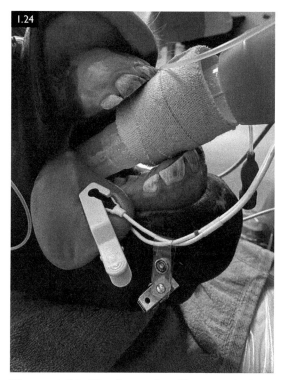

Figure 1.24 Mouth gag placed between incisors

- The head and neck are extended maximally (**Figure 1.25**), and the lubricated endotracheal tube is advanced over the tongue and between the molars. Some resistance will be felt when the endotracheal tube reaches the larynx. The tube is gently withdrawn a few centimeters, rotated 45° and advanced toward the larynx again, repeating this process until the endotracheal tube advances smoothly into the trachea.

- Confirmation that the endotracheal tube is in the trachea can be achieved via several methods:
  - Palpation of the neck to ensure the tube is not in the esophagus.
  - Appreciation of the flow of air through the endotracheal tube on spontaneous respiration with the hand.
  - Condensation on the inside of the endotracheal tube during expiration.
  - Movement of the rebreathing bag in coordination with breathing if the horse is connected to the anesthesia machine.
  - Detection of carbon dioxide in the expired gases.

- Horses can be intubated nasotracheally to allow for surgical procedures in the oral cavity without the endotracheal tube in the field. Nasotracheal intubation is performed with a smaller size endotracheal tube and preferably a tube with an LVHP cuff due to the smooth inert surface of the tube when the cuff is deflated. It has been recommended to use a tube that is one size smaller than what would be used orally (i.e., a horse that would normally be intubated with a 26-mm tube should accommodate a 24-mm tube nasotracheally). Smaller tubes should be available in the event that the originally selected tube is too large to be used nasotracheally.

- Due to the development of edema in the nasal passages with prolonged recumbency (especially dorsal recumbency),

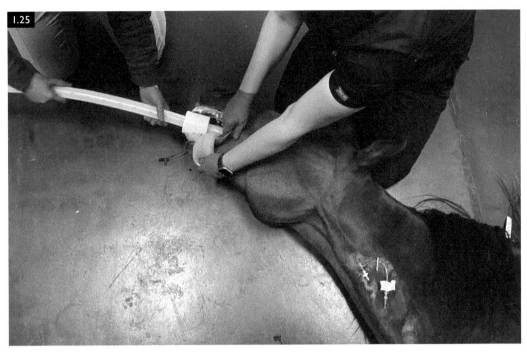

Figure 1.25 Head and neck extended

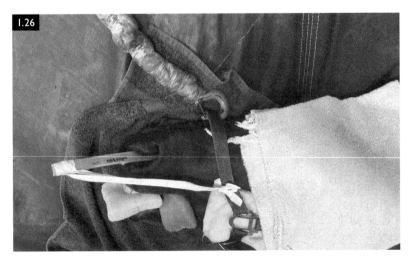

Figure 1.26 Nasal tube in recovery

it is sometimes necessary to place a nasopharyngeal tube during the recovery period to ensure that a patent airway is maintained. This is commonly accomplished by using smaller 10–14-mm internal diameter endotracheal tubes in the nasal passages (**Figure 1.26**).

- When nasal edema is present, approximately 0.5–0.75 ml of phenylephrine 10 mg/ml (0.01–0.015 mg/kg for a 500 kg horse) diluted in 5 ml of saline (total volume 5.5 ml) can be instilled in each nostril (total dose per horse 0.02–0.03 mg/kg) to decrease the edema in adult horses.

- See also Chapter 4.

1.8 VENTILATORS

- Ventilators are used to provide positive pressure ventilation in patients that are under anesthesia. They are indicated in several situations: the presence of apnea, hypoventilation (hypercapnia), hypoxemia, and/or excessive work of breathing.
- Ventilators accurately control the patient's alveolar ventilation to manage CO_2 levels, ensure oxygen delivery to the alveoli, and prevent or resolve pulmonary atelectasis.
- Mechanical ventilators are commonly used in horses under gas anesthesia.
- Ventilators are classified based on a number of different variables:
  - Major control variable.
  - Power source.
  - Drive mechanism.
  - Cycling mechanism.
  - Type of bellows.

1.8.1 Major Control Variable

- This is the limiting variable that the ventilator uses to determine the tidal volume delivered to the patient. Most ventilators are either pressure- or volume-controlled ventilators.
- In a volume-limited ventilator, the tidal volume is predetermined and will be delivered regardless of the associated pressures required.
- With a pressure-limited ventilator, a peak inspiratory pressure is used to determine the tidal volume delivered to the patient.
- The volume delivered by the ventilator can be affected by changes in patient respiratory or circuit compliance/resistance, inspiratory flow rates, leaks, inspiratory time, and the location of the pressure sensor.

1.8.2 Power Source

- The power source can be either compressed gas or electricity.
- Some ventilators employ both compressed gas and electricity.

1.8.3 Drive Mechanism/Circuit

- The drive mechanism refers to the force that generates the positive pressure breath. This is usually compressed gas or an electronically driven piston. Ventilators that use compressed gas for the drive mechanism are called "dual circuit" ventilators as there are two gas systems—the driving gas and the gas delivered to the patient.
- Ventilators that do not use compressed gas to power ventilation are referred to as "single-circuit" ventilators.

1.8.4 Cycling Mechanism

- The cycling mechanism is the means by which the ventilator cycles from inspiration to expiration. In most ventilators, the cycling mechanism is a timer.
- Some ventilators (i.e. Bird Mark ventilators) use a pressure cycling mechanism. In this style of ventilator, the buildup of airway pressure causes the ventilator to cycle.

1.8.5 Bellows

- Ventilator units with compressible bellows are classified as either "ascending" (**Figure 1.27**) or "descending" (**Figure 1.28**) type bellows.
- These titles are assigned based on the action of the bellows during the expiratory phase of the respiratory cycle. If the bellows rise on expiration, then the bellows are "ascending". If the bellows fall on expiration, then the bellows are "descending".
- Some ventilators (i.e., Tafonius ventilators) use piston-style bellows, which are not generally classified as ascending or descending.

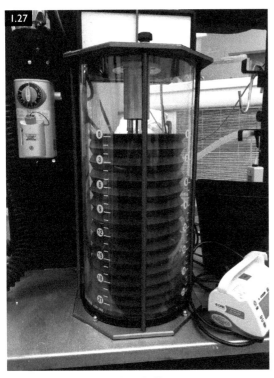

Figure 1.27 **Ascending bellows**

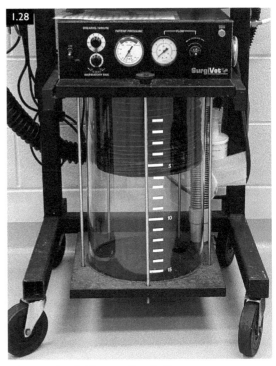

Figure 1.28 **Descending bellows**

1.9 GENERAL CONSIDERATIONS FOR LARGE ANIMAL VENTILATORS

- Most ventilators used in large animal anesthesia are electronically time-cycled and can be classified as either a dual-circuit gas-driven ventilator or single-circuit piston-driven ventilator.
- Dual-circuit gas-driven ventilators:
  - They have two separate gas sources: the patient airway gas and the ventilator driving gas.
  - The patient airway gas is housed within the anesthesia circuit and the ventilator bellows. Driving gas surrounds the ventilator bellows (between the bellows and the housing). As the ventilator fires, the pressure of driving gas around the ventilator bellows increases, forcing the bellows to compress and administer a breath to the patient.

- The ventilator bellows replaces the rebreathing bag and APL valve of the anesthetic circuit.
- The bellows configuration contains the following elements: the bellows, the bellows housing, the spill valve, the exhaust valve, and the ventilator hose connection.
- The bellows can be either ascending or descending, as described above. Ascending bellows provide some amount of positive end expiratory pressure (PEEP) based on the weight of the bellows. The spill valve allows gas to leave the bellows during the expiratory phase of ventilation if the pressure in the airway overcomes the valve. This pressure is usually 2–4 cmH$_2$O. Descending bellows can cause some amount of negative airway pressure on expiration as the bellows fall.

- The driving pressure component of the ventilator is the air inside the bellows housing surrounding the bellows. The driving gas generally comes from the intermediate pressure zone of the anesthetic machine with a pressure of 35–55 psi. The flow rate of the driving gas is specified by the ventilator to administer the desired tidal volume over the desired inspiratory period.
- On inspiration, pressure increases in the bellows housing, administering a positive pressure inspiration to the patient. Upon expiration, the exhaust valve allows the driving gas to be ventilated from the bellows housing.
- With some variation between ventilators, the anesthetist generally has the opportunity to control respiratory rate, inspiratory flow rate (driving gas flow), and/or inspiratory to expiratory time ratio (I:E ratio).
- Single-circuit piston driven ventilators:
  - They employ an electronically controlled piston to increase airway pressure, administering a positive pressure breath. These ventilators usually require electric power and may have a battery back-up to be used during transport or in situations where electrical outlets are not available.
  - These ventilators are more efficient with regard to the use of gas, as a driving gas source is not required.
  - Additional advantages of this type of ventilator include to the ability to use various advanced ventilation strategies including PEEP, continuous positive airway pressure (CPAP), assisted ventilation, and gas mixtures.
  - The most commonly used example of this style of ventilator in large animal anesthesia is the Tafonius ventilator (**Figure 1.29**).

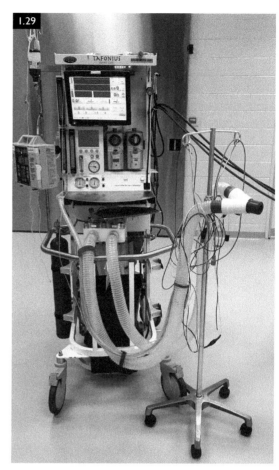

Figure 1.29 Tafonius ventilator

- There are several factors that affect delivered tidal volume in anesthetic ventilators:
  - *Fresh Gas Flow*: Fresh gas continues to flow into the anesthesia circuit throughout the inspiratory phase of ventilation. Most veterinary ventilators do not account for this additional volume contribution to the patient's tidal volume.
  - *Compliance and Compression Volumes*: Hoses used in breathing circuits have varying degrees of compliance. Stretch of these hoses during the inspiratory phase of ventilation can lead to changes in tidal volume delivered to

the patient. Therefore, the volume of gas administered as indicated by the compression of the ventilator bellows is not entirely accurate, as some volume is lost to expansion of the airway hose.

- *Leaks*: Any leaks within the anesthesia circuit will impact the delivered tidal volume as airway gas is lost through the leak during positive pressure inspiration. Depending on the bellows style, detection of a large leak while the patient is anesthetized can be quite easy or not obvious at all. Ascending bellows will collapse when there is a large leak in the circuit, making the presence of a leak obvious to the anesthetist. Conversely, descending bellows can entrain room air or driving gas during the expiratory phase, making detection of the large leak difficult. This poses the additional hazard that entrainment of room air or driving gas can result in lower than expected inspired inhalant anesthetic concentrations and lower than expected inspired oxygen concentration in the case of room air entrainment.

1.10   SELECTED LARGE ANIMAL VENTILATOR MODELS

1.10.1 Mallard Medical Anesthesia Ventilator

- The Mallard ventilator (**Figure 1.30**) is classified as a dual-circuit ventilator. They have electric power and are pneumatically driven. These ventilators are electronically time-cycled and volume-limited.
- Depending on the model, tidal volume can be adjusted by moving a cylinder and plate within the bellows housing to coincide with the desired setting. Tidal volume can also be changed by adjusting the inspiratory flow setting.

- Due to the ascending bellows, inherent PEEP of 2–3 cmH$_2$O is present. Additionally, an optional PEEP valve can be added to the system with the ability of incorporating up to 20 cmH$_2$O of PEEP.

1.10.2 Drager Large Animal Anesthesia Ventilator

- The Drager large animal ventilator (**Figure 1.31**) is a component of the Narkovet-E Large Animal Anesthesia Machine; the entire system is called the Narkovet-E Large Animal Anesthesia Control Center. This ventilator is classified as dual-circuit, tidal volume present, time-cycled, and pneumatically driven. The bellows are descending.

1.10.3 Hallowell Tafonius

- The Tafonius (**Figure 1.29**) is a fully programmable large animal anesthesia workstation.
- The benefit of the Tafonius is that it can be used on animals weighing between approximately 50–1000 kg by simply changing the Y-tubes and airway settings.
- It is compatible with most modern-day vaporizers.
- It offers touchscreen monitoring (**Figure 1.32**) and ventilation control PC (**Figure 1.33**) with the option to bypass the PC and program ventilator settings in auxiliary mode.
- The PC and touchscreen manifold can provide electronic recording of intra-anesthetic physiologic values with the option for the user to add significant events to the anesthetic record (i.e. induction time, surgery start time).
- Upon startup, the Tafonius will perform a system check which includes initialization of the piston in a machine leak and compliance test.

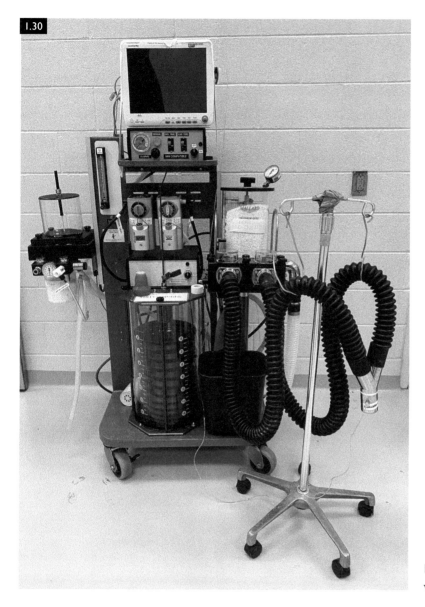

Figure 1.30 Mallard ventilator

Ventilator and Ventilation

- It is equipped with a piston-driven ventilator that can be used on patients of various sizes and can accommodate a wide range of tidal volumes.
- The piston-driven ventilator eliminates the need for a driving gas and decreases the amount of wasted gas.

- The ventilator can be used for both controlled and assisted modes of ventilation.
- Additionally, it has the ability to provide PEEP and CPAP.
- It is also equipped with a mount for a reservoir bag; however, the piston and cylinder allow for spontaneous ventilation.

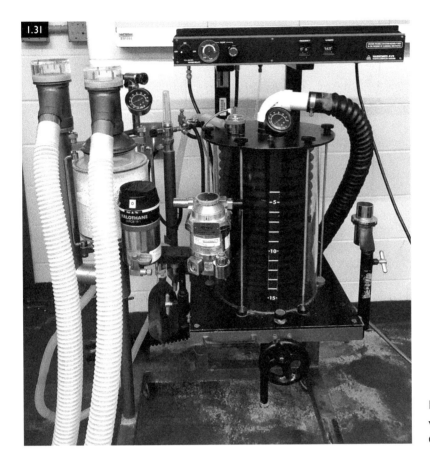

Figure 1.31 Drager ventilator
Courtesy of Dr. Ann Weil

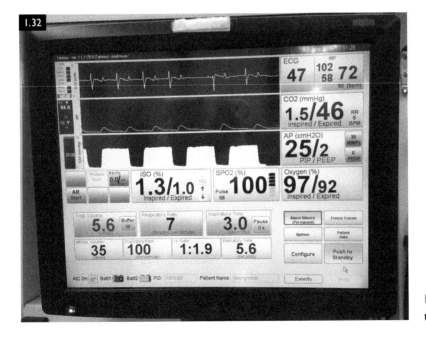

Figure 1.32 Tafonius touchscreen monitoring

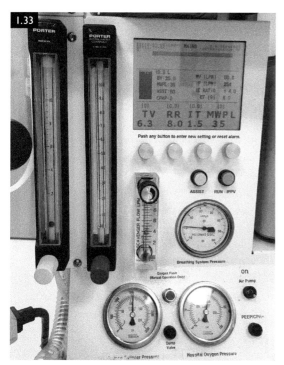

Figure 1.33 Ventilation control PC

- Airway pressure is measured at the Y-piece and can detect changes in airway pressure greater than 0.5 cmH_2O.
- When a change in airway pressure is detected, the piston alters its position, minimizing resistance to breathing.

Touchscreen Controls

1) Ventilator settings
   - Assist or control ventilation can be selected. Additionally, CPAP or PEEP can also be set.
   - Tidal volume (range 0.1–20 l in 0.1 l increments), respiratory rate (range 1–30 breath/min), and inspiratory time (range 0.5–4 seconds in 0.1 seconds increments) can be modified on the touchscreen.
   - It is possible to enter the inspiratory pause (IP) in fractions of seconds or as a percentage of the total inspiratory time.
   - The maximum working pressure limit (MWPL), which ranges from 10 to 80 cmH_2O in 1 cmH_2O increments, can be set. This is the airway pressure above which ventilation is prevented.
   - The fraction of inspired oxygen (FiO_2) can be modified from 0.2 to 1.

2) Monitoring
   - The PC touchscreen displays temperature, heart rate, and respiratory rate.
   - Pulse oximetry and associated plethysmography are displayed.
   - Direct arterial blood pressure monitoring is available. Systolic, mean, and diastolic values and arterial waveforms are displayed.
   - Inspiratory and expiratory CO_2 values are reported, along with a capnograph.
   - Inspired and expired inhalational anesthetic concentration (volume %) are measured and displayed.
   - Values for minute volume, inspiratory flow, I:E ratio, and expiratory time are calculated and displayed based on preselected values for tidal volume, respiratory rate, and inspiratory time.
   - Additionally, airway pressure, flow, and volume versus time graphs can be selected and displayed.

3) Scavenging
   - Waste anesthetic gases are collected and diverted to a manifold on the back of the machine.
   - The scavenging manifold can be used with both a passive and an active scavenging system.
   - When utilizing an active scavenging system, a flowmeter on the front of the machine controls the flow of the vacuum within the scavenging manifold.

1.10.4 Tafonius Junior

- The Tafonius Junior is an anesthesia machine similar to the Tafonius without the PC and touchscreen monitoring system and their associated cost.
- It is a piston-driven ventilator that is controlled similarly to the auxiliary control on the Tafonius.

1.10.5 Surgivet Dhv1000/Anesco Large Animal Ventilator

- This ventilator (**Figure 1.34**) is classified as dual-circuit, tidal volume limited, and time-cycled. It is pneumatically driven and electronically controlled. The bellows are descending.
- This unit can be purchased as a stand-alone ventilator that can be used with various anesthesia machines, or it can be purchased as a component of an anesthesia workstation.

1.10.6 Bird Mark Respirator-Driven Ventilators

- Bird Mark ventilators (**Figure 1.35**) have been used for many years in large animal anesthesia. This ventilator was originally designed for use in humans but was modified to attach to a "bag-in-a-barrel" bellows system for use in large animal anesthesia.
- These units are robust, and many units that were manufactured decades ago are still in working order, being used routinely.
- Depending on the configuration, these units are either single-circuit or dual-circuit.

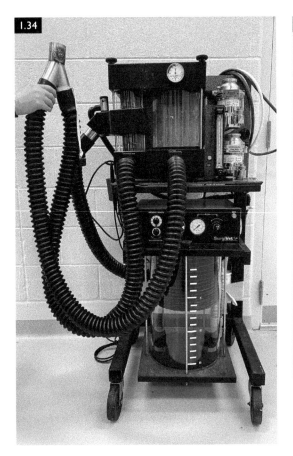

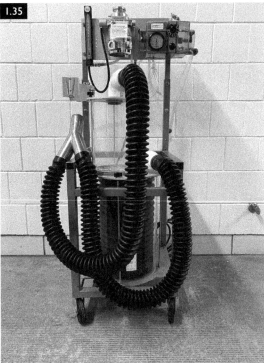

Figure 1.35 Bird Mark ventilator

Figure 1.34 Anesco ventilator

When used with a bag-in-a-barrel design for large animal anesthesia, the configuration is dual-circuit.

- These ventilators are classified as pressure-cycled, pressure-limited, and pneumatically powered. They are also capable of assist modes of ventilation, firing when the patient generates enough negative pressure with spontaneous ventilation.
- These ventilators are also designed to entrain room air to administer gas with a lower oxygen concentration if desired by the user.

FURTHER READING

Bednarski RM (2009) Anesthesia equipment. In: *Equine Anesthesia Monitoring and Emergency Therapy*, 2nd edn. (eds Muir WW, Hubbell JAE), Saunders Elsevier, St Louis, pp. 315–331.

Dorsch JA, Dorsch SE (2008) *Understanding Anesthesia Equipment*, 5th edn., Lippincott Williams & Wilkins, Philadelphia.

Mosley CA (2015) Anesthesia equipment. In: *Veterinary Anesthesia and Analgesia: The Fifth Edition of Lumb and Jones*, 5th edn. (eds Grimm KA, Lamont LA, Tranquilli WJ et al), Wiley Blackwell, Ames, pp. 23–85.

CHAPTER 2

PREANESTHETIC EVALUATION

Cynthia Trim

2.1   INTRODUCTION

- Preanesthetic evaluation is an essential component of clinical anesthesia practice. Achieving satisfactory sedation or anesthesia without problems can be difficult even when horses are healthy.
- Evaluation of the patient before drug administration can identify factors, such as specific behavior, anatomical features or ill health, that may influence the animal's response to sedative or anesthetic agents and provide direction for the choice or exclusion of anesthetic agents and management.
- Identifying potential problems may allow changes in routine anesthetic management that prevent problems, to the benefit of the patient, the veterinarian and the relationship with the owner.
- An evaluation should be performed even when a procedure is to be conducted with the horse standing. Furthermore, it is not uncommon that the need arises to convert sedation to general anesthesia to be able to complete the procedure.
- A full evaluation requires not only knowledge of anesthetic practice and details of the procedure to be performed but also the skills of a behaviorist, knowledge of animal management of the species, expertise in internal medicine and, in specific cases, training in critical care, surgery, lameness diagnosis and other specialties.
- The duration of the evaluation may be extensive for animals with many problems

or short in apparently healthy animals scheduled for elective procedures.
- Nonetheless, an evaluation appropriate to the patient is valuable. Many anecdotal cases come to mind where following protocol has revealed an unexpected complication, for example, when an aged pony was resisting dental treatment and brief general anesthesia was suggested. No health issue was identified from the owner's history or a physical examination, yet submitting a blood sample for laboratory tests (decision based on age of the animal and protocol) revealed a creatinine of 13 mg/dl, resulting in a subsequent change in the medical plan.
- In the event of an unexpected complication, confirmation of a preanesthetic evaluation written in the medical record provides support in a litigation case.

2.2   GENERAL PLAN

A format for the evaluation is recommended to ensure that nothing is forgotten, as follows:
- A review of the history and any available laboratory test results.
- Obtaining information from the owner or handler to assess the animal's mental state and observation of the animal without interaction.
- A physical examination, specifically cardiovascular and respiratory systems and any system associated with the proposed procedure.

DOI: 10.1201/9780429190940-2

- Further laboratory or diagnostic tests based on the information gathered thus far.
- Consideration of the impact of the proposed procedure on anesthetic management, such as animal position, access for monitoring, and risk for complications (e.g. blood loss).

Example of preanesthetic evaluation form

CLINICIAN APPROVAL_____

EQUINE ANESTHESIA: PREANESTHETIC EVALUATION

Date:_____   Case# _____   Owner Name _____

Patient Info

Breed:_____   Age:_____   Wt: _____   Sex/Repro Status: _____

Temperament: _____

Summary of Vital Signs and Lab Data: _____

_____

Current/Concurrent Disease: _____

Current Meds: _____

ASA Status: 1   2   3   4   5   E

Estimated Anesthesia Time: _____   Estimated Sx Time: _____

Patient Position: _____

Potential Complications: _____

_____

What aspects of the sx procedure will alter the patient's anesthetic management?

_____

_____

How could you alter anesthetic management to minimize potential complications for the patient?

_____

_____

2.3   HISTORY: WHAT INFORMATION IS USEFUL?

- An adverse response to previous administration of sedative agent(s) or anesthetics, allowing the current plan to be modified to circumvent a repeat of the complication.
- The animal's work use may provide an indication for anticipated response to restraint or recumbency.

- Training as a racehorse creates a different temperament from a trail-riding pleasure horse or an animal used to pull a cart or carriage on a street.
- Animals that are hyperexcitable, trained to exhibit exaggerated movements when showing or with minimal experience of interaction with unfamiliar personnel may not be sedated to the expected degree after administration of specific drugs at usual dose rates, may be anticipated to attempt jumping out of stocks or to run away, and may be difficult to achieve an adequate depth of general anesthesia followed by an unsatisfactory recovery from anesthesia.
- Pregnancy (**Figure 2.1**).
  - Recommend confirming pregnancy by rectal examination or some other means before inducing general anesthesia, for clarification in the event that the mare is not in foal at a later date.

- An abortion can occur after stress, decreased arterial oxygenation (hypoxemia) and low arterial blood pressure (hypotension), which may be associated with exposure to an unfamiliar environment or general anesthesia.
- A positive outcome is more likely when the mare is ≤ 15 years old and at ≥ 40 days of gestation.
- Risk of abortion associated with anesthesia is 3.5 times more likely in mares with colic, significantly associated with anesthesia duration ≥ 3 hours and intraoperative hypotension.
- History of previous ill health or surgeries. Depending on the disease, new laboratory or diagnostic tests may be indicated to reassess current status. Anesthesia should be managed to prevent worsening of disease.
- Hyperkalemic periodic paralysis (HYPP) carries a risk for fatal outcome.

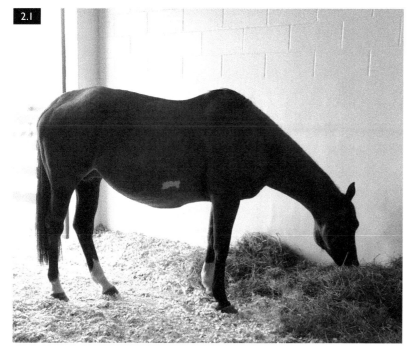

Figure 2.1 **Pregnant mare**

- Serum potassium may increase during anesthesia, with or without classic ECG changes (loss of P waves and high T waves), and may be accompanied by tachycardia and muscle fasciculations.
- Alternatively, potassium concentration may be normal during anesthesia, and the horse recovers normally from anesthesia but then collapses a few hours later.
  - If confirmed before anesthesia, be prepared to measure serum potassium at intervals during anesthesia and to infuse calcium gluconate (**Figure 2.2**) or borogluconate and 5% dextrose in water IV when an episode is suspected.
- Polysaccharide storage myopathy Type 1 (glycogen storage disease) is characterized by intermittent exertional rhabdomyolysis and gait abnormalities, especially in Quarter Horses and draft horses. This disease may be implicated in horses unable to rise after anesthesia.
- Current administration of drugs.
  - Organophosphate compounds, oral or topical, administered within two weeks of general anesthesia may significantly decrease the anesthetic dose requirement. The depolarizing muscle relaxant succinylcholine is contraindicated in these animals.
  - Sodium or potassium penicillin injected intravenously may result in an acute decrease in blood pressure for about 40 minutes as a result of decreased myocardial contractility. Induction of anesthesia should be delayed after administration of this drug.
- Time of recent feeding of hay or grain.
  - There are some differences of opinion, but withholding grain for 24 hours and hay for 12 hours before induction of heavy sedation or general anesthesia is recommended to decrease risk of post-anesthetic colic.
  - Horses that have been on grass pasture are also at risk for developing severe bloat during general anesthesia. Grass should be withheld for several hours before induction of anesthesia.

2.4   OBSERVATION OF BEHAVIOR

- Behavior observations are added to information from the physical examination and laboratory test results for the assessment of health status in sick animals and, for some patients, an indication for adjusting drug dose rates.
- Obtain a description from the client of the animal's behavior in its own environment.
  - Listen to information offered by the client because it may be useful; do not assume that you know what they are going to say.

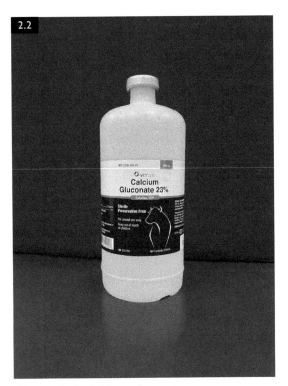

Figure 2.2 Calcium gluconate

- Observe the animal in the treatment area to assess the animal's mental status before your interactive examination.
  - Presence of muscle movement such as pacing, startling, circling or tail swishing may indicate the need for sedation even before examination and predicts an unsatisfactory response to drug administration.
  - Increased muscle tension in the neck and limbs and presence of muscle tremors must be interpreted in context.
    - Horse may be anxious. Approach slowly. Horse may startle into action by an abrupt action or noise. An anxious horse is at increased risk for hypotension (decreased circulating blood volume) during anesthesia or myopathy (decreased peripheral perfusion) after inhalation general anesthesia.
    - Muscle tremors in a horse with colic may be associated with gastrointestinal strangulation or ischemia.
  - Facial expression and ear position may indicate anxiety or pain. Signs of pain are discussed in Chapter 12.
  - The degree of interaction with the person holding the lead rope may suggest whether the animal will walk all over you when you get close or if it will avoid treading on you even when it is anxious.
  - Character of breathing. If rapid or labored, the cause should be determined.
  - Animals with neurologic disease and a significant degree of ataxia must be managed differently from healthy animals (see Chapter 11).
  - Although infrequent, rabies must be considered as a differential diagnosis in horses that are depressed and will not eat or drink. Other signs of this disease including aggressiveness, increased sensitivity to touch and convulsions are easier to recognize.

2.5 PHYSICAL EXAMINATION RELATING TO ANESTHESIA

2.5.1 Species and Breed

- Differences in temperament vary among species.
  - Temperament may be a major obstacle to overcome in feral horses and ponies, mustangs, Przewalski's horses and zebras and often precludes the possibility of a physical examination.
  - In domesticated horses, donkeys and mules, work use and handling have a large impact on individual temperament regardless of species, so that animals accustomed to discipline, close contact with many people and exposure to different sights and sounds may be easier to handle in the hospital environment.
- Breeds of horses certainly differ in their responses to anesthesia, partly a result of differing temperaments and partly influenced by physiological differences, such as circulating blood volume.
  - Thoroughbred (**Figure 2.3**), Warmblood and Arabian (**Figure 2.4**) horses are typically more hot-tempered than some other breeds, may require larger drug dose rates to achieve satisfactory anesthesia and may have less desirable quality of recovery from anesthesia.
  - The differences in depth and duration of anesthesia may also be related to larger circulating blood volumes, resulting in lower blood concentrations from a given drug dose rate than in horses with smaller blood volumes.
  - An example of breed differences was documented for xylazine-ketamine anesthesia, where the duration of anesthesia was significantly shorter in Thoroughbred horses than in Quarter horses.
  - Draft horses (**Figure 2.5**) have been documented to have a smaller blood

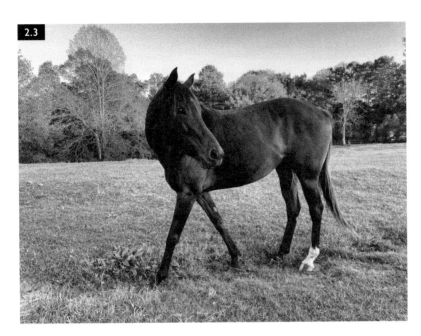

Figure 2.3
Thoroughbred
Courtesy of Dr. Valerie
Moorman

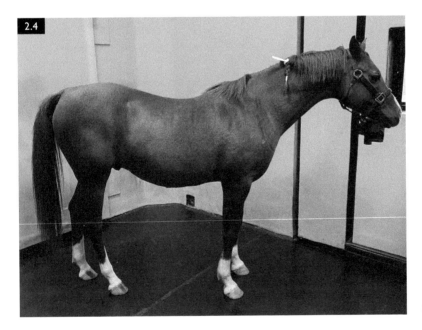

Figure 2.4 Arabian

volume than Thoroughbred horses. Lower dose rates frequently are sufficient for induction of anesthesia in Draft horses.

- Anatomical differences between breeds may have to be considered; for example, orotracheal intubation is more difficult in donkeys than in horses.

- Breed requirements may present additional management problems.
- Performance Tennessee Walking (TWH) horses frequently have stacked shoes on the forefeet (**Figure 2.6**). During anesthesia, create support for the hooves so the

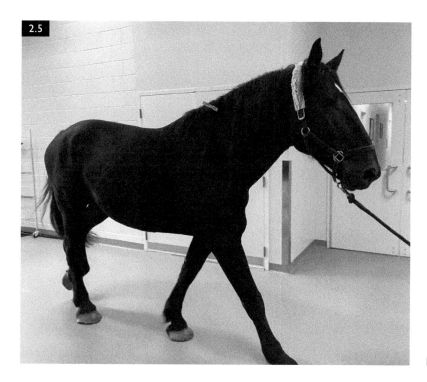

Figure 2.5 Draft horse

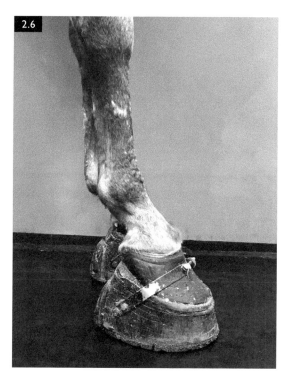

Figure 2.6 Stacked shoes on a Tennessee Walking horse

weight does not drag on the muscles and tendons of the limbs. Fortunately, horses of this breed are usually level-headed, and the shoes should not be a problem during recovery from anesthesia.

- American Saddlebred horses, Morgans and Hackneys may have had their tails cut to improve the tail set (**Figure 2.7**). These animals must not have a rope tied to their tail for support or assistance to stand.
- Test results differ among laboratories (different equipment, sample preparation), but ranges of normal values also differ among species and breeds.

2.5.2 Body Conformation, Size

- Body condition scores lower or greater than normal impact distribution of administered drugs, adequacy of ventilation and strength when attempting to stand in recovery.

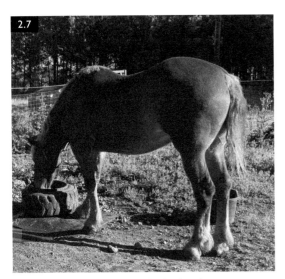

Figure 2.7 Horse with docked tail
Courtesy of Karissa Carpenter

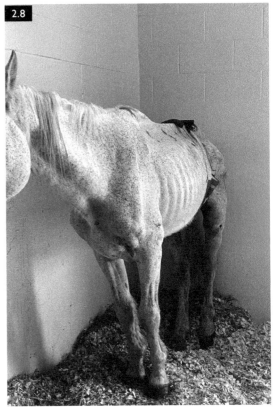

Figure 2.8 Thin horse

- Assess body condition. Body condition scoring system 1–9 for horses is available from Kentucky Equine Research (https://1kwz3b48jpiz1wph1oe7jzew-wpengine.netdna-ssl.com/wp-content/uploads/2015/07/body-condition-score-chart.pdf).
  - This system describes a horse with a moderate score of 5/9 as having a flat back (no crease or ridge), ribs easily felt but not visually distinguishable, fat around the tailhead slightly spongy, withers rounded over the spine, and shoulders and neck that blend smoothly into the body. A score of 1 is extremely emaciated, and 9 is excessively fat.
- Horses that are thin or emaciated (**Figure 2.8**) may have trouble standing after general anesthesia (prolonged dog-sitting, stumbling, multiple attempts to stand). Plan to provide assistance, e.g. upward lifting on the tail and steadying the head once standing.
- Animals that are large or have a large abdomen (**Figure 2.9**) are more likely to develop lower arterial oxygenation

during general anesthesia than lighter or leaner horses. This results from greater compression by the abdominal contents on the diaphragm during recumbency, which impairs ventilation. Plan to supplement inspired oxygen concentration above 21% (air):
- Attaching a pulse oximeter probe to the tongue of the anesthetized horse may provide a measure of hemoglobin oxygenation (SpO_2). Supplement with oxygen if SpO_2 < 93%. Readings may be inconsistent from a pulse oximeter probe.
- Insufflation of oxygen, 15 l/min for an adult horse, from a tube inserted 14 cm (6 inches) into a ventral nasal meatus or into the endotracheal tube (**Figure 2.10**). Oxygen supply from a cylinder and a

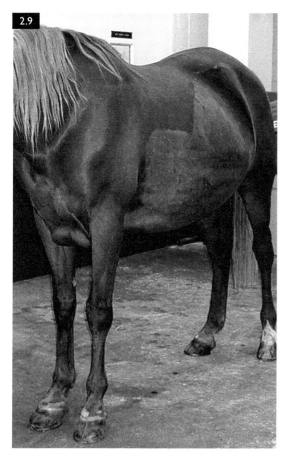

Figure 2.9 **Distended abdomen**
Courtesy of Dr. Michelle Barton

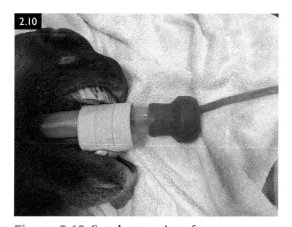

Figure 2.10 **Supplementation of oxygen through an endotracheal tube**

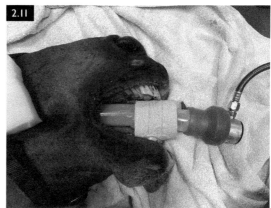

Figure 2.11 **Connecting demand valve to endotracheal tube**

flowmeter or from the house oxygen supply in a clinic.

- Insert an endotracheal tube and use a demand valve connected to a pressurized oxygen supply (**Figure 2.11**). Trigger the demand valve to deliver 4–6 breath/min, inspiratory time 1.5–2 seconds. A small 'E' size cylinder containing 625 liters will supply oxygen at 15 l/min for approximately 40 minutes or 5 l/breath from a demand valve for 10–20 minutes.
- When planning ahead for procedures to be performed in the hospital, an anesthetic delivery system (anesthesia machine circle) can be connected to an endotracheal tube to deliver > 90% oxygen (or an air/oxygen mixture). This technique can be implemented when insufflation is ineffective or used from the beginning of anesthesia in large horses or when total intravenous anesthesia (TIVA) is anticipated to last longer than 90 minutes.
- Horses that are heavily muscled have an increased risk for postanesthetic myopathy after general anesthesia. Take precautions:
  - Keep duration of anesthesia < 2 hours if possible.

- Monitor arterial blood pressure and keep mean arterial pressure > 70 mmHg.
- Foam padding 24 cm (10 inches) thick under the horse (**Figure 2.12**).

- For lateral recumbency, elevate upper fore and hind limbs to a position at least parallel to the ground (**Figure 2.13**).

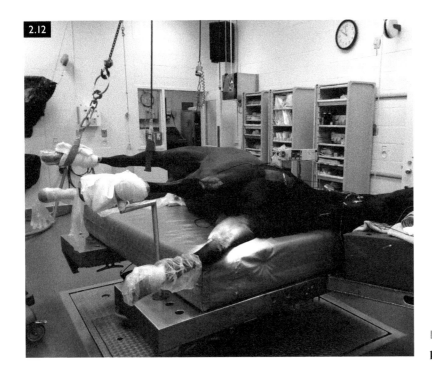

Figure 2.12 Foam padding under the horse

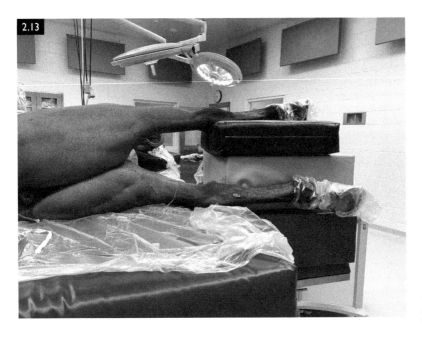

Figure 2.13 Elevation of upper limbs to make parallel to the ground

- Animals weighing < 140 kg (approximately 300 lb) will require small versions of large animal anesthesia equipment.
  - Endotracheal tubes manufactured specifically for foals, ponies and miniature horses are longer than those used in dogs to account for the long nose.
  - The length is necessary to avoid accidental extubation when moving these small animals or flexing the head and neck.
  - A selection of endotracheal tube sizes must include a few dog tubes of internal diameter 7–9 mm (**Figure 2.14**) and foal tubes sizes 10–20 mm with lengths of 40–57 cm (16–24 inches) (**Figure 2.15**).

- A resuscitator bag (Ambu bag) should be included for assisted or controlled ventilation when breathing is inadequate (**Figure 2.16**).
- Animals with an (appropriately fitting) endotracheal tube that is ≤ 16 mm internal diameter can be connected to a small animal circle delivery system.
- Examples of modifications to the weight cutoff guideline would be a heavy older pony that has a small trachea and small lung volume that could be managed using a large dog circle system, and a young foal of a large breed that can be intubated with an 18-mm internal diameter endotracheal tube; this animal should be connected to a large-animal-size circle delivery system.

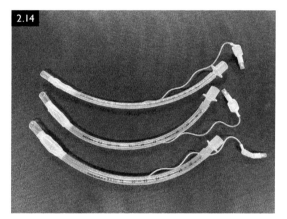

Figure 2.14 Range of dog endotracheal tubes, 7–9 mm internal diameter (ID)

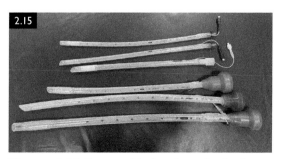

Figure 2.15 Range of foal endotracheal tubes, 10–18 mm internal diameter (ID)

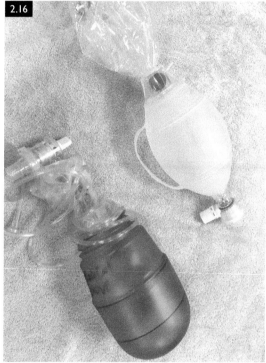

Figure 2.16 Ambu bags

2.5.3 Age

- Requirements for young (2–4 years), healthy adults with an athletic conformation provide the standard by which response to anesthetic agents by age is compared.
- Neonatal foals 1–7 days old have specific differences from this standard. Heart rate and cardiac output are high, and myocardial contractility and vagal reflex are low at birth.
- Avoid inducing bradycardia with sedatives, e.g. alpha$_2$-agonist sedative, because the cardiac output will be more severely decreased.
- Maintain an adequate blood volume to maintain adequate blood pressure.
- Pediatric animals are 7–10 days up to 3–4 months of age.
- Minimize risk of milk reflux into the pharynx and pulmonary aspiration by preventing nursing for 30 minutes before heavy sedation or anesthesia.
- Measure blood glucose (**Figure 2.17**) before anesthesia and every 30–60 minutes during anesthesia because neonatal and pediatric animals (**Figure 2.18**) are at risk for hypoglycemia. Infuse intravenously dextrose 5% in water during anesthesia at 3–5 ml/kg/hour and the rate adjusted to maintain blood glucose > 100 mg/dL (5.55 mmol/L). Balanced electrolyte solution should also be infused.
- Administer low dose rates of anesthetic agents for animals up to 2–3 weeks of age. Thereafter the anesthetic requirement progressively increases.
- Horses ≥ 15 years of age are seniors.
    - At this age, requirement for anesthetic drugs decreases.
    - Hypotension occurs more frequently during anesthesia.
    - Assistance to standing after anesthesia needed for some old animals.

2.5.4 Sex

- Differences in anesthetic requirements between the sexes have been identified in laboratory animals and for some anesthetics in dogs but are not really appreciable for horses once the temperament and body condition are accounted for.
    - Duration of action of guaifenesin documented as longer in male horses.

2.5.5 Cardiovascular System

- Since sedative and general anesthetic agents may significantly change cardiopulmonary function, it is essential that the cardiovascular system be evaluated for abnormalities.

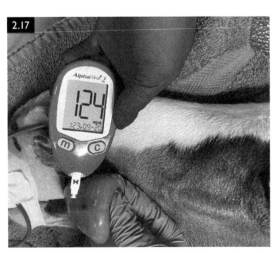

Figure 2.17 Glucometer

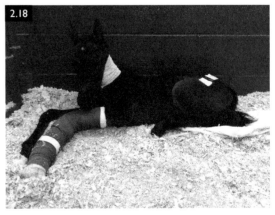

Figure 2.18 Neonatal patient

- Observe mucous membrane color; check that capillary refill time is < 2 seconds; palpate peripheral pulse for strength, rhythm and quality.
- Measure heart rate.
- Auscultate cardiac and lung sounds with a stethoscope to obtain baseline information.
- Irregular cardiac rhythms should be identified.
  - Listen for a pattern; is the rhythm regular or irregular?
  - Palpate the facial or median artery while auscultating cardiac sounds to identify any heartbeats unaccompanied by a peripheral pulse.
  - An electrocardiogram (ECG) may be advisable, if available.
- Second-degree atrioventricular (AV) heart block is a normal dysrhythmia in many horses (**Figure 2.19**).
  - Rhythm is regular with 2–4 beats separated by a pause, repeated.
  - The increase in activity involved when turning the horse in a circle twice may decrease vagal tone. If the dysrhythmia is absent on re-auscultation, it is likely to be second-degree atrioventricular block of little significance.
  - ECG appearance of several normal cardiac complexes followed by a P wave without an associated QRST complex.
  - Diseases associated with second-degree AV block include septic joint(s) with hyperpyrexia, ruptured urinary bladder and recent history of infectious disease.
- Second-degree AV block has the potential to develop into advanced or third-degree atrioventricular block during anesthesia.
  - If severe and non-treated, could result in cardiac arrest.
- Irregular cardiac rhythms include sinoatrial block, atrial fibrillation and premature ventricular depolarizations. These can be difficult to identify without an ECG.
  - Sinoatrial block is not common and on auscultation can be mistaken for second-degree atrioventricular heart block. When sinoatrial block is present before anesthesia, heart rates of < 15 beats/min may be present immediately after induction of anesthesia. Treatment at that time is atropine, 0.005–0.01 mg/kg, IV.
  - Atrial fibrillation usually results in hypotension during anesthesia. It is better to identify atrial fibrillation before general anesthesia, and potential consequences of proceeding should be discussed with the client.
    - ECG reveals no P waves, a baseline ripple effect that may be fine or coarse, relatively normal QRST complexes that are irregularly irregular, and a normal or fast heart rate (**Figure 2.20**).

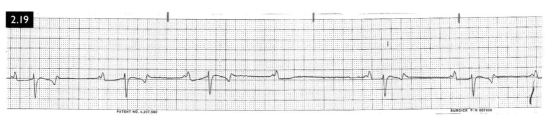

Figure 2.19 Second degree atrioventricular (AV) block
Courtesy of Dr. Michelle Barton

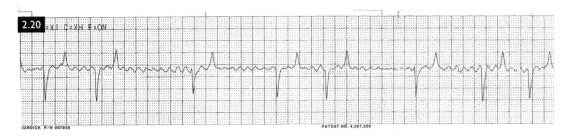

Figure 2.20 Atrial fibrillation
Courtesy of Dr. Michelle Barton

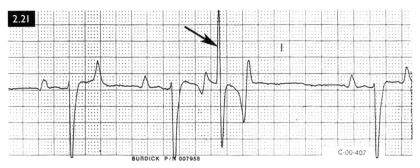

Figure 2.21 Ventricular premature complex
Courtesy of Dr. Michelle Barton

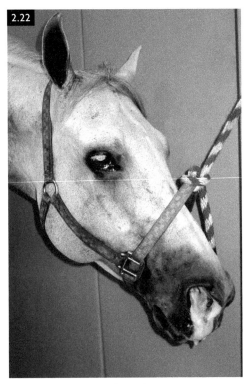

Figure 2.22 Nasal discharge
Courtesy of Dr. Michelle Barton

- Plan to treat hypotension using a dobutamine infusion.
- Premature ventricular depolarizations or complexes (VPC) can be heard as an irregular rhythm. If auscultated in a horse with colic, the likely initiating factor is endotoxemia. ECG characteristically shows large abnormal QRST complexes followed by a pause before a normal cardiac complex (**Figure 2.21**).

2.5.6 Respiratory System

- Conducting anesthesia safely can be significantly challenged in animals with evidence of infectious respiratory disease or pulmonary dysfunction. Most of these conditions impact arterial oxygenation during sedation or anesthesia.
  - Evaluation should identify:
  - Evidence of nasal discharge (**Figure 2.22**) and enlarged lymph nodes.

- Presence of a cough.
- Mucous membrane color.
- Character and rate of breathing.
- Auscultation of the airflow in the lungs, with and without the use of a rebreathing bag (**Figure 2.23**).
- Inflammatory disease may worsen after anesthesia because anesthetic agents, injectable and inhalation, depress the immune system.

- Prevent transmission of infectious disease to another animal by appropriate cleaning of equipment, the operative surroundings and personal clothing.
- Horses with recurrent airway obstruction (equine asthma, recurrent airway obstruction [RAO], chronic obstructive pulmonary disease [COPD]) are usually hypoxemic during anesthesia.
  - Plan to supplement with oxygen.

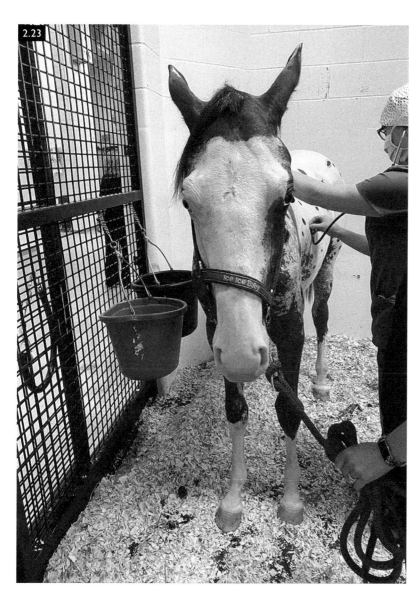

Figure 2.23
Auscultation of airflow in the lungs of standing horse

- Administration of albuterol/salbutamol may provide sufficient bronchodilation to counteract the hypoxemia.
- Atropine, 0.01 mg/kg, IV before anesthesia may prevent bronchoconstriction for about one hour, but after anesthesia check for presence of gastrointestinal sounds before feeding.
- It has been noted that horses given IV alpha-2 agonists for sedation that immediately develop an increased respiratory rate should have their body temperature checked for the presence of fever.

2.5.7 Temperature

- Normal rectal temperature is 37.0–38.0°C (99.5–101.0°F).
- Increased rectal temperature above the upper limit of normal range is a flag to further evaluate the patient for evidence of pulmonary or other disease.

2.5.8 Other Factors that Impact on Anesthetic Management

- Note animals with lameness or any orthopedic abnormality of a limb that would interfere with muscle strength or stability. Make plans to assist at induction of anesthesia so that the animal becomes recumbent without compounding the injury. Likewise, plan for assisted recovery during attempts to stand after anesthesia.
  - Examples:
    - Animal with excessively overgrown or laminitic feet.
    - Fractures and luxations requiring noninvasive (casting/splinting) (**Figure 2.24**) or invasive surgical procedures.
- Note evidence of partial upper airway obstruction, such as laryngeal hemiplegia, nasal or pharyngeal neoplasia or guttural pouch disease.
  - Make plans before anesthesia to manage complications such as airway obstruction.
  - Endotracheal intubation may be difficult in these animals and may require use of an endotracheal tube with a smaller internal diameter than ideal. If an endoscope is available, it can be inserted inside the endotracheal tube and used to

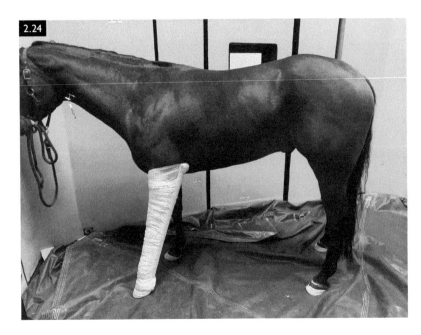

2.24

Figure 2.24 Limb with a splint

visually guide the tube into the larynx.

- A tracheotomy may be indicated either before induction of anesthesia, immediately after induction of anesthesia, or during anesthesia and before recovery.
- Obstruction of sight in one eye by a hood with an eye cup for protection may be associated with a difficult recovery, with the horse exhibiting apparent anxiety, early attempts to stand and ataxia, particularly when the hood had not been worn or the animal was not completely blind before anesthesia.
- Trauma occurring within the previous 24 hours. The scope of the impact of trauma on the various components of anesthesia is too great to discuss in full.
  - Examples:
    - Moderate hemorrhage, e.g., from a laceration or after castration. Circulating blood volume will be restored within a few hours by influx of fluid from the intracellular space; however, if the animal requires general anesthesia the same day or the following day, it is at risk for hypotension or decreased anesthetic requirement during anesthesia, even for TIVA.
    - Trauma resulting from collision with a fence may appear to involve superficial lacerations, but always investigate the possibility of thoracic penetration.

2.6   DIAGNOSTIC TESTS

2.6.1 Hematology and Biochemical Tests

- Controversy exists concerning the value of preanesthetic hematologic and biochemical laboratory tests on every animal before general anesthesia.
- May not be practical for procedures to be performed outside a clinic. One option is to collect blood at the first visit and review the results before returning for a second visit to conduct the surgical procedure.
- Common practice is to measure only packed cell volume (PCV) and total protein (TP) in young healthy animals < 5 years of age. Further hematology and tests for electrolytes, liver enzymes and renal function are performed in animals ≥ 5 years.

2.7   WHY INCLUDE THE MEDICAL OR SURGICAL PROCEDURE

- The preanesthetic evaluation described thus far has assessed the health status of the animal. There are several classifications of health status used for human patients.
- The American Society of Anesthesiologists classification is frequently applied to veterinary patients:
  - Class I, healthy.
  - Class II, healthy with a minor abnormality.
  - Class III, horses with a disease that is not immediately life-threatening.
  - Class IV, horses with severe diseases that require life-saving surgery.
  - Class V, horses that are severely ill, and cardiopulmonary collapse is present or imminent.ny of these class assignments can be preceded by E that denotes an emergency situation.
- Although complications are more likely to occur during and after anesthesia of animals in classes III-V, these classes do not provide an accurate prediction of risk because the procedure may also carry risk.
- Location and time of day, hospital *versus* field anesthesia and daily working hours *versus* out-of-hours may limit the personnel and equipment available. Anesthesia performed out-of-hours has been associated with increased mortality rate in a retrospective study.

- Access to the site of the procedure on the animal may dictate the position of the animal, thus the type of anesthesia and altered risk.
- Procedure may have associated adverse effects, e.g., hemorrhage, increased pain, airway obstruction, impaired strength in one or more limbs or long duration, that increase overall risk of complications.

2.8 SUMMARIZE, PLAN AND EXECUTE

- Summarize points from the preanesthetic evaluation, including requirements for the procedure.
- List drugs or management that should be excluded.
- List suitable drugs and required management, including appropriate locoregional nerve blocks.
- List anticipated complications and make plans for treatment. Communicate these plans with involved personnel.
- Communication with the owner or representative is advisable after the evaluation and before anesthesia. Risks of anesthesia include possibility of myopathy, neuropathy, spinal myelomalacia and limb fracture. Suggest insisting on a quiet environment without patient stimulation during recovery from anesthesia.
- Recommended practices:
  - Develop checklists for equipment needed for specific types of anesthesia and procedures. Write a list of drugs and dosages for *each* animal, including calculations in ml, to avoid mistakes arising from the need to make quick calculations during the procedure.
  - Insertion of a jugular venous catheter with a cap, secured to the animal to avoid accidental dislodging.
  - Include a person with anesthesia training for monitoring animals during general anesthesia. This person should make a written record of the timeline with drug administration (drug, dose, route) and recorded heart and respiratory rates and any other measurements.
  - Mental practice before administering drugs. This involves thinking through the sedation or anesthesia process, thinking through the medical or surgical process, and making plans for treating expected or potential complications.

FURTHER READING

Chenier TS, Whitehead AE (2009) Foaling rates for abortion in pregnant mares presented for medical or surgical treatment of colic: 153 cases (1993–2005). *Can Vet J* **50**:481–485.

Pang DSJ, Panizzi L, Paterson JM (2011) Successful treatment of hyperkalaemic periodic paralysis in a horse during isoflurane anaesthesia. *Vet Anaesth Analg* **38**:113–120.

Wohlfender FD, Doherr MG, Driessen B et al (2015) International online survey to assess current practice in equine anesthesia. *Equine Vet J* **47**:65–71.

CHAPTER 3

SEDATION AND RESTRAINT FOR STANDING PROCEDURES

Jesse Tyma

3.1 INTRODUCTION

Performing procedures using standing sedation should always be preferred to general anesthesia in horses when the patient and procedure allow for this approach. This is due to the high morbidity and mortality associated with general anesthesia in this species. Many procedures can be safely performed with sedation and a good local block technique in cooperative patients.

3.2 PHYSICAL RESTRAINT

- Take into account:
  - Horse's signalment (age, sex, breed), temperament, the planned procedure, the qualifications of the handler, the environment, and the equipment available.
- Select an ideal environment (**Figure 3.1**), preferably devoid of distractions and obstacles.
  - It should be free of bright or changing light, loud noises, and/or other horses or animals.
- Using the least restraint required is the best practice for the safety of the horse, handler, and attendant.
- Stressed or fractious horses are unlikely to tolerate any manual restraint or handling.
  - High sympathetic drive causes resistance to standard doses of sedative agents (e.g. alpha-2 adrenergic agonists).
- "Plan for the worst!"

- A general rule that should be honored in any situation or procedure requiring restraint and/or sedation of the horse.
- Prepare for prompt intervention in the possible occurrence of any complication.
- The ability to perform procedures while standing is more important than in other species because of the increased risk of general anesthesia-associated complications in the horse.

3.2.1 Halter and Lead

- Basic and essential equipment for controlling a horse:
  - Halter (**Figure 3.2**).
    - Well-fitting and made of nylon.
    - If a horse is ever to be tied via the halter or turned out with the halter in place, having at least a small piece of leather is imperative as a "breakaway" mechanism (**Figure 3.3**) should the horse become entrapped.
- Lead rope (**Figure 3.4**).
  - Should be made of a soft material that will not harm the handler's hands.
  - Never wrap a lead rope around a hand or fingers while handling (**Figure 3.5**).
- Horses are customarily led from the left side (**Figure 3.6**).
- Horses should be handled from the same side as the operator during a procedure.
  - If the horse reacts to a stimulus, it can be swiftly turned away from the operator from this position.

DOI: 10.1201/9780429190940-3

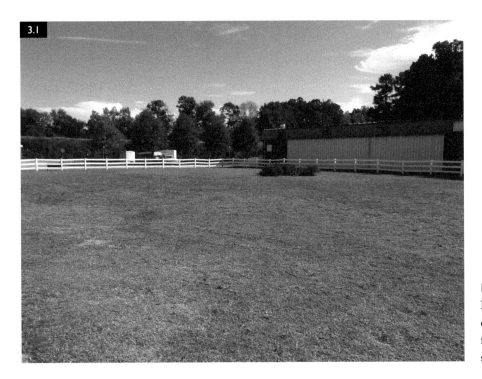

Figure 3.1
Ideal
environment
for standing
sedation

- The handler should always remain attentive to the horse and attendant, and horse should be maintained on a short lead.
- Horses are not customarily tied for procedures; however, in a well-broken animal that has been trained to stand at a tie, a quick-release knot may be utilized (**Figure 3.7**).

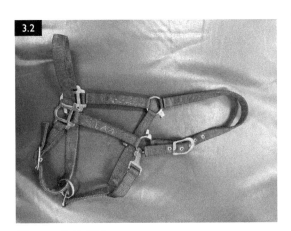

Figure 3.2 Halter

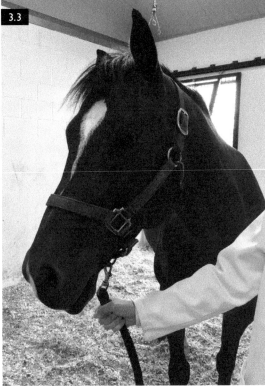

Figure 3.3 Leather breakaway strap on a halter

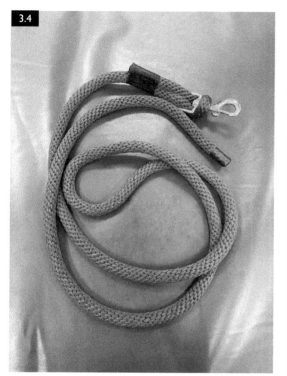

Figure 3.4 Lead rope

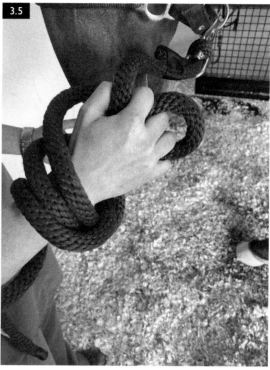

Figure 3.5 Lead rope wrapped around hand/ fingers (showing what not to do)

3.2.2 Chain Lead

- A chain lead is a lead rope with a chain affixed to the proximal portion of the lead (**Figure 3.8**).
- Placement techniques:
  - Over the nose (**Figure 3.9**).
  - Under the jaw (**Figure 3.10**).
  - Through the mouth (**Figure 3.11**).
  - Across the superior gingiva (**Figure 3.12**).
  - Note: If there is excess chain, position the chain snap on a higher halter ring on the cheek such that the handler will not have to grasp the chain.
- Proper method of use:
  - Gentle, abrupt tugs on lead during unwanted behavior.
  - Release pressure when behavior ceases.
- Always use judiciously and with caution.
  - Horses that are unfamiliar with chain leads may initially be alarmed by their use.
  - The behavior of some unruly horses may deteriorate with the use of negative reinforcement.
  - An unskilled handler should be assisted in placing the chain and instructed on its proper use.
  - A chain can injure a horse if used with too much force.
  - Never tie a horse with a chain.
  - Avoid continuous pressure, which often produces the opposite (undesired) effect (the horse will resist more adamantly).

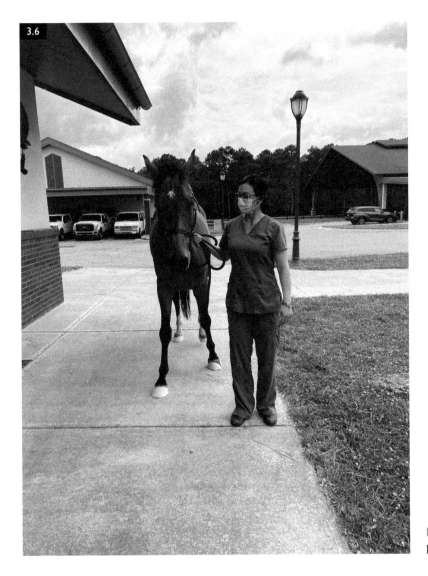

Figure 3.6 Leading horse from left side

3.2.3 Twitch

- A restraint device applied to the horse's superior lip to provide distraction during a procedure.
- Most devices have a long (20–100 cm), sturdy handle (wooden or plastic) and either a rope loop or a chain attached at the end; they need to be held and controlled by the handler (**Figure 3.13**).
- The "humane twitch" is a smaller, self-retaining metal device that can be affixed to the halter (**Figure 3.14**).

- Application: Grasp the horse's superior lip with one hand (**Figure 3.15**) and position the chain/rope around the grasped lip with the other (**Figure 3.16**), then twist the device until both secure and tight (**Figure 3.17**).
  - Helpful tip: Leave at least one finger out of the rope loop while placing the twitch so that the rope does not fall back onto the handler's wrist.
- Effects on horse:

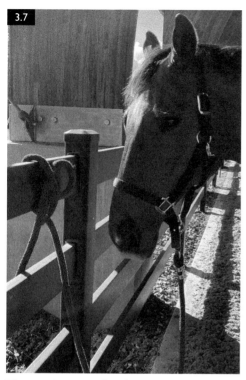

Figure 3.7 Quick-release knot used to tie horse

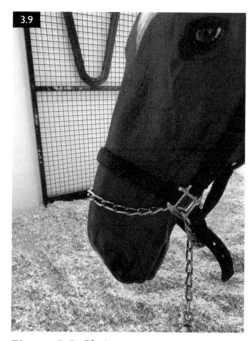

Figure 3.9 Chain over nose

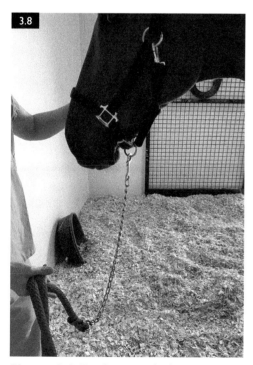

Figure 3.8 Lead rope with chain

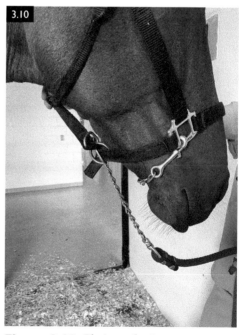

Figure 3.10 Chain under jaw

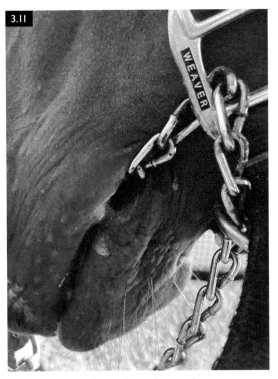

Figure 3.11 Chain through mouth

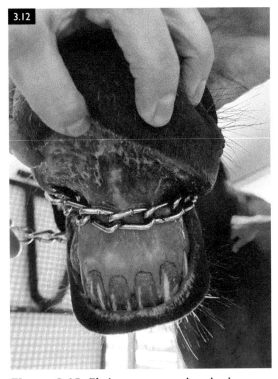

Figure 3.12 Chain across superior gingiva

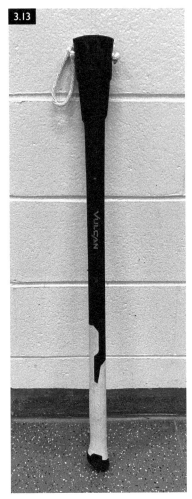

Figure 3.13 Twitch

- The horse becomes quieter with an eyelid droop, and it loses interest in its surroundings.
- The tolerance and acceptance of pain increases.
- The pain elicited upon tightening the twitch serves as a distraction.
- There is suspected endorphin release from the stimulation of acupuncture points (mechanoreceptors) on the upper lip.
- Gentle tapping/twisting of the device accentuates these effects.
- Always use judiciously and with caution:
  - The handler must stay alert and aware.

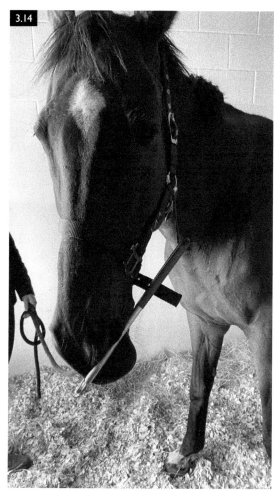

Figure 3.14 **Humane twitch**

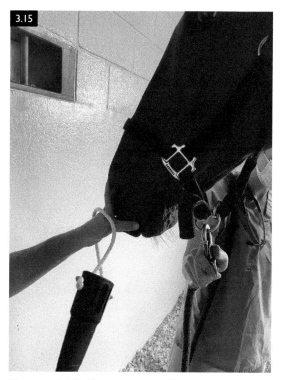

Figure 3.15 **Grasp superior lip**

- The twitch should remain held between the horse and the handler.
- The operator should be notified immediately if the twitch is displaced.
- The twitch should not be applied until it is needed because the aforementioned effects are attenuated with the duration of application.
- Alternative methods ("twitches") if no device available:
  - Firm grasp of the upper lip (**Figure 3.18**).
  - Ear twitch (grasping and twisting an ear) (**Figure 3.19**).
    - Do not pull down on the ear, as this may damage the motor nerves of the ear.

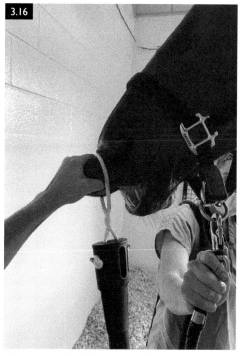

Figure 3.16 **Wrap rope/chain around lip**

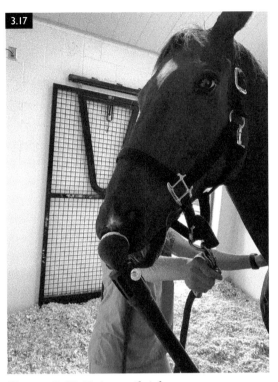

Figure 3.17 Twist until tight

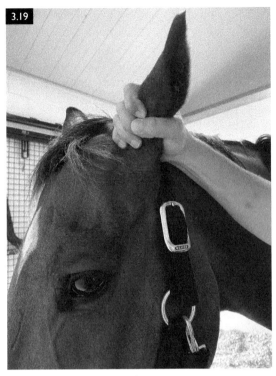

Figure 3.19 Ear twitch

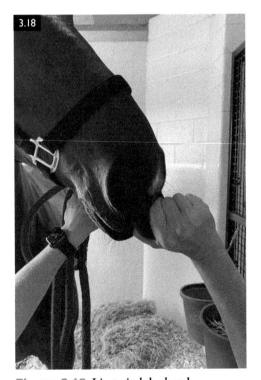

Figure 3.18 Lip twitch by hand

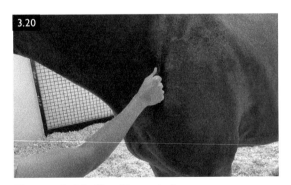

Figure 3.20 Shoulder twitch

- Head- and/or ear-shy horses are poor candidates for an ear twitch.
- Shoulder twitch.
  - Grasping and tightly holding the loose skin cranial to the scapula and rolling the skin into the wrist (**Figure 3.20**).
- Particularly useful in young horses.

3.2.4 Lifting a Foot

- Helpful when trying to immobilize a horse (**Figure 3.21**).
- Useful to encourage weight-bearing on the contralateral limb.
- Not helpful when attempting a procedure on a raised limb.
- May be used in conjunction with other forms of restraint.
- Indications:
  - Procedures to be performed on the contralateral limb in which the limb needs to remain still, including diagnostic regional anesthesia for lameness exams, repair of distal limb wounds, and/or arthrocentesis.
- Precautions:
  - The limb holder should be aware of their own foot placement if the horse suddenly slams down its foot.

3.2.5 Stocks

- Used to confine a horse and maintain a stationary patient for diagnostic and therapeutic procedures (**Figure 3.22**).
- If ropes are used to enclose the animal at the front end of the stocks, they should be secured with a quick-release knot.

- An attendant should remain at the horse's head while the horse is restrained in the stocks.
- Useful setup to perform standing surgical procedures in which the horse will require sedation and application of local anesthesia.
- Precautions:
  - Limbs are not immobilized within stocks.
  - Horses are capable of jumping out the front or sides of stocks.
  - Should be avoided in horses unaccustomed to confinement.
  - Those working with stocks should avoid positioning their limbs between the horse and the frame of the stocks to avoid injury.

3.3 CHEMICAL RESTRAINT

- Of the drugs approved for use in horses for standing chemical restraint, five

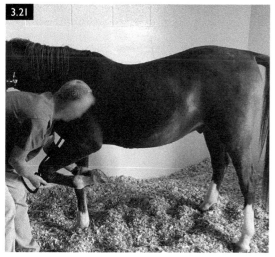

Figure 3.21 Lifting a foot to facilitate immobilization

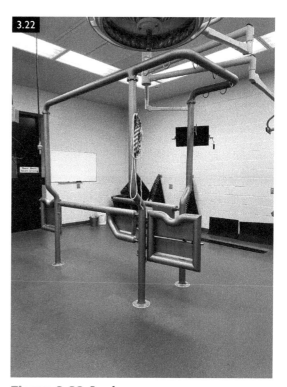

Figure 3.22 Stock

(acepromazine, butorphanol, detomidine, romifidine, and xylazine) are commercially available.

- No single drug produces ideal, repeatable standing chemical restraint in every horse. Combination of different drugs (**Table 3.1**) allows for enhanced sedation and analgesia-decreased dose of each drug.

3.3.1 Alpha-2 Agonists

- Sedative and analgesic.
- Sedation with muscle relaxation, ataxia, and analgesia.
- Xylazine, romifidine, and detomidine are approved for use in the horse in the United States.
- Intravenous administration of alpha-2 adrenergic receptor agonists is the basis for most drug combinations for moderate to profound standing sedation.
- Mechanism of action.
  - Agonism of alpha-2 adrenoreceptors in the central nervous system (CNS).
    - Inhibition of norepinephrine and dopamine storage and release.
    - Decrease in firing rate of central and peripheral neurons.
  - Decrease in CNS sympathetic output and peripheral sympathetic tone; increase in parasympathetic tone.
  - Alpha-1 effects functionally antagonize the hypnotic effects of alpha-2 antagonism.
- Applied pharmacology.
  - Relatively predictable levels of sedation and muscle relaxation.
  - Sedation is dose-dependent.
  - Increase in tolerance to painful stimuli.
  - Depression of cardiovascular function.
  - Excellent muscle relaxation of the front end, causing a head droop.

Table 3.1 **Example of drug combinations used for standing procedures**

COMBINATIONS	INITIAL BOLUS (IV)	MAINTENANCE (IV)
Xylazine + butorphanol	(X) 0.22–0.66 mg/kg + (B) 0.02 mg/kg	Repeat 1/3 X as needed.
Detomidine + butorphanol	(D) 2.5–5 µg/kg + (B) 0.02 mg/kg	Repeat 1/3 D as needed.
Xylazine + acepromazine	(X) 0.22–0.5 mg/kg + (A) 0.02 mg/kg	Repeat 1/3 D as needed.
Xylazine + butorphanol + acepromazine	(X) 0.22–0.66 mg/kg + (B) 0.02 mg/kg + (A) 0.02 mg/kg	Repeat 1/3 D as needed.
Xylazine + morphine	(X) 0.1–0.5 mg/kg + (M) 0.1 mg/kg (IM or IV slowly)	(X) 0.65 mg/kg/hour +/- (M) 0.03 mg/kg/hour
Detomidine + butorphanol	(D) 6 µg/kg + (B) 0.02 mg/kg	(D) 0.5 µg/kg/min for 15 min 0.3 µg/kg/min for next 15 min 0.1 µg/kg/min for next 15 min +/- (B) 0.01–0.02 mg/kg/h
Detomidine + morphine +/- Acepromazine	(D) 6 µg/kg + (M) 0.1–0.15 mg/kg +/- (A) 0.01–0.02 mg/kg	(D) 0.5 µg/kg/min for 15 min 0.3 µg/kg/min for next 15 min 0.1 µg/kg/min for next 15 min +/- (M) 0.02 mg/kg/h

- During standing procedures, the head should be supported with a headstand (**Figure 3.23**).
- The head should be kept at a higher level than the heart.
- Elevating the head prevents congestion of the nasal turbinates, which can cause obstruction to airflow and difficulty breathing.
- The respiratory depressant effects are clinically irrelevant in most horses.
  - Respiration rate decreases, but tidal volume increases.
- Decrease in heart rate with subsequent decrease in cardiac output (up to 50% decrease from pre-drug values) with no change in cardiac contractility.

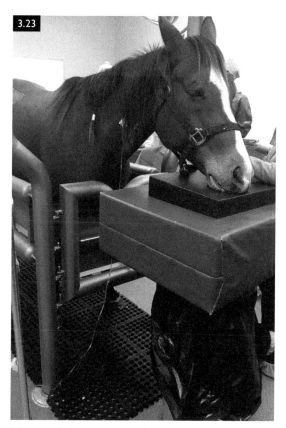

Figure 3.23 Headstand for standing procedures

- Initially peripherally mediated reflex bradycardia due to vasoconstriction and increased blood pressure.
- Later, centrally mediated bradycardia due to enhanced parasympathetic tone.
- Initial increase in blood pressure is followed by hypotension as bradycardia persists in the face of resolving vasoconstriction.
- Induction of hyperglycemia (adult horses > foals).
  - Stimulation of alpha-2 adreno-receptors on pancreatic beta cells, inhibiting insulin secretion.
- Increase in urine output; maximum flow is 30–60 minutes after drug administration.
- Thermoregulation is altered, causing sweating.
- Depression of the swallowing mechanism. Passing a nasogastric tube may be more difficult after administering these drugs.
- Biodisposition.
  - Metabolized by liver; metabolites excreted in urine.
- Clinical use.
  - More profound sedation than that produced by phenothiazines.
  - Predictable sedative—most horses respond as expected.
  - Horses will drop head (**Figure 3.24**) and shift weight from side to side, becoming indifferent to surroundings.
  - The knees or hind legs may buckle; horses may stumble or become profoundly ataxic.
  - There is potential for the horse to be startled and kick out behind.
  - Potential for unprovoked aggression (Rompun rage) reported with both xylazine and detomidine.
  - Draft horses and foals are particularly sensitive to alpha-2 agonist sedation. Use cautiously if at all in neonates and pediatric patients.

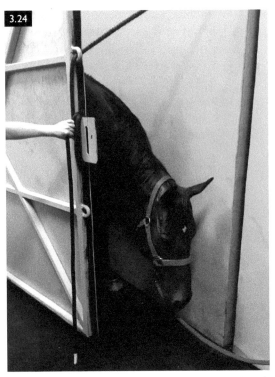

Figure 3.24 Horse with head dropped, sedated

- Complications, side effects, and clinical toxicity.
  - Inadequate sedation, analgesia, and ataxia.
  - Sweating, piloerection.
  - Bradycardia.
  - Sinus arrhythmia.
  - First-degree AV block.
  - Second-degree AV block.
  - Initial hypertension followed by hypotension.
  - Decreased respiratory rate with compensatory increase in tidal volume.
  - Relaxation of the muscles of the upper airway, which can cause stridor.
  - Decreased salivation and gastric secretions.
  - Reduction or cessation of gastrointestinal motility for at least one hour after administration.

- Increased urine volume production within 30–60 minutes of administration.
- Incidental effects include increase in intrauterine pressure, hyperglycemia, and hypoinsulinemia.
- Antagonism.
  - These agents can be antagonized by alpha-2 adrenoreceptor antagonists. When the antagonist is administered IV, it should be injected slowly to avoid adverse effects (excitatory awakening, pain, hypotension, and arrhythmias).
  - Atipamezole (0.05–0.2 mg/kg IM or slow IV).
    - Most selective for alpha-2 receptor antagonism, avoiding unwanted effects of alpha-1 antagonism, including profound hypotension.
  - Yohimbine (0.04–0.15 mg/kg IM or slow IV).
    - Mildly selective for alpha-2 receptors.
  - Tolazoline (0.5–4.0 mg/kg IM or slow IV).
    - Not selective.

3.3.1.1 Xylazine
- Dose-related sedation.
- Quick onset of action (1–2 minutes) and duration of 20–30 minutes.
- As a solo agent:
  - Good for restraint for procedures on the front half of the horse.
  - Potential for the horse to startle and kick behind.
  - Often generates a head-down posture; horse is more apt to exhibit hind end aggression than in a state of sedation in which the horse is standing more squarely on all feet.
- Dose: 0.2–1 mg/kg IV.
- Use in conjunction with other sedatives (opioid and/or longer-acting alpha-2 agonist) for longer duration of and/or more potent sedation.

- Sanctioned drug usage.
  - United States Equestrian Federation (USEF)/Federation Equestre International (FEI) has not established withdrawal and/or detection time.

3.3.1.2 Detomidine
- Dose-related sedation.
- More specific alpha-2 receptor agonist than xylazine.
- Approximately 100 times more potent than xylazine with duration of action twice as long.
- Moderate onset of action (3–5 minutes) and duration of 45–60 minutes.
- Dose: 0.01–0.02 mg/kg IV or IM.
- Sanctioned drug usage.
  - USEF/FEI: detention time of 48 hours.
- Detectable in urine up to 3 days following administration (any route).
- Oral transmucosal gel.
  - Dormosedan Gel (Zoetis, Florham Park, NJ, USA).
  - Designed to be administered by veterinarians and/or prescribed for use to qualified laypersons.
  - For patient that is not amenable to injections and/or owner who is not skilled at injections.
  - Inconsistent effects and long duration to onset.
  - Dose 0.04 mg/kg sublingually in an oromucosal gel containing 7.6 mg detomidine/ml.
  - Sublingual application is ideal.
  - In a field study, it was effective in facilitating the completion of routine veterinary and husbandry procedures in horses known to require sedation for such procedures.

3.3.1.3 Romifidine
- Dose-related sedation.
- More specific alpha-2 receptor agonist than xylazine and detomidine.

- Quick onset of action (1–2 minutes) and duration of 30–40 minutes.
- Depth of maximal sedation reported to be lower than that of detomidine (as determined by lowering of the head).
- Less reported ataxia than with other alpha-2 agonists.
- Analgesic effects are controversial and are shorter in duration than sedative effects.
- Dose: 0.04–0.12 mg/kg IV.
- Sanctioned drug usage.
  - USEF/FEI—detention time of 60 hours.

3.3.2 Opioids
- Mechanism of action.
  - Bind to opioid receptors in the CNS and peripheral organs.
  - Opioid receptors include mu (μ), kappa (κ), and delta (δ) receptors.
  - Alterations in autonomic tone.
  - Increases in dopamine release/brain dopamine receptor sensitivity.
    - Behavioral changes.
    - Increased locomotor activity.
  - Inhibition of ascending transmission of nociception from the dorsal horns of the spinal cord.
  - Activation of descending pain control circuits from the midbrain.
- Applied pharmacology.
  - Most relevant effects on CNS and gastrointestinal (GI) tract.
    - Analgesia.
    - Mild sedation or excitement.
    - Increased locomotor activity.
    - Mild cardiovascular depression (bradycardia).
    - Mild increase in body temperature.
  - Excitatory effects and increased locomotor activity more likely to occur in patients that are not in pain at the time of administration.
  - Increased pain tolerance when administered alone or in combination with alpha-2 agonists or NSAIDs.

- Potential to mildly depress ventilation.
- Cough suppressant effect.
- Clinical doses do not produce major effects on the cardiovascular system.
- Clinical importance of the effect on GI motility is controversial.
  - Pronounced and prolonged decreases in propulsive motility can occur.
- Biodisposition.
  - Metabolism and elimination are complex and dose-related.
  - Extensively metabolized in the liver.
  - Metabolites can be active and have the potential to be cumulative. Repeated dosing could produce unwanted side effects.
- Clinical use.
  - Opioid agonists, partial agonists, and agonist-antagonists are most useful when co-administered with sedative-hypnotics to provide additional analgesia for standing chemical restraint.
  - Thought to help "keep the feet on the ground".
  - When administered alone in non-painful horses: unpredictable, inability to produce desired effects, development of side effects.
  - Can be administered alone to treat pain.
    - Colic, trauma, post-surgical pain, laminitis, etc.
- Complications, side effects, and clinical toxicity.
  - Most complications are observed in horses that are non-painful at the time of administration. These effects are unlikely to occur in horses that are painful.
    - Disorientation.
    - Increased locomotor activity.
    - Hyper-responsiveness to touch and sounds.
    - Development of ataxia.
  - Horses can appear sedate but can be startled easily.

- Constipation and impaction colic can occur after repeated administration of opioid agonists.
- Extremely large doses can cause seizures.
- Some agents are frequently associated with histamine release, especially when given IV (e.g. morphine, meperidine). In the case of morphine, the incidence is not clinically relevant when administered slowly IV.
- Antagonism.
  - Reversible with opioid antagonists, such as naloxone.
    - Prompt reversal of both central and peripheral effects of opioid agonists.
    - Also antagonism of endogenous opioid ligands (e.g. endorphin, dynorphin).

3.3.2.1 Butorphanol
- Opioid mixed agonist-antagonist; agonist at kappa receptors and antagonist at mu receptors.
- Classified by the United States Drug Enforcement Administration (DEA) as a controlled schedule IV substance.
- Minimal effect on intestinal transit time and gut sounds.
- Dose: 0.01–0.02 mg/kg IV or IM.
- Sanctioned drug usage.
  - USEF/FEI: detention time of 72 hours.
  - Detectable in urine up to 3 days following administration (any route).

3.3.2.2 Morphine
- Full mu agonist.
- Classified by the DEA as a controlled schedule II substance.
- Intestinal transit time is decreased.
- Can be used for standing procedures in combination with an alpha-2 agonist. It is recommended to wait until the horse is sedated before administering morphine.
- Can be administered IM or IV. When used as IV bolus, it should be injected slowly to

decrease the incidence of histamine release. Can also be administered as a constant rate infusion (CRI) (**Table 3.1**).
- Can be used epidurally to provide analgesia for standing procedures.
- Dose: 0.1–0.2 mg/kg IM, IV, intra-articular, and epidural.

3.3.3 Phenothiazine Tranquilizers
- Produce calming, indifference, and decreased locomotion.
- Mild sedation.
- No analgesia.
  - Thought to enhance the analgesic and CNS depressive activity of other drugs used for standing sedation (alpha-2 agonists and opioids).
- Arousability and avoidance behaviors are maintained. The horse remains able to respond to stimuli and react spontaneously and potentially violently.
- Mechanism of action.
  - Dopamine antagonist. It blocks the action of dopamine centrally and peripherally.
  - Alpha-1 adrenergic blockade that can lead to arterial hypotension.
- Applied pharmacology.
  - Most common hemodynamic effect is a decrease in arterial blood pressure.
- Clinically used doses reduce arterial blood pressure by 15–20 mmHg.
  - Dose-dependent, may produce reflex tachycardia.
- Biodisposition.
  - Metabolized by the liver, excreted in the urine.
- Clinical use.
  - In the United States, available as a 1% injectable solution (10 mg/ml).
  - Also available in an oral gel form in the United Kingdom.
  - Onset of action is approximately 15–30 minutes, although peak effect may take up to 45 minutes to achieve.

- Duration of effect depends on dose administered and the metabolic state of the horse but can last as long as 6–10 hours.
- Increasing the dose will not increase the intensity of sedation, only the duration of action.
- Effects of drug administration.
  - Produces a calmer demeanor.
  - Will not make an aggressive or rambunctious horse an acquiescent patient.
  - Decrease in respiratory rate observed, although drug does not directly affect respiration.
  - In stallions and geldings: rarely causes paraphimosis (flaccid paralysis of the retractor penis muscle).
  - To assess degree of sedation: monitor for protrusion of the flaccid penis in male horses, eyelid droop, and protrusion of the nictitans (third eyelid).
  - If horse is hypovolemic, may cause acute hypotension and recumbency.
  - Treatment: large volumes of intravenous fluids.
  - Paradoxical excitement is rare but has been reported.
  - Reduction in packed cell volume and total protein concentration.
    - Dose-dependent.
    - May last up to 12 hours.
    - Attributed to sequestration of red blood cells in the spleen and subsequent hemodilution of the circulating blood secondary to vasodilation in the spleen and peripheral circulation.
  - Reduction in platelet activity and prolonged clotting times.
- Complications, side effects, and toxicity.
  - Inadequate sedation.
  - Ataxia, hypotension, and reflex tachycardia are the most common side effects.

- Especially in excited horses, may cause a profound decrease in systemic blood pressure leading to collapse.
  - Impending signs include profuse sweating, hyperpnea, tachycardia, and marked ataxia within 5 minutes of intravenous drug administration.
  - Treatment is symptomatic: intravenous fluid replacement (5–20 ml/kg IV).
- Paraphimosis (**Figure 3.25**).
  - Devastating, potentially life-threatening side effect.
  - The mechanism responsible is unknown.
  - Incidence is estimated to be less than 1 in 10,000.
  - Treatment: conservative therapy includes reduction of edema with massage, placing the penis in a sling to maintain it within the preputial sheath, cold water hydrotherapy, and administration of analgesic drugs.
- Extrapyramidal effects

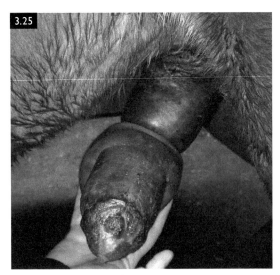

Figure 3.25 **Paraphimosis**
Courtesy of Dr. Brittany Cheesman

- Large doses (> 0.2 mg/kg) can cause abnormal behavior, reluctance to move, slight rigidity, mild muscle tremors, and restlessness.
- Severe ataxia at high doses.
- Contraindications.
  - Stallions used for breeding purposes due to potential for paraphimosis. However, the incidence is very low.
  - Patients with thrombocytopathia due to inhibitory effect on platelets.
  - Hypovolemic patients are more likely to develop severe hypotension.
  - Septic patients.
  - When testing for allergens.
- Acepromazine has antihistaminic properties.
  - Rarely, can cause sudden collapse in excited horses.
- In animals with high circulating levels of catecholamines.
  - Peripheral alpha-1 receptors are blocked by acepromazine. This will unmask the vasodilation caused by the circulating epinephrine on beta-2 receptors, resulting in profound secondary hypotension (epinephrine reversal).
- Antagonism.
  - No specific antagonist.

3.3.3.1 Acepromazine

- Dose: 0.02–0.1 mg/kg IV, IM, PO. It is recommended not to exceed 30 mg total.
- Sanctioned drug usage.
  - USEF/FEI: Prohibited substance.
- Detectable in urine up to 7 days following administration (any route).
- May be used for legitimate therapeutic purpose, but horse will be withdrawn from competition for 24 hours, and a written medication form must be filed documenting the therapeutic indication and application.

3.4 CASE EXAMPLES

3.4.1 Twelve-Year-Old Quarter Horse Mare with a Superficial Right Antebrachial Laceration

- The mare (body weight: 500 kg) is administered romifidine (10 mg) and acepromazine (10 mg) intravenously for examination.
- Following a physical examination in which the mare is held with a halter and lead rope, the mare's plane of sedation is deemed inadequate as she begins moving around more during removal of a pressure bandage.
- Detomidine (2 mg) and butorphanol (5 mg) are administered intravenously.
- A shoulder twitch is applied to the horse through bandage removal.
- The mare remains sedate but aware throughout the remainder of the evaluation and laceration repair.

3.4.2 An Eight-Year-Old Warmblood Gelding Presents for a Lameness Evaluation

- The horse has a history of routine empirical treatment of the distal hock joints with steroids and hyaluronic acid prior to the show season.
- A moderate left hindlimb lameness is detected on baseline gait analysis, and the horse has a positive response to hock/stifle (proximal limb) flexion of the lame limb.
- It is elected to perform intra-articular anesthesia of the left distal intertarsal and tarsometatarsal joints.
- The horse is sensitive to palpation of the hindlimbs, has a history of kicking, and is generally high-strung.
- No sedation can be administered due to the necessity of repeat gait analysis very shortly following the procedure.
- For the procedure, the horse is restrained by an experienced handler standing on the left side of the horse with a chain lead positioned over the nose and a lip twitch in place.
  - The twitch is tightened rhythmically with a twist of the handler's wrist to maintain the horse's attention.
- An additional assistant holds up the left forelimb for the intra-articular deposition of local anesthetic.

3.4.3 A Twenty-Two-Year-Old Thoroughbred Gelding Presents to a Referral Center for Colic

- The horse is approximately 500 kg in weight and was refractory to medical management in the field.
- Prior medical therapy included:
  - Non-steroidal anti-inflammatory administration (flunixin meglumine, 1.1 mg/kg IV)
  - Sedation with xylazine (150 mg IV, twice).
- Signs of colic have been present for eight hours and have been worsening in severity along with progressive abdominal distention.
- Upon arrival, the horse is down in the trailer but able to rise. It has a heart rate of 64 beats/minute and is quiet but responsive.
- The gelding is restrained with a lead rope and is positioned in a set of stocks for examination and diagnostics.
- The horse immediately begins pawing and buckling on the contralateral forelimb. Intravenous sedation (detomidine, 5 mg, and butorphanol, 5 mg) is administered, the horse relaxes, and signs of colic dissipate.
- A lip twitch is placed for passage of a nasogastric tube and palpation per rectum.
  - Three liters of net reflux are obtained from the stomach, and a large, gas-distended viscus is palpated in the right caudal abdomen, extending across midline.
- Bloodwork demonstrates mild elevation of peripheral lactate (3.4 mmol/L) but is otherwise generally unremarkable.

- Thirty minutes into the evaluation, signs of colic return; the aforementioned sedation is repeated, in addition to an additional dose administered intramuscularly.
- Surgical management of the colic is discussed with the owner based on progression of clinical signs and persistent, refractory pain.

3.4.4 A Fourteen-Month-Old Tennessee Walking Horse with a Right Front Pastern Laceration

- The unhandled and unbroken filly weighs approximately 350 kg.
- A halter is in place but is not useful as a leading device.
- The filly is corralled into a small examination area free of additional objects and in a quiet area.
- While lightly restraining the filly, an experienced horse person swiftly administers acepromazine (10 mg) and detomidine (3 mg) intramuscularly prior to any examination; the filly is allowed to rest without stimulation for 20 minutes.
- Following this period of sedative onset, the filly is more amenable to handling.
- Additional sedation is administered intravenously (xylazine, 100 mg, and butorphanol, 5 mg).
  - This produces profound sedation with a head-down stance.
- The filly is positioned against a wall with the affected limb away from the wall and lightly restrained with a halter and lead rope by an experienced handler.
- The limb is clipped and cleaned, and peri-neural anesthesia is administered for exploration and closure of the wound and bandaging of the limb.
- The filly is discharged with oral detomidine gel for administration prior to subsequent bandage changes by the owner.

3.4.5 A Three-Year-Old Holsteiner Mare Presents for Management of Fistulous Withers

- The mare weighs approximately 450 kg.
- Although the mare has been ground-broken, she is needle-shy, unruly, and anxious and strikes without warning.
- The mare is sensitive to palpation and manipulation of the draining wound tract over her withers.
- The mare's condition requires frequent cleanings and topical application to the affected site and surrounding skin, which has become irritated and inflamed.
- The mare is administered oral acepromazine (30 mg) twice daily in her feed, and an intravenous catheter is placed with a long extension set to facilitate ease drug administration when needed.
  - The catheter is flushed every 6 hours to maintain patency.
- For procedures, the mare is sedated with intravenous detomidine (5 mg) and butorphanol (5 mg) in the stall and is walked into the exam room with a chain lead rope placed over the nose.
- The mare's withers are examined while the mare is in the stocks for the safety of the operators.

3.4.6 A Four-Month-Old Colt with Bilateral Forelimb Flexural Limb Deformity

- The colt is stalled with his healthy companion mare, an eighteen-year-old Quarter horse broodmare weighing approximately 500 kg.
- A bilateral inferior check ligament desmotomy is planned.
- Prior to removing the foal from the stall for the procedure, the mare is held with a lead rope and sedated intravenously with detomidine (5 mg) and acepromazine (5 mg),

and intramuscularly with detomidine (5 mg) and acepromazine (5 mg).

- A muzzle is placed to prevent the mare from choking on feed available while sedate. The mare does not react to the foal's departure and remains quiet in the stall for 1.5 hours throughout the procedure.

FURTHER READING

Bettschart-Wolfensbberger R (2015) Horses. In: *Veterinary Anesthesia and Analgesia: The Fifth Edition of Lumb and Jones*, 5th edn. (eds Grimm KA, Lamont LA, Tranquilli WJ et al), Wiley Blackwell, Ames, pp. 857–866.

Fédération Equestre Inrenationale (2018) *FEI List of Detection Times*. https://inside.fei.org/system/files/FEI%20Detection%20Times%202018_0.pdf. Accessed 14 April 2019.

Gardner R, White GW, Ramsey DS et al (2010) Efficacy of detomidine oromucosal gel in horses for procedures requiring sedation. *Proceedings of the 56th Annual Convention of the American Association of Equine Practitioners*, Baltimore, pp. 50–52.

Guedes A (2013) How to maximize standing chemical restraint. *Proceedings of the 59th Annual Convention of the American Association of Equine Practitioners*, Nashville, pp. 461–463.

Hubbell JAE (2009) Practical standing chemical restraint in the horse. *Proceedings of the 55th Annual Convention of the American Association of Equine Practitioners*, Las Vegas, pp. 2–6.

Lagerweij E, Nelis PC, Wiegant VM et al (1984) The twitch in horses: A variant of acupuncture. *Science* **225**:1172–1174.

Muir WW (2009) Anxiolytics, nonopioid sedative-analgesics, and opioid analgesics. In: *Equine Anesthesia Monitoring and Emergency Therapy*, 2nd edn. (eds Muir WW, Hubbell JAE), Saunders Elsevier, St. Louis, pp. 185–209.

Robertson JT, Muir WW (2009) Physical restraint. In: *Equine Anesthesia Monitoring and Emergency Therapy*, 2nd edn. (eds Muir WW, Hubbell JAE), Saunders Elsevier, St. Louis, pp. 109–120.

Valverde A (2010) Alpha-2 agonists as pain therapy in horses. *Vet Clin North Am Equine Pract* **26**:515–532.

Vigani A, Garcia-Pereira FL (2014) Anesthesia and analgesia for standing equine surgery. *Vet Clin North Am Equine Pract* **30**:1–17.

CHAPTER 4

INDUCTION OF ANESTHESIA

Kristen Messenger and Rachel Reed

4.1 INTRODUCTION

Induction of anesthesia in the horse is a multi-step process that begins with preparation of the patient and ends with initiation of anesthetic maintenance agents. Equine anesthetic induction is hazardous and requires trained personnel and specialized equipment.

4.2 PREPARATION OF THE HORSE FOR INDUCTION OF ANESTHESIA

- Fasting: Horses are commonly fasted for 12 hours prior to anesthesia. Fasting reduces the gastrointestinal contents, which results in decreased incidence of regurgitation and increased ventilatory compliance while under anesthesia.
  - A soft grazing muzzle can be placed on the horse to prevent it from eating shavings or grass (**Figure 4.1**).
  - Fasting is not necessary for emergency cases.
  - Aspiration pneumonia is less common in horses compared to dogs and cats, since horses do not actively vomit. They can, however, regurgitate and aspirate.
- Intravenous catheter placement: A 14- or 16-gauge IV catheter should be aseptically placed in the jugular vein prior to anesthesia. Catheter placement can be facilitated with a lidocaine local block and a low dose of xylazine (0.2 mg/kg IV) if needed. The catheter should be secured with suture and a locking port (**Figure 4.2**).

- Premedications: Ensure that any pre-operative medications such as antibiotics or NSAIDs have been administered. Premedications used for sedation and as part of the induction protocol will be discussed below.
  - Pre-anesthesia checklists are utilized by many practices to ensure all necessary tasks have been completed prior to anesthesia. A checklist should include:
    - Identification of the animal (e.g. case number).
    - Client consent obtained.
    - Physical evaluation.
    - Bloodwork.
    - Type of procedure and surgical site.
    - Recumbency.
    - Administration of pre-operative drugs (e.g. NSAIDs and antibiotics).
    - Patient preparation (e.g. mouth rinsed and feet cleaned).
    - IV catheter placement.
- Mouth rinsing: The oral cavity is rinsed of any debris (grass, hay, feed material) prior to induction of anesthesia to prevent passage of debris into the airway during intubation.
  - Horses can be sedated with a small dose of xylazine (0.2 mg/kg) if necessary to facilitate rinsing of the oral cavity (**Figure 4.3**).
- Other pre-anesthetic considerations: Correction of dehydration and existing electrolyte abnormalities (e.g., calcium, potassium), provision of pre-emptive analgesia.

DOI: 10.1201/9780429190940-4

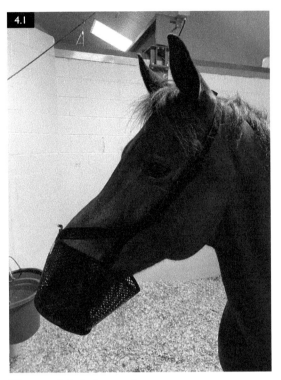

Figure 4.1 **Soft muzzle**

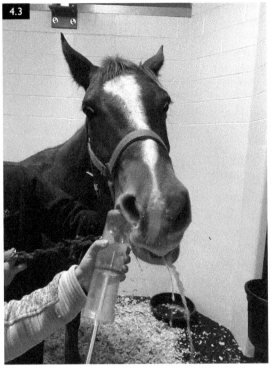

Figure 4.3 **Rinsing of mouth**

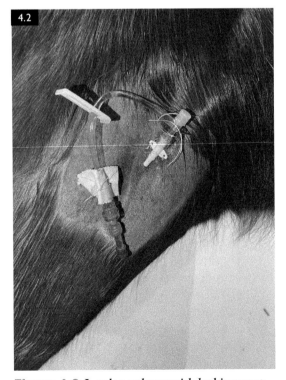

Figure 4.2 **Jugular catheter with locking port**

4.3 COMPONENTS NECESSARY FOR THE INDUCTION OF ANESTHESIA

- Induction area: Ideally, anesthesia should be induced in a quiet area free of obstacles and with an exit route for personnel.
  - Most large-animal hospitals are equipped with padded induction stalls with swinging gates to confine the horse to a small area prior to anesthesia (**Figure 4.4**). This situation is ideal to protect the horse and the personnel involved with the anesthetic event.
  - Some hospitals are equipped with tilt tables, allowing for horses to be strapped to the table prior to induction and then tilted into lateral recumbency after anesthesia has been induced (**Figure 4.5**).
  - Anesthesia can also be induced in open outside areas. The anesthetist should be cognizant of nearby hazards such as

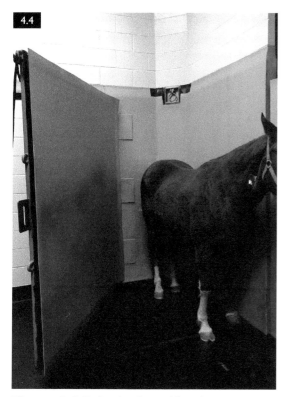

Figure 4.4 **Induction box with swing gate**

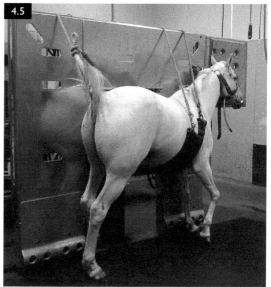

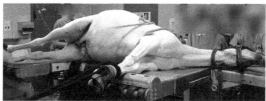

Figure 4.5 **Tilt table**
Courtesy of Dr. Wei-Chen Kuo

fences, holes, buildings, equipment, and other debris.
- Halters and leads: The horse should be restrained with a snug-fitting nylon or leather halter (**Figure 4.6**).
  - Rope halters should be avoided for anesthetic induction.
  - A lead rope can be used to bring the horse to the induction area and throughout the induction event. However, in some scenarios, it may be preferable to remove the lead rope and proceed just holding the halter.
- Tools for intubation: Endotracheal tubes, sterile lubrication, and speculum/bite block should be present in the induction area in order to rapidly intubate the horse after intubation (**Figure 4.7**).
  - Additional supplies such as endoscopes or nasogastric tubes may be necessary if a difficult intubation is expected.

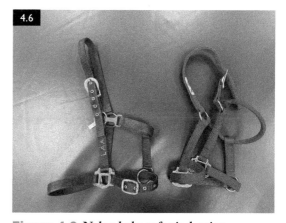

Figure 4.6 **Nylon halters for induction**

- Eye lubrication should be available to lubricate and protect the cornea after induction.
- Tail ropes: The authors have seen some facilities (usually those without induction

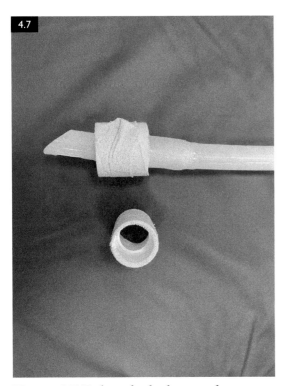

Figure 4.7 Endotracheal tube, speculum

doors/walls) utilize a tail rope during the induction process.

- The tail rope may be controversial but can be used to assist the horse in falling backwards instead of forwards, where it is more likely to injure both itself and personnel.
- A slip-knot is applied to the tail once the horse has been sedated. It is then run through a ring or bar securely attached to the wall behind the horse. A separate person involved in induction pulls on the tail rope as the horse is being induced to encourage backward movement of the animal.
- Complications of a tail rope include personnel injury and broken tail.
- A tracheotomy kit should be available in the area of induction and recovery; items that should be present in the kit include scalpel, temporary tracheotomy tube, lidocaine,

syringes, alcohol preparation, 4x4" gauze sponges, clippers, and sedation/anesthesia drugs.

4.4 DRUGS FOR THE INDUCTION OF ANESTHESIA

Premedications/sedatives are used as part of the induction protocol. No horse should ever be administered an induction agent without being adequately sedated, except for specific emergency cases (e.g., catastrophic recovery events or horses recumbent in a trailer without an intravenous catheter).

- Drugs commonly used for provision of sedation prior to induction of anesthesia in horses include alpha-2 adrenergic agonists and acepromazine.
- Opioids are commonly administered prior to induction of anesthesia in order to provide pre-emptive analgesia. A detailed discussion of drugs used for sedation in horses can be found in Chapter 3.

4.4.1 Drugs

- *Ketamine*: The most commonly used drug for the induction of anesthesia in horses. It is a phencyclidine derivative, and its mechanism of action is via antagonism of the N-methyl-D-aspartate (NMDA) receptor.
  - Ketamine provides smooth induction of anesthesia with a large margin of safety.
  - It is a sympathomimetic drug, so induction of anesthesia is associated with an increase in heart rate and cardiac output in patients that have an intact sympathetic nervous system at the time of induction.
  - Furthermore, it is long lasting, with a single induction dose providing 15–20 minutes of recumbency time.

- Ketamine also has analgesic effects via NMDA receptor antagonism and opioid receptor agonism.
- Additionally, the drug is cost-effective and capable of inducing general anesthesia in a horse with reasonable volumes.
- Ketamine does not provide good muscle relaxation; therefore, it is often combined with a benzodiazepine in a co-induction protocol.
- *Benzodiazepines*: These agents are commonly used during induction of anesthesia in co-induction agents in combination with ketamine.
  - The mechanism of action of these agents is agonism of the GABA-A receptor.
  - The commonly used benzodiazepines in equine anesthesia include diazepam and midazolam.
  - These drugs can be used interchangeably, because there is no difference from a clinical perspective in the effect of these drugs. The most common adverse effect in the horse is muscle weakness.
  - Benzodiazepines can be used to cause sedation prior to induction of anesthesia in foals.
- *Tiletamine and zolazepam:* These two drugs come pre-mixed under the trade names of Telazol and Zoletil. The induction has similar attributes compared to ketamine and midazolam but has been associated with prolonged recoveries.
- *Propofol*: This agent is an agonist at the GABA receptor and provides hypnosis and muscle relaxation.
  - Propofol may be used in the place of a benzodiazepine, with ketamine, to provide some muscle relaxation during induction.
  - The dose is 0.4–0.5 mg/kg, although anecdotally 20 ml to the average-sized 450–500 kg horse is acceptable.

- Recovery has been reported to be faster and smoother with propofol compared to midazolam.
- Propofol can be used alone as an induction agent for horses at a dose of 1.5–2 mg/kg.
  - As a solo agent, there are some disadvantages including paddling at induction, hypoventilation/apnea, a large volume required, and cost.
  - This technique is not recommended for standard-size adult horses. Can be used for foals and miniature horses.
- *Alfaxalone*: This agent is an agonist at the GABA receptor, providing hypnosis and muscle relaxation similar to that of propofol.
  - Similar to propofol, it can be used in combination with ketamine.
  - Use of alfaxalone alone is quite costly, requires a large volume, and can cause myoclonus in the induction and recovery periods; therefore, it is not recommended.
- *Barbiturates*: The most common barbiturate used for the induction of anesthesia in horses is thiopental.
  - At present, this drug is not commercially available in the United States.
  - Thiopental must be administered via an indwelling intravenous catheter, as perivascular administration is associated with severe tissue necrosis and sloughing, which is caused by the very basic pH of the solution (pH > 10).
- *Inhalants*: Induction using only an inhalant is rarely performed.
  - If and/or when it is indicated in adult horses, special equipment such as a tilt table is required to prevent injury to personnel and the patient.
  - It can be performed more safely in a neonate.
  - Sevoflurane is generally recommended because of rapid onset and less airway

Table 4.1 **Induction agents**

INDUCTION AGENT(S) AND DOSE	COMMENTS
Ketamine 2.2 mg/kg IV	Patients remain cardiovascularly stable, continue to protect their own airway, and breathe spontaneously. Poor muscle relaxation.
Ketamine 2.2mg/kg IV + Midazolam/diazepam 0.05mg/kg IV	Patients remain cardiovascularly stable, continue to protect their own airway, and breathe spontaneously.
Tiletamine-zolazepam 1.1 mg/kg IV	Similar qualities to ketamine induction. Associated with prolonged recoveries.
Propofol 1.5–2 mg/kg IV	Associated with poor recoveries; patients often become apneic immediately after induction and require IPPV; patients may develop myoclonus. Can be used in foals and miniature horses
Ketamine 2 mg/kg IV + Propofol 0.4 mg/kg IV	Improved induction quality compared to propofol alone

irritation. It is also easily titrated to effect due to low solubility of the agent. However, it is more expensive compared to isoflurane.

- Drugs and protocols commonly used for induction of general anesthesia are summarized in **Table 4.1**

4.5 OROTRACHEAL INTUBATION

- Intubation provides a means to deliver oxygen and inhaled anesthetic gasses without exposing staff to potentially harmful waste anesthetic gasses.
- Intubation allows the anesthetist to provide positive pressure ventilation to the horse, which is often required for invasive procedures or procedures lasting longer than ~60 minutes. Hypoxemia secondary to ventilation/perfusion mismatch is very common in anesthetized horses, necessitating positive pressure ventilation during anesthesia in many cases.
- The airway (trachea and lungs) is protected from aspiration of gastric contents. Regurgitation is rare in equine anesthesia; however, it is possible especially in colic cases.

4.5.1 How to Place an Endotracheal Tube

- Endotracheal intubation is performed "blindly" in most cases.
- Once the horse is in lateral recumbency, a bite block or speculum can be placed between the horse's upper and lower incisors (**Figure 4.8**).
- The tongue should be manually pulled forward through the interdental space (**Figure 4.8**).
- The horse's head and neck can be gently extended to create a straighter path from the tip of the teeth to the trachea.
  - Make sure to protect the dependent eye as you are extending the head/neck.
- An appropriate-size endotracheal tube is then introduced into the oral cavity, past the molar teeth, and VERY GENTLY advanced into the trachea (**Figure 4.9**).
  - This step is very important and must be performed gently and without trauma to the horse's airway.
  - If the endotracheal tube does not advance into the trachea immediately, which is very common, then the tube should be withdrawn a few inches, rotated approximately 60–90 degrees, and then advanced again.

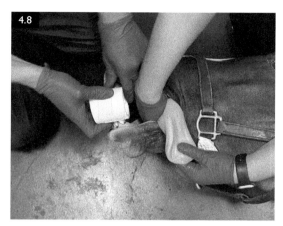

Figure 4.8 Speculum in place, pulling tongue out

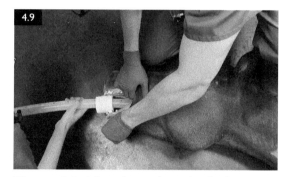

Figure 4.9 Advancing endotracheal tube

- This procedure is repeated (keep rotating the tube in the same direction) until the endotracheal tube easily enters the trachea in a smooth motion.
- If any resistance is met during this process, do not force the tube forward! This will cause trauma to the arytenoid cartilages, which can lead to swelling and airway obstruction.
- When intubation is performed correctly, the tube slides into the trachea easily.
- An assistant can push on the horse's thorax, and airflow can be easily felt coming through the tube for confirmation.
- Once confirmed, the endotracheal tube cuff should be inflated until gentle resistance is felt in the pilot balloon.

- Do not over-inflate the endotracheal tube cuff. Over-inflation can lead to several problems, including:
  - Necrosis of the tracheal mucosa.
  - Obstruction of the endotracheal tube.
  - Often, over-inflation of the cuff goes unnoticed until after the procedure, when the horse could have clinical signs associated with tracheal necrosis or irritation (coughing, hemorrhagic sputum, dyspnea).
  - Tracheoscopy can confirm mucosal injury.
- Conversely, the cuff must be inflated to a volume that creates an air-tight seal between the cuff and the walls of the trachea, to ensure that:
  - Positive pressure ventilation can be performed.
  - No pollution of anesthetic gasses into the environment/theater will occur, which would unnecessarily expose personnel.
    - The anesthetist can confirm the seal is appropriate by placing their hands over the horse's nares once the horse is connected to an anesthesia machine or a mechanical ventilator.
  - When a manual breath is administered, no airflow should be felt exiting the horse's nares on expiration.
- In some scenarios, it is desirable to intubate the horse in sternal recumbency just after induction.
  - This is often done in order to minimize the chance of aspiration reflux in the case of colic patients or fluid retained in the esophagus in choke patients.
  - The same procedure is followed as outlined above with the horse in sternal, and when the endotracheal tube cuff is inflated, the horse is allowed to roll into lateral recumbency.
- See also Chapter 1.

4.5.2 Endotracheal Tube Size Selection

- For the average 450 kg horse, a 26 mm endotracheal tube is usually an appropriate size; however, it is good anesthesia practice to have one size below and one size above the anticipated "correct" size (**Figure 4.10**). Remember to check the cuff for leaks *prior to* induction of the horse.
- For procedures involving the airway, when the tube may or may not be temporarily removed, a smaller endotracheal tube may be used (22 or 24 mm).
- If the horse has a known history of laryngeal paralysis, then a smaller tube is recommended.
- For foals, specialized silicone tubes are commercially available in sizes ranging from 8 to 16 mm internal diameter (**Figure 4.11**).
- See also Chapter 1.

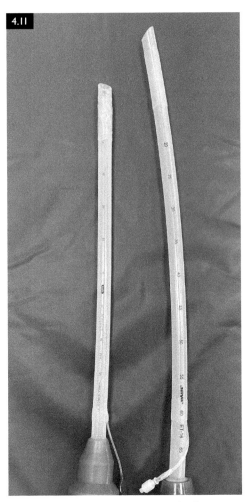

Figure 4.11 Foal endotracheal tubes

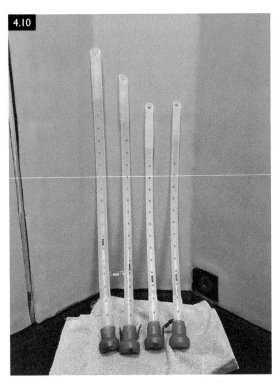

Figure 4.10 Multiple endotracheal tube sizes prepared for induction

4.6   NASOTRACHEAL INTUBATION

- Performed if orotracheal intubation is contraindicated (**Figure 4.12**), which may occur in unusual circumstances in adult horses.
- Can be used to facilitate access to the oral cavity during dental procedures.
- Nasotracheal intubation can be performed in foals, although orotracheal intubation is generally recommended.

4.6.1   How to Place a Nasotracheal Tube

- An appropriately sized endotracheal tube is vital to successful nasotracheal intubation.

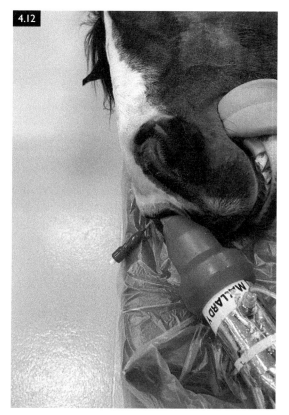

Figure 4.12 Nasotracheal intubation

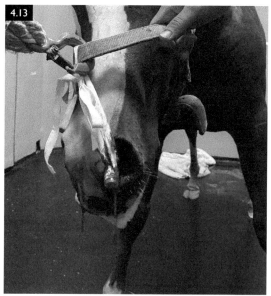

Figure 4.13 Nasal hemorrhage

Size 14–16 mm endotracheal tubes are generally the appropriate size for an adult horse.
- With the horse in lateral recumbency, adjust the head and neck so an almost straight line can be created from the tip of the nose to the trachea.
  - Make sure to protect the dependent eye as you are extending the head/neck.
- Apply sterile lubricant around the patient end of the endotracheal tube. This procedure is generally performed blindly.
  - The anesthetist will be aiming for the ventro-medial meatus of the nasal cavity and will gently advance the tube towards the pharynx.
- If any resistance is felt, stop advancement, remove the tube, and attempt replacement to avoid complications (see next section).

- When correctly placed, the tube will continue to easily advance into the nasopharynx and ultimately into the trachea.
- This procedure can be difficult at first, as the tube tends to advance into the esophagus rather than the trachea. The anesthetist can attempt to advance the tube during inspiration, which may increase the chance of successful placement.
- As with orotracheal intubation, backing the tube out a few inches, rotating ~60 degrees, and re-advancing the tube is recommended if necessary.
- Confirmation of a successfully placed nasotracheal tube is via confirmation of airflow through the tube during expiration.

4.6.2 Complications of Nasotracheal Intubation
- The most common complication of nasotracheal intubation is hemorrhage (**Figure 4.13**). The sinuses are very delicate and heavily vascularized, thus easily irritated.

- To minimize the chance of this complication, a nasotracheal tube should never be roughly placed in a horse.
- Traumatic hemorrhage is a common enough complication that if a horse has a known coagulopathy, this procedure should not be attempted without specialized equipment (scope) and/or available replacement blood products.
- Trauma to the larynx can occur with nasotracheal intubation, just as in orotracheal intubation, which can lead to swelling, irritation, and potentially fatal airway obstruction.
- Because the nasotracheal tubes are often small in diameter, it can be difficult to obtain an appropriate seal on the cuff.
- See also Chapter 1.

4.7 MANAGEMENT OF DIFFICULT AIRWAYS

- If there is difficulty with intubation, often a smaller endotracheal tube can be successfully placed using the technique described above. However, there can be functional or anatomic abnormalities that preclude a successful orotracheal intubation.
- In the case of unexpected difficulty with orotracheal intubation, an endoscope is recommended to visualize the arytenoids and successfully intubate, perhaps with a smaller tube.
  - The endoscope can be inserted into the endotracheal tube lumen before the intubation and used to guide the tube between the arytenoids.
  - Once the endoscope passes in place in the glottis, the endotracheal tube can then be gently moved forward over the scope.
- If a complete obstruction occurs (e.g., swelling, laryngeal nerve dysfunction), an emergency tracheotomy can be performed.

- The authors recommend an emergency tracheotomy kit be available for any procedure involving equine anesthesia. The contents of the kit should be labeled and dated, audited at least bi-annually, and replaced every time the kit is used.

4.7.1 Temporary Tracheostomy

- Ideally, a tracheotomy is performed by a surgeon in a non-emergent setting. It can be performed prior to anesthesia as a standing procedure with sedation and local anesthesia if upper airway obstruction is anticipated as a complication (recommended).
- How to perform a tracheotomy:
  - Clip the hair and aseptically prepare the skin on the ventral aspect of the neck, approximately 1/3–1/2 the length of the neck distal to the mandible.
  - Perform local block with lidocaine over the area to be incised.
  - Using sterile technique, make a vertical incision with a #10 blade.
  - Bluntly dissect and separate the muscles.
  - Identify the trachea.
  - Make a horizontal incision between two tracheal rings.
  - Insert and secure temporary tracheostomy tube.
  - Provide supplemental oxygen as needed.

4.8 PERSONNEL SAFETY DURING THE INDUCTION OF ANESTHESIA

- The induction process is second only to recovery in terms of risk to personnel and patients.
- Larger equine hospitals may have special induction walls/doors available for use. These walls are recommended to protect personnel from harm during induction, but they are not always available or practical.
- The number of individuals required for induction will depend on several factors,

including equipment and facility setup. At minimum, two experienced anesthetists should be present at all times. Ideally, three, four, or more individuals should be present.

- Individuals involved in the induction process should be kept up to date in regard to the progress of the induction.
  - For example, after administering induction drugs, the anesthetist should say, "drugs have been administered." This allows all individuals in the room to be aware the horse will become ataxic and recumbent shortly.

4.9 CASE EXAMPLES

4.9.1 Field Castration in a Colt (ASA Status I)

- Xylazine 1 mg/kg IV to heavily sedate.
- Induce with 2.5–3 mg/kg ketamine IV.
- Note: 50% of each of these drugs and doses can be drawn up and used for "top off" if the horse is light during the procedure.
- The horse is restrained by two individuals, one at the head, serving to guide the head down as the horse becomes recumbent, and one at the tail, serving to pull backward, encouraging the horse to sit and then lay down.
- After the horse is recumbent, it is rolled into lateral recumbency, and the eyes are lubricated and covered with a towel for the procedure.
- As this is a field procedure that is anticipated to be short, the horse is not intubated and is allowed to breathe ambient air spontaneously.

4.9.2 Arthroscopy in a Healthy Horse (ASA Status II)

- Xylazine 1 mg/kg IV to heavily sedate + butorphanol 0.02 mg/kg.
- Propofol 0.4 mg/kg IV, followed by ketamine 2.5 mg/kg IV.
  - Alternatively, midazolam 0.05 mg/kg can be substituted for propofol if desired.

- The horse is restrained behind an induction swing door. One anesthetist stands at the horse's head and holds it elevated to encourage the horse to sit and then lay down.
- After the horse goes down into sternal recumbency, the swing door is opened, and the horse is pulled into lateral recumbency.
- The eyes are lubricated, and the dependent eye is closed.
- A PVC mouth gag is placed between the horse's incisors and the head and neck extended; the tongue is pulled out to the non-dependent side.
- The orotracheal tube is inserted over the tongue and gently advanced toward the larynx. Resistance is met at the level of the larynx, so the tube is pulled back 5–10 cm, rotated, and advanced forward again, this time entering the trachea.
- An assistant presses on the horse's chest as the anesthetist feels for air movement in and out of the endotracheal tube to confirm correct placement.

4.9.3 Exploratory Laparotomy for Emergency Colic (ASA Status IV)

- The horse has been actively refluxing and is currently quite painful.
- Xylazine 0.5–1.0 mg/kg IV (start with the lowest possible dose and titrate up as needed) + hydromorphone 0.04 mg/kg.
- Propofol 0.4 mg/kg + Ketamine 2.5 mg/kg IV for induction.
- The horse is restrained behind an induction swing door for the induction.
- One anesthetist stands at the horse's head and holds it elevated to encourage the horse to sit and then lay down.
- After the horse goes down, the mouth gag is placed between the incisors and the head and neck extended for intubation in sternal recumbency due to the active reflux.
  - The tongue is pulled out and to one side, and the endotracheal tube is inserted

into the mouth, over the tongue, and through the larynx to the trachea.

- After the endotracheal tube is in place, the cuff is inflated, the swing door is opened, and the horse is now rolled into lateral recumbency. Special attention is paid to protecting the corneas, and lubrication is applied.

4.9.4 Emergency Laparotomy for Uroabdomen in a Neonate (ASA Status IV)

- Note: The foal should be moderately stabilized if possible prior to anesthesia, and electrolyte abnormalities should be addressed prior to the induction of anesthesia.
- Sedation: Midazolam 0.05 mg/kg + butorphanol 0.02 mg/kg.
- Induction: Ketamine 2 mg/kg + propofol 0.4 mg/kg IV.
- The foal is restrained by hand in the prep area and induced adjacent to the surgery table. The anesthetist holds the head with special attention paid to protecting the eyes. Other personnel present serve to restrain the rest of the body as the foal goes down.
- A mouth gag is placed between the incisors and the head and neck extended. The tongue is pulled out of the mouth, and the foal is intubated in the same manner as an adult.

FURTHER READING

Benson GJ, Thurmon JC (1990) Intravenous anesthesia. *Vet Clin North Am Equine Practice* **6**:513–528.

Doherty T, Valverde A (2006) *Manual of Equine Anesthesia and Analgesia*, Blackwell Publishing, Ames, pp. 212–216.

Yamashita K, Muir WW (2009) Intravenous anesthetic and analgesic adjuncts to inhalation anesthesia. In: *Equine Anesthesia Monitoring and Emergency Therapy*, 2nd edn. (eds Muir WW, Hubbell JAE), Saunders Elsevier, St. Louis, pp. 260–276.

CHAPTER 5

TOTAL INTRAVENOUS ANESTHESIA

Rachel Reed

5.1   INTRODUCTION

- Total intravenous anesthesia (TIVA) is the provision of all the desired qualities of general anesthesia including unconsciousness, muscle relaxation, amnesia, analgesia, and attenuation of autonomic responses via the administration of only intravenous anesthetic agents.
- TIVA is most commonly used in field anesthesia where the anesthetic equipment used for inhalant anesthesia is generally unavailable.
- TIVA is well-suited to field anesthesia due to several specific advantages:
  - Expensive and cumbersome vaporizers and anesthetic machines are not required.
  - Minimal cardiorespiratory depression, which provides some comfort to the anesthetist when there are limited monitoring capabilities available in field anesthesia environments.
  - Better recovery scores in comparison to inhalant anesthesia. This is especially beneficial in field anesthesia, where padded recovery stalls are not available, and patients are recovered by hand with a halter and lead rope.
  - The analgesic nature of most drugs used provides superior pain prevention and relief compared to use of inhalant anesthetics alone.
  - There is no concern for exposure of personnel to inhalant anesthetics and no need for scavenging.

- No contribution to greenhouse gases that accompanies the use of volatile anesthetics.
- The potential disadvantages associated with TIVA include:
  - Accumulation of the drug in the body tissues with prolonged anesthesia resulting delayed recovery.
  - The potential need for a syringe pump to deliver precise volumes over time.
  - There is currently no real-time method of monitoring plasma concentration of injectable agents, and therefore the infusion rate must be adjusted based on patient responses to depth assessment and known pharmacokinetic data.
    - This is in contrast to inhalant agent use, where end tidal agent concentrations accurately reflect the amount of the inhalant circulating in the blood.
- It is recommended that field anesthesia with TIVA procedures be limited to 60–90 minutes for several reasons:
  - Accumulation of the drug in the tissues with prolonged infusions.
  - Inability to provide proper ventilation.
  - Inability to provide extensive monitoring.
  - Lack of adequate padding and positioning aids.
  - Limited access to emergency equipment, drugs, and personnel.
  - Expense of anesthetic maintenance drugs when used for long periods.

DOI: 10.1201/9780429190940-5

5.2 PRE-ANESTHETIC CONSIDERATIONS AND TREATMENTS

- Similar to those undergoing inhalational anesthesia, patients receiving TIVA should receive a physical exam, and a full history should be obtained prior to anesthesia. A minimum data base is also recommended but is often unavailable.
- An eight-hour fast is recommended.
  - It has been shown that ingesta moves out of the equine stomach within a matter of hours, and spontaneous reflux or regurgitation is unlikely to occur in healthy anesthetized horses.
  - A decreased ability to spontaneously ventilate due to the volume of ingesta in the GI tract is one reason to fast horses pre-operatively despite the insignificant risk of regurgitation and aspiration.
- Significant attention and preparation should be paid to choosing and preparing the location of anesthetic induction and maintenance.
  - A large space free of equipment, obstacles, and debris should be chosen.
  - The area should be well-padded but with a surface providing good footing for recovery.
  - The safety of personnel must also be considered with the provision of multiple escape routes.

5.3 DRUG ADMINISTRATION: BOLUS ADMINISTRATION VERSUS INFUSION

- TIVA is accomplished by the administration of either intermittent boluses of anesthetic or a continuous infusion of the anesthetic drugs. There are several ways to administer a continuous infusion.
- The major difference between most infusion schemes is whether or not the pharmacokinetic characteristics of the drug are taken into consideration (**Table 5.1**).
  - The plasma concentration associated with most drugs administered at a constant rate will continue to rise over time, and the patient will progress through deeper planes of anesthesia as the concentration rises.
  - In order to avoid this unnecessary rise in plasma concentrations, the anesthetist can decrease the infusion rate in accordance with the time, patient response, and known pharmacokinetics for the drug in that species.
- The rate-controlled infusion style of TIVA is used for field anesthesia in horses (**Table 5.1**).
  - This method is simple, requires minimal knowledge of the pharmacokinetics of the drugs used, is easy to administer, and patients generally remain cardiovascularly stable.

Table 5.1 **Continuous rate infusion strategies**

NON-PHARMACOKINETIC DEPENDENT		PHARMACOKINETIC DEPENDENT	
Constant rate infusion: Infusion rate does not change throughout procedure	*Rate-controlled infusion:* Infusion rate is adjusted based on observed needs of patient	*Stepped infusion:* Initial rapid infusion rate is decreased over time according to PK data	*Electronically controlled:* A computer administers the drug at an initial high rate and titrates the infusion down in accordance with PK data

- The anesthetist continuously monitors the patient's anesthetic depth via assessment of the palpebral reflex, eye movement (nystagmus), eye position, and response to painful stimuli as a guide to titration of the anesthetic drugs via infusion or intermittent boluses.
- Equipment used for infusions can be very simple or quite complex.
  - The simplest form is to administer the anesthetic drugs as a large volume (either diluted in saline or a combination employing guaifenesin, which is formulated in large volumes) through an IV drip set (**Figure 5.1**). The drip rate can then be adjusted to administer the anesthetic at a rate obtaining the desired plane of anesthesia. A disadvantage of this approach is that the actual rate of administration is difficult to ascertain. Additionally, if the infusion is being administered simultaneously with other fluids (i.e. isotonic crystalloid replacement fluids, lidocaine, etc.), adjustment in the rate of one drip set will affect the rate of the competing drip sets. Therefore, it is necessary to constantly assess the drip rates of all infusions.
- Drip counters (**Figure 5.2**) are an inexpensive means of delivering more

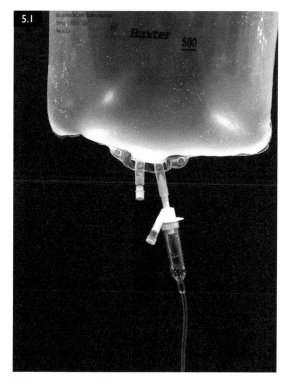

Figure 5.1 IV drip set

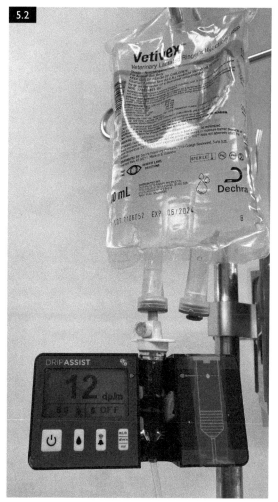

Figure 5.2 Drip counter

accurate infusion rates. The drip rate is still manually adjusted, but the drip counter will provide the user with exact infusion rates and the ability to set alarms if the infusion rate changes.

- More advanced means of drug delivery include syringe pumps (**Figure 5.3**) and inline pumps (**Figure 5.4**) that attach to the fluid administration set. These types of pumps deliver the exact infusion rate programmed by the user and can be adjusted throughout the anesthetic event. Although very precise and user-friendly, these pumps can be quite expensive.

5.4 DRUG PROTOCOLS AND DOSAGES

- Premedication and induction of anesthesia for TIVA is similar to the protocols used for inhalant anesthesia (**Table 5.2**). It is helpful if the patient has an intravenous catheter already in place prior to beginning the anesthetic event, but this is not always possible.
  - In addition to ensuring continuous intravenous access, some anesthetic agents used for TIVA, guaifenesin in particular, can cause significant irritation and tissue damage if administered extravascularly. Therefore, it is ideal to place a catheter for administration of infusions.
- The traditional mainstay of equine premedication has been the administration of alpha-2 adrenergic agonists (i.e. xylazine, detomidine, romifidine). These agents provide dose-dependent sedation in addition to analgesia.
  - The ability to reverse these drugs with alpha-2 adrenergic antagonists, such as yohimbine, tolazoline, and atipamezole, is another advantage of their use.
- Opioids are often administered to provide additional analgesia but do not provide enough sedation to be used as the only premedication. At high doses, opioids have even been shown to cause excitement in healthy horses. They are often used in addition to an alpha-2 adrenergic agonist at the time of premedication. Although rarely necessary, these agents are also reversible with opioid antagonists such as naloxone or naltrexone.
- Acepromazine, a phenothiazine sedative, has been used for decades in horses.

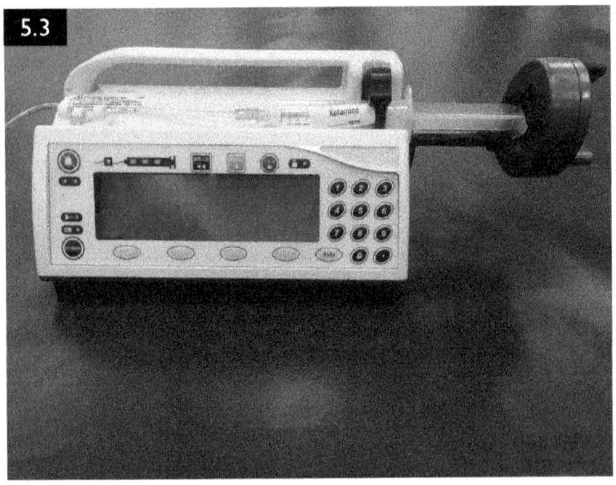

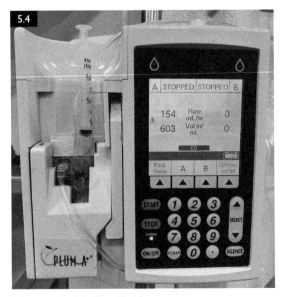

Figure 5.3 Syringe pump

Figure 5.4 Inline fluid pump

Table 5.2 **Pre-anesthetic agents**

DRUG	DOSAGE	COMMENTS
Xylazine	0.8–1.1 mg/kg IV or IM	Fastest onset time; most commonly used
Romifidine	0.08–0.1 mg/kg IV or IM	Associated with less ataxia than other alpha-2 agonists
Detomidine	0.005–0.02 mg/kg IV or IM	More likely to cause AV block than other alpha-2 agonists
Acepromazine	0.01–0.02 mg/kg IV or IM	Has been associated with persistent penile prolapse; minimal sedation, may predispose to hypotension; improves recovery quality
Butorphanol	0.02–0.05 mg/kg IV or IM	Provides analgesia with minimal sedation
Morphine	0.1 mg/kg IV or IM	May cause histamine release

The sedation afforded by acepromazine is long-lasting but less profound than that of alpha-2 adrenergic agonists. Acepromazine can lead to intraoperative hypotension at high doses, is not reversible, and has been associated with persistent penile prolapse with an incidence of approximately 0.02%.

5.5 INDUCTION AND MAINTENANCE

- Induction of horses in field conditions can be challenging in comparison to the controlled environment of an induction room. It is important to make sure that all individuals involved in the anesthetic event understand the risks associated with equine anesthesia and are accustomed to working with horses.
- Induction agents should only be given once the horse is showing obvious signs of sedation including hanging head, droopy lip, relative unresponsiveness to stimulation, and ears in a relaxed position. Drugs and drug combinations are discussed in Chapter 4.
- The horse is generally induced in a field with one person controlling the head via the halter and lead rope. If available, another person should hold the tail, and additional handlers on the sides support the horse's fall to sternal and then lateral recumbency (**Figure 5.5**).
- Once the patient is recumbent it is important to provide adequate padding as the patient is moved to the desired recumbency for the procedure (i.e. dorsal vs lateral).
  - Equine anesthesia presents specific concerns for myopathy and neuropathy, and these complications can be avoided by providing ample padding, special attention to positioning, and maintenance of adequate blood pressure throughout the procedure.
  - Special attention should be placed to the dependent forelimb if in lateral recumbency, and this limb should be pulled cranially to avoid radial nerve injury (**Figure 5.6**).
  - Additionally, the anesthetist should assess the position of the tail and penis (if the patient is male) and ensure that neither are tucked under the patient.
  - The anesthetist should evaluate the position of the head, ensuring that it is well-padded, that both eyes are well-lubricated, and that the dependent eye is kept closed. During the anesthetic period, placing a towel over the horse's head will decrease stimulation from the environment (**Figure 5.7**).

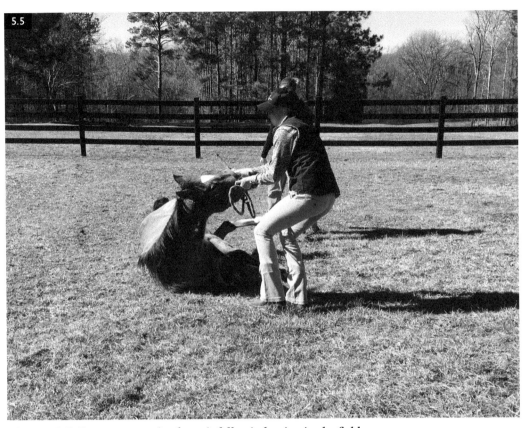

Figure 5.5 Person supporting horse's fall at induction in the field

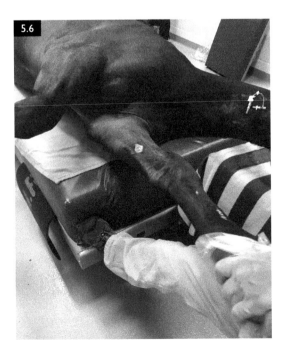

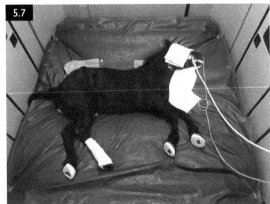

Figure 5.7 Towel placed over head to decrease environmental stimulation

Figure 5.6 Dependent forelimb pulled forward

- Once the patient is in the desired position, the maintenance infusion or intermittent boluses to maintain general anesthesia can be initiated.
  - Unfortunately, there is no single injectable agent capable of providing all of the components of general anesthesia (unconsciousness, muscle relaxation, amnesia, analgesia, attenuation of autonomic reflexes); therefore, multiple anesthetic agents are employed simultaneously.
  - Drugs most commonly used to extend the period of anesthesia include ketamine, xylazine, guaifenesin, and midazolam.
- If intermittent boluses are used, two parts ketamine to one part xylazine is usually administered as needed to maintain anesthesia. A maintenance mixture (or "top-up") can be made with 1 mg/kg ketamine and 0.5 mg/kg xylazine, and approximately 1/4–1/3 of this mixture is given as needed to maintain anesthesia.
- TIVA using infusion of specific anesthetic mixtures provides a more precise and stable plane of anesthesia in comparison to intermittent boluses.
  - As with standing sedation, the rate of administration of these infusions is adjusted throughout the procedure to maintain an acceptable plane of anesthesia.
  - Some examples of TIVA maintenance infusions are provided (**Table 5.3**). It is wise to keep a top-up dose of ketamine and xylazine available in case of unexpected lightening of the anesthetic plane.
- Guaifenesin has been the mainstay for provision of muscle relaxation in equine TIVA protocols for many years.
  - It is a centrally acting muscle relaxant and provides no analgesia. It is available in several concentrations, generally in volumes of 500 ml to 1000 ml.
  - Concentrations greater than 10% should be avoided due to the risk of lysis of red blood cells caused by the high osmolality of the solution.
  - Prolonged infusions or high doses of guaifenesin have been associated with muscle weakness in recovery.
- Although not a complete anesthetic on its own, ketamine is commonly used in TIVA maintenance solutions to provide unconsciousness and analgesia.
- Alpha-2 adrenergic agonists contribute sedation, muscle relaxation, anxiolysis, and analgesia.
- In the case that guaifenesin is not available or preferred, a benzodiazepine can be used in its place to provide muscle relaxation and amnesia. In this case, all drugs can be added to a liter bag of saline to form the maintenance infusion.
- Lidocaine can be used as an adjunct to the maintenance infusion for TIVA. Lidocaine provides several beneficial effects to the patient including analgesia, an anti-inflammatory effect, free-radical scavenging, decreased required infusion rate of TIVA agents, an anti-arrhythmic effect, and an intestinal pro-kinetic effect.
  - Its use has been associated with ataxia in recovery, and therefore it is recommended to discontinue the infusion 20 minutes prior to cessation of anesthesia.
- As with standing procedures, local anesthesia should be provided whenever necessary, and pre-emptive administration of an NSAID is ideal.

5.6 SUPPORTIVE CARE AND MONITORING

- If possible, oxygen supplementation should be provided. This will maximize

Table 5.3 **Maintenance Infusions**

DRUGS	DOSAGES	COMMENTS
"Triple Drip" (Figure 5.8) Ketamine Xylazine Guaifenesin 5%	1000–2000 mg 500–650 mg 1000 ml	Most commonly used means for maintaining TIVA. Should last about 60 minutes in most average horses (500 kg).
Ketamine Xylazine Midazolam	1000 mg 500 mg 25 mg	Add to 1 L bag of 0.9% saline for infusion. Should last about 60 minutes in most average horses (500 kg)
Ketamine Detomidine Guaifenesin 5%	1000 mg 10 mg 1000 ml	Similar to triple drip. May see more AV block.
Lidocaine (as an adjunct to above)	Bolus: 2 mg/kg CRI: 2–4 mg/ kg/h	Not to be used as only maintenance agent. Decreases necessary maintenance infusions. Discontinue 20 minutes prior to end of anesthesia.

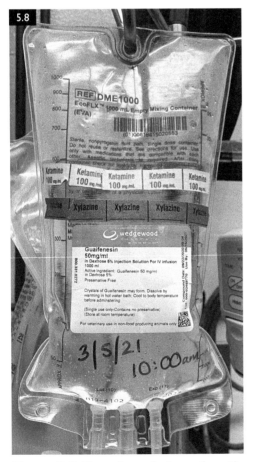

Figure 5.8 Ketamine, xylazine and guaifenesin (triple drip)

delivery of oxygen to the tissues and decrease the incidence of anesthesia-related hypoxemia.

- Anesthesia of horses is associated with a significant degree of ventilation perfusion mismatch and hypoventilation.
- In field anesthesia, supplementation of oxygen generally requires the foresight to bring the equipment for oxygen supplementation. This requires a compressed gas oxygen cylinder (i.e. a full E or H cylinder), a regulator (**Figure 5.9**), an appropriately sized endotracheal tube (**Figure 5.10**), a flowmeter with fresh gas tubing, and/or a demand valve (**Figure 5.11**). For information on how to transport compressed gas cylinders, see the OSHA website (www.osha.gov).
- Portable oxygen concentrators are also available that extract oxygen from ambient air (**Figure 5.12**). These units are generally capable of creating 90–95% oxygen.
- Oxygen can be supplemented in two ways:

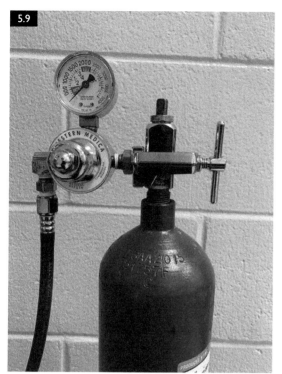

Figure 5.9 Compressed gas cylinder and regulator

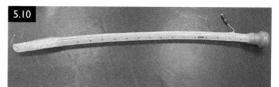

Figure 5.10 Endotracheal tube

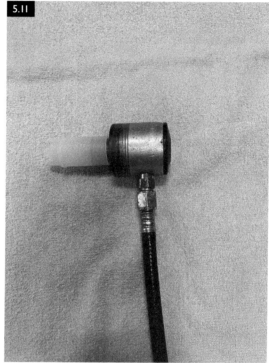

Figure 5.11 Demand valve

- *Tracheal insufflation:* This requires a flowmeter assembly and fresh gas infusion line to be placed in the patient's trachea. It is recommended to administer 100% oxygen at 15 L/min at the level of the mid-trachea to have a positive effect on arterial oxygen partial pressure.
- *Positive pressure ventilation*: This requires intubation of the patient with an endotracheal tube and a demand valve to administer positive pressure breaths (endotracheal intubation is described in Chapters 1 and 4).
  - The ability to administer positive pressure breaths is particularly advantageous if the anesthetist has chosen to use a protocol involving propofol, which is frequently associated with post-induction apnea.
  - This technique should be employed when the horse is placed in dorsal recumbency, due to increased intrathoracic pressure (caused by the abdominal content pressing on the diaphragm).
  - It is possible to leave the demand valve attached to the endotracheal tube and allow the patient to breathe through the valve.

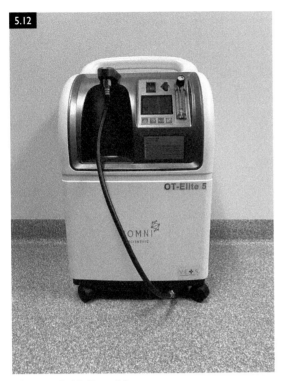

Figure 5.12 Portable oxygen concentrator

The negative pressure associated with inspiration activates the valve, assisting the breath with positive pressure oxygen. This method has the disadvantage that it does add some resistance to expiration through the endotracheal tube.

- Intravenous fluid support can be provided in the form of an isotonic crystalloid replacement fluid. The administration of intravenous fluids while under anesthesia provides basal metabolic fluid requirements, counters the vascular relaxation caused by some anesthetics, and replaces insensible losses throughout the procedure, promoting a more stable cardiovascular state. An infusion rate of 5 ml/kg/h has been recommended in healthy individuals.

- Some forethought should be given to environmental factors associated with temperature. Patients under anesthesia have a decreased ability to thermoregulate, and environmental factors can exacerbate this issue.
  - If it is a hot day, it is best to plan the surgery early in the morning and find a shady area for the anesthetic event. Conversely, if temperatures are cold and ice or snow are present, it is best to find an area free of obstacles within an indoor facility to perform the procedure (e.g., indoor arena). The area would be preferably soft (i.e. shavings, sand) but with good footing for recovery.
- In most field anesthesia environments, minimal monitoring equipment is available to the anesthetist. The anesthetist should be diligent in monitoring subjective visual indications of patient status. One can easily monitor heart rate, pulse quality, respiratory rate and depth, mucous membrane color, and capillary refill time without the aid of an electronic monitor. These simple observations can provide a wealth of information in regard to the physiologic status of the patient.
  - Hand-held pulse oximetry units are available and helpful to the anesthetist in monitoring heart rate and saturation of hemoglobin with oxygen (**Figure 5.13**).
  - Most ECG units are cumbersome and expensive, making them unlikely to be available in the field. Smaller, inexpensive units that attach to smart phones have been developed and work well in a variety of species (**Figure 5.14**). This ECG design is much more conducive to field anesthesia use.
  - Small oscillometric blood pressure monitors are also available for field anesthesia monitoring (**Figure 5.15**).

These units are fairly expensive, and accuracy in equine patients is variable.

- Anesthetic depth should also be continuously monitored by assessing the patient for nystagmus, spontaneous blinking, the strength of the palpebral reflex, and movement in response to a noxious stimulus. Patients maintained on TIVA at an adequate

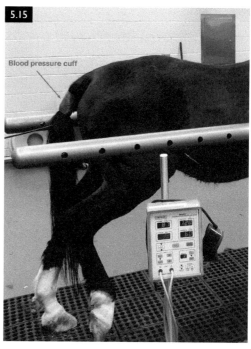

Figure 5.15 Portable oscillometric blood pressure monitor

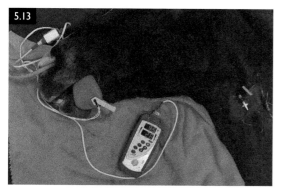

Figure 5.13 Hand-held pulse oximetry unit

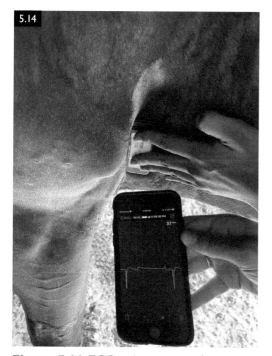

Figure 5.14 ECG unit on smart phone

plane generally do not have nystagmus, do not blink spontaneously, do not move in response to a noxious stimulus, but do maintain a slow palpebral reflex and strong corneal reflex. These parameters are used as a guide to anesthetic titration.

5.7 RECOVERY

- The recovery period can be quite dangerous in field anesthesia conditions, and therefore skilled individuals with equine experience are preferred to assist in recovery.
- The maintenance infusion and replacement fluids should be discontinued. All equipment and debris should be removed from the recovery area.
- At least one experienced person should be present for recovery. This person should be at the head, guiding the horse to standing

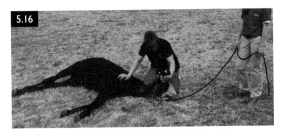

Figure 5.16 At recovery, one person at the head and one holding the lead rope

with a halter and lead rope. If available, one additional person should be at the tail to help prevent the horse from swaying too far to one side or the other once standing (**Figure 5.16**).

- The horse should be allowed to lie quietly for as long as possible before attempting to rise. Once standing, the horse should stand quietly for several minutes to allow any residual ataxia to resolve before attempting to walk.

5.8   CASE EXAMPLES

5.8.1 A 15-Year-Old Arabian Mare Presents for Left Eye Enucleation

- The mare (body weight = 520 kg) is otherwise healthy, and pre-anesthetic bloodwork is normal. She has already received a single dose of flunixin meglumine. The surgery will be performed in lateral recumbency and is expected to take 20–30 minutes.
  - The patient is premedicated with acepromazine 0.01 mg/kg IM and morphine 0.1mg/kg IM 30 minutes prior to the planned start of the procedure.
  - A catheter is placed in the left jugular vein.
  - The patient is premedicated with xylazine 1.1 mg/kg and induced with ketamine 2.2 mg/kg and midazolam 0.1 mg/kg.
  - The horse is placed in lateral recumbency on the operating table.

- Prior to the first incision, the patient receives a retrobulbar block to desensitize the orbit, an auriculopalpebral nerve block to prevent motor movement of the eyelids, and a ring block around the eye to desensitize the eyelids.
- A top-up of 1 mg/kg ketamine and 0.5 mg/kg xylazine is prepared and administered in small boluses (approximately 2–2.5 ml every 10 minutes) to maintain adequate anesthetic depth for the procedure.
- Throughout the procedure, the anesthetist monitors heart rate, respiratory rate, mucous membrane color, and capillary refill time.
- Once the procedure is completed, the patient is placed on a pad in a quiet recovery stall and allowed to stand un-aided.

5.8.2 A Five-Year-Old Quarter Horse Gelding with a Laceration

- The horse presents for debridement and closure of a laceration over the medial aspect of the right hind cannon bone. The horse is otherwise healthy but poorly behaved. Pre-anesthetic bloodwork is normal.
  - Attempts to debride and close the wound with standing sedation have failed. The patient has already received a single dose of flunixin meglumine.
- The patient is premedicated with detomidine 20 µg/kg IM in order to achieve enough relaxation to place an intravenous jugular catheter.
- With the catheter in place, the patient receives an additional 1 mg/kg of xylazine to achieve a deeper plane of sedation prior to induction.
- Induction of anesthesia is achieved with ketamine 2.2 mg/kg and midazolam 0.05 mg/kg intravenously.

- Once the patient is positioned for the procedure, an infusion of isotonic crystalloid replacement fluid is started at 5 ml/kg/h.
- Triple drip containing 500 ml of 5% guaifenesin, 1000 mg ketamine, and 500 mg xylazine is administered intravenously to maintain anesthesia.
  - With constant assessment of anesthetic depth, the anesthetist titrates the triple drip to maintain an adequate plane of anesthesia.
  - The anesthetist continuously monitors heart rate, respiratory rate, pulse quality, and hemoglobin saturation with oxygen via pulse oximetry.
  - The patient is intubated, and oxygen is supplemented via a portable oxygen cylinder and demand valve.
- When the procedure is complete, the infusion is discontinued, and the patient is allowed to recover to standing with the guidance of a handler at the halter and at the tail.
- Once there is no further evidence of ataxia, the horse is led back to his enclosure.

FURTHER READING

Doherty TJ, Valverde A (2006) *Manual of Equine Anesthesia and Analgesia*, Blackwell Publishing, Ames, pp. 212–216.

Driessen B, Zarucco L et al (2011) Contemporary use of acepromazine in the anesthetic management of male horses and ponies: A retrospective study and opinion poll. *Equine Vet J* **43**:88–98.

Hubbel JA, Aarnes TK et al (2002) Evaluation of a midazolam-ketamine-xylazine infusion for total intravenous anesthesia in horses. *Am J Vet Res* **73**:470–475.

Lerche, P (2013) Total intravenous anesthesia in horses. *Vet Clin Equine* **29**:123–129.

Lin HC, Branson KR et al (1992) Ketamine, telazol, xylazine, and detomidine: A comparative anesthetic drug combinations study in ponies. *Acta Vet Scand* **33**:109–115.

Lohmann KL, Roussel AJ et al (1999) Comparison of nuclear scintigraphy and acetaminophen absorption as a means of studying gastric emptying in horses. *Am J Vet Res* **61**:310–315.

Marntell S, Nyman G, Funkquist P (2006) Dissociative anesthesia during field and hospital conditions for castration of colts. *Acta Vet Scand* **47**:1–11.

Moyer W, Schumacher J, Schumacher JR. (2011) *Equine Joint Injection and Regional Anesthesia*, Academic Veterinary Solutions, Chadds Ford.

Valverde, A (2013) Balanced anesthesia and constant-rate infusions in horses. *Vet Clin North Am Equine Pract* **29**:89–122.

Yamashita K, Muir WW (2009) Intravenous anesthetic and analgesic adjuncts to inhalation anesthesia. In: *Equine Anesthesia Monitoring and Emergency Therapy*, 2nd edn. (eds Muir WW, Hubbell JAE), Saunders Elsevier, St. Louis, pp. 260–276.

CHAPTER 6

INHALANT ANESTHESIA AND PARTIAL INTRAVENOUS ANESTHESIA

Ann Weil

6.1 INTRODUCTION

Maintenance of anesthesia in horses can be achieved with inhalant alone, combined with injectable drugs (partial intravenous anesthesia or PIVA), or with injectable drugs alone (total intravenous anesthesia or TIVA). The anesthetic maintenance plan should be based on the patient, the procedure to be performed, and the resources available to the anesthetist. In this chapter, only inhalant anesthesia and PIVA will be discussed. Refer to Chapter 5 for TIVA.

6.2 CHOOSING WHICH TECHNIQUE

- Advantages of inhalant anesthesia:
  - Provides ventilation support and protects the airway.
  - Improves oxygenation (this is debatable in the horse).
  - Improves control over movement.
  - Increases muscle relaxation and improves operative conditions.
  - Very little drug metabolism is needed to wake up from the procedure.
  - Easy to adjust and titrate depth of anesthesia.
  - More suitable for procedures of long duration because of the ability to support respiratory function and the ability to be rapidly eliminated by the lung for recovery.
- Disadvantages of inhalant anesthesia:
  - Need for expensive equipment.
  - Not practical for doing procedures other than in a hospital.

- Enhanced risk of recovery problems such as muscle weakness, excitement and delirium.
- No analgesia provided by the inhalant.
- When faced with the decision to pick a technique, many anesthesiologists have elected to combine the best of both worlds. In other words, use inhalant anesthesia, but augment that anesthetic protocol with some injectable anesthetics and adjunctive drugs to improve conditions for the equine patient.
- Almost every adult horse is induced to anesthesia with injectable anesthetics.
- Maintenance can be done with inhalant anesthetics, injectable anesthetics or both.
- Foals are the exception to this. Many young foals can be easily induced with inhalants via mask (**Figure 6.1**) or nasotracheal intubation.

6.3 INHALANTS

- Inhalant anesthetics require a machine with a vaporizer and a carrier gas in order to be used (**Figure 6.2**). Please see Chapter 1 for details on the anesthetic machine and equipment necessary to perform inhalant anesthesia. Each different inhalant should be administered in a vaporizer calibrated for that particular agent.
- Inhalant anesthetics are delivered via the lung to the target tissues of general anesthesia, namely the central nervous system, which includes the brain and spinal cord.
  - A more detailed description of the fundamentals of inhalant anesthesia

DOI: 10.1201/9780429190940-6

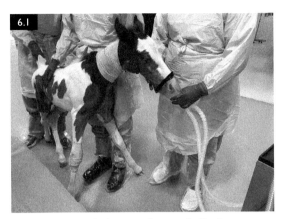

Figure 6.1 Inhalant via facemask (foal)

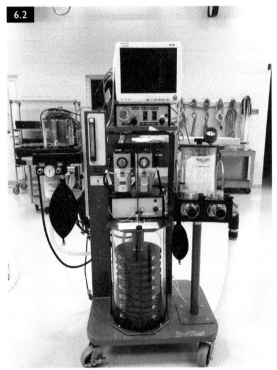

Figure 6.2 Anesthesia machine

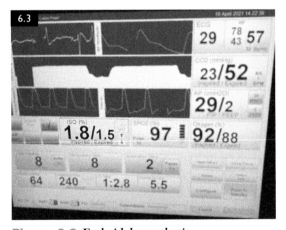

Figure 6.3 End-tidal anesthetic

can be found in many comprehensive textbooks of anesthesiology. The intention of this chapter is to provide some practical information on the use of inhalant anesthetics in the horse.

- Inhalation anesthetics are administered as a vaporized gas. It is the partial pressure of this gas in the central nervous system that produces general anesthesia.
  - The partial pressure of the gas must reach the lung via ventilation.
  - From the lung, the gas travels to the target tissues (central nervous system) primarily by means of the vascular system.
- The partial pressure of inhalant in the lung (alveolar partial pressure) parallels the partial pressure of inhaled anesthetic in tissues like the brain.
  - One great advantage of inhaled anesthesia is the ability to measure the amount of anesthetic-producing effect at any given time. This is done by measuring the amount of expired (end-tidal) anesthetic, which is an estimate of alveolar concentration (**Figure 6.3**).
  - The end-tidal concentration of anesthetic gives the anesthetist the ability to know how much inhalant anesthetic is available in tissues like the central nervous system, thus the ability to track the amount of anesthetic in the animal in real time. This cannot be done with injectable anesthetics.
- In order to achieve a desired level of alveolar partial pressure (and thus a desired level

of brain or target tissue partial pressure), the anesthetic must be delivered to the lung. There are two basic things that must happen in order for this to be achieved:
- The anesthetic machine must be able to deliver the desired level of anesthetic.
- The lungs must be able to exchange gases (ventilation must occur).
- Large-animal anesthetic machines (rebreathing, circle) and ventilators have a huge circuit volume to overcome (**Figure 6.4**). Therefore, at the beginning of the anesthetic period, an overpressure technique is used to deliver an adequate amount of inhalant to transition the horse to inhalant anesthesia while still anesthetized with the injectable induction drugs.
  - The overpressure technique implies high oxygen flow rate will be used at the beginning of the anesthesia (8–10 l/min) and the vaporizer set at the maximum concentration (5% for isoflurane). This is done to fill the circuit rapidly with a high concentration of anesthetic. Care must be taken to monitor the animal for signs of increasing depth, so the vaporizer can be turned down to a maintenance level.
  - The oxygen flow rate can be reduced once the desired concentration of anesthetic is being delivered (≈ 10 ml/kg/min).
- A mechanical ventilator can be very helpful at the beginning of the anesthetic period to help present the inhaled anesthetic to the lung.
  - This eliminates the reliance on spontaneous ventilation at the beginning of the anesthetic period, when the horse may be experiencing respiratory depression from the injectable anesthetics.
  - The use of a ventilator helps the anesthetist to achieve the desired degree of inhaled anesthetic more rapidly.
- Once the inhaled anesthetic reaches the lung, the inhaled drug must reach the target tissues. It does this by being carried by the vascular circulation. "Uptake" factors describe what happens to the alveolar partial pressure of anesthetic. There are three classic uptake factors:
1. Blood:gas solubility or partition coefficients.
   - Modern inhalant anesthetics are relatively insoluble. The more insoluble the agent, the quicker it will reach a partial pressure capable of producing general anesthesia. Thus, use of insoluble inhalant agents will induce an animal more quickly. The reverse is also true in that the more insoluble the agent, the more quickly recovery will occur.

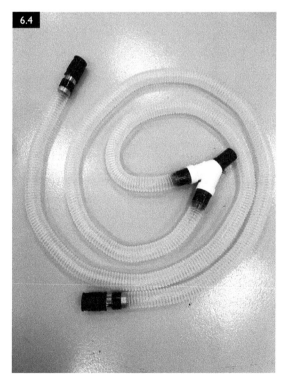

Figure 6.4 **Large-animal rebreathing circuit**

2. Cardiac output.
   - It is patient-dependent. The larger the cardiac output of the patient, the longer it will take to reach the partial pressure necessary to produce general anesthesia.
3. Alveolar-venous partial pressure difference.
   - As long as there are tissues in the body that have a lower partial pressure of gas than the lung, gases will move to equilibrate partial pressure. The alveolar-venous partial pressure difference represents the concentration gradient down which the inhalant will move.

- Characteristics of the modern inhalant anesthetics in the horse (isoflurane, sevoflurane, desflurane) can be found in **Table 6.1**.

6.4   MINIMUM ALVEOLAR CONCENTRATION (MAC)

- Refers to the amount of anesthetic gas (at 1 atm) at which 50% of a patient population will not have gross movement when exposed to a supramaximal noxious stimulus.
- Is used as a measure of potency of inhaled anesthetics. The higher the MAC, the more inhalant it takes to anesthetize the patient.

- Each inhalant has its own unique MAC.
- MAC tends to be similar across most domestic species.
- A surgical plane of anesthesia is considered to be 1.5 x MAC.
- Factors that reduce the MAC requirement:
  - Hypothermia.
  - Pregnancy.
  - Age (younger animals require less).
  - Severe hypotension.
  - Severe hypoxemia.
  - Metabolic acidosis.
  - The use of analgesics, tranquilizers, sedatives, injectables or local anesthetics, etc.
- Factors that increase the MAC requirement:
  - Hyperthermia.
  - Hypernatremia.
  - Neurostimulants (i.e. ephedrine).
- Factors that do not influence MAC:
  - Hypertension.
  - Metabolic alkalosis.
  - Duration of anesthesia.
  - Type of surgical stimulus.

6.5   INHALANTS

- All inhalant anesthetics act as significant respiratory depressants.
- None of the modern inhalants provide significant anti-nociceptive activity.

Table 6.1 **Characteristics of modern inhalant agents in the horse**

	ISOFLURANE	SEVOFLURANE	DESFLURANE
Molecular weight (g)	185	200	168
Boiling point (°C)	49	59	23.5
Vapor pressure at 20°C	240	160	700
Preservative	none	none	none
Blood:gas partition coefficient	1.13	0.65	0.58
MAC (%)	1.31	2.84	8.06
Biotransformation (%)	0.2	3	0.02

- The horse is more prone to myocardial depression than other common domestic species at equipotent vaporizer settings; in other words, a horse will experience a greater degree of cardiac output depression at a certain vaporizer setting than other animals.
- Many anesthetized horses will require inotropic support as a result.
- Isoflurane, sevoflurane and desflurane all support vital organ blood flow in a similar manner.
- All inhalants produce dose-dependent cardiovascular depression.

6.5.1 Isoflurane

- Isoflurane (**Figure 6.5**) is the most commonly used inhalant in the horse, due to its wide availability and low cost.
- Has a more pungent odor than sevoflurane or desflurane.

- Considered to be an agent of intermediate solubility, but one can still predict a relatively quick recovery in a short duration procedure.
- Undergoes very little metabolism.
- Does not contain preservatives.

6.5.2 Sevoflurane

- Sevoflurane (**Figure 6.6**) is considered an insoluble inhalant, which gives it faster induction and recovery characteristics than isoflurane.
- Changes in depth can be made quickly.
- The odor is not as objectionable if used to induce anesthesia via mask.
- Sevoflurane is less potent than isoflurane, so more is required to anesthetize a patient.

6.5.3 Desflurane

- Desflurane (**Figure 6.7**) has a very high vapor pressure, so it requires an electronic

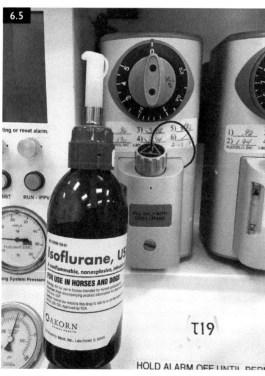

Figure 6.5 Isoflurane

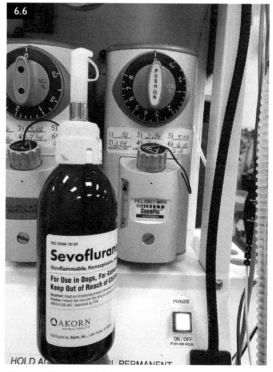

Figure 6.6 Sevoflurane

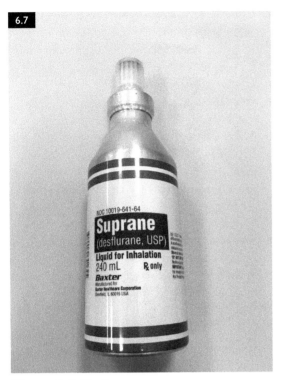

Figure 6.7 Desflurane

(temperature-controlled, pressurized) vaporizer to control vaporization.
- High degree of insolubility means that patients induce, recover and change depth very quickly.
- Is the least potent of the inhalants, so more is required to produce anesthesia.
- Not very practical in adult horses due to the specialized equipment needed to use it.

6.5.4 Halothane
- No longer available.

6.6   INHALANT INDUCTION IN FOALS

- Most young foals can be intubated with a nasotracheal tube whilst standing (**Figure 6.8**).
- Inhalants can be used to induce anesthesia, thus eliminating the need to metabolize drugs in very young foals.

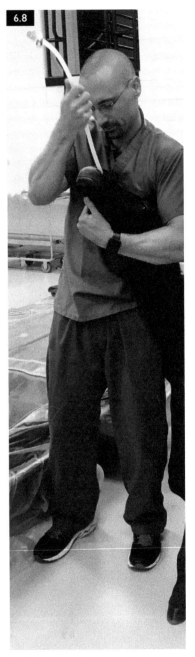

Figure 6.8 Nasotracheal intubation foal

- High oxygen flow rates and vaporizer settings are used in an overpressure technique to achieve recumbency in the foal and then reduced to levels needed to maintain anesthesia.

- The nasotracheal tube can be switched to an oral endotracheal tube of larger diameter once the foal has been anesthetized.

6.7 PARTIAL INTRAVENOUS ANESTHESIA (PIVA)

- Has been defined as "a form of balanced anaesthesia that implies the use of low concentrations of inhalation anaesthetics in combination with injectable agents in order to reduce the cardiorespiratory depressant effects of the inhalants and to improve analgesia and anaesthetic stability" (Nannarone and Spadavecchia 2012).
- Advantages:
  - Analgesia.
  - A more stable plane of anesthesia.
  - MAC-sparing effect or reduction of the amount of inhalant anesthesia required, which may improve cardiovascular performance of the anesthetized horse.
- Disadvantages:
  - Accumulation of drug in the plasma and tissues.

- Prolonged recovery.
- Potential for drug interactions.
- Please see Chapters 4 and 5 for the variety of injectable anesthetics that can be used prior to maintenance with an inhalant.
- Useful adjuncts to inhalant anesthesia include bolus or CRI administration of opioids, lidocaine, ketamine or alpha-2 agents (**Table 6.2**).

Sample protocols:

- Guaifenesin with xylazine and ketamine.
- Lidocaine with butorphanol and dexmedetomidine.
- Lidocaine alone in colic.

6.7.1 Ketamine

- Dissociative anesthetic.
- NMDA antagonist that is considered anti-nociceptive.
- Produces some indirect stimulation of the cardiovascular system via the sympathetic nervous system.

Table 6.2 Doses of different drugs used for PIVA (see example of protocols after the table)

	LOADING DOSE (IV)	CRI (IV)
Xylazine	0.5–0.75 mg/kg	1–4 mg/kg/hour
Romifidine	80 µg/kg	18 µg/kg/hour
Detomidine	10 µg/kg	5–10 µg/kg/hour
Dexmedetomidine	3.5 µg/kg	1–1.75 µg/kg/hour
Lidocaine	1.5–3 mg/kg	25–50 µg/kg/min
Ketamine	2–3 mg/kg	1–3 mg/kg/hour
Morphine	0.15 mg/kg	0.1 mg/kg/hour
Butorphanol	25 µg/kg	25 µg/kg/hour
Guaifenesin	None	25 mg/kg/hour
Diazepam	None	0.1 mg/kg/hour
Midazolam	20 µg/kg	20 µg/kg/hour

- Can produce excitement when used at high doses or for prolonged periods.
- Can be combined with an opioid, lidocaine, or an alpha-2 agent to provide PIVA.

6.7.2 Opioids

- Sedation is seen with some opioids, but potential exists for excitement and increased locomotor activity, depending on particular drug and dose used.
- Impaired GI motility can also be a concern.
- Inconsistent effects on inhalant MAC in the horse, so may not decrease the amount of inhalant necessary for surgery.
- Nevertheless, they are commonly used as part of a balanced partial intravenous anesthetic technique.
- Butorphanol.
  - Kappa agonist, mu antagonist.
  - May be administered as a bolus periodically throughout anesthesia (bolus dose 0.01–0.03 mg/kg).
  - CRI can also be used (25 µg/kg/hour).
  - Should limit total cumulative dose to 50 mg in an adult horse to decrease the potential for excited recovery.
- Fentanyl.
  - Mu agonist.
  - May produce excitable and/or violent recovery.
- Morphine.
  - Mu agonist.
  - Bolus dose 0.1–0.2 mg/kg IV with CRI 0.1 mg/kg/hour.
  - Give IV slowly to decrease possible histamine release.

6.7.3 Alpha-2 Agonists

- Provide substantial sedation and analgesia in the horse.
- Produce significant cardiovascular depression and increased systemic vascular resistance.
- Can greatly reduce MAC needed for inhalants.

- Choices of alpha-2 agents include:
  - Detomidine (10 µg/kg IV bolus), 5 µg/kg/hour CRI.
  - Romifidine (80 µg/kg IV bolus), 18 µg/kg/hour CRI.
  - Dexmedetomidine (3.5 µg/kg IV bolus), 1.75 µg/kg/hour CRI.
  - Medetomidine (7 µg/kg IV bolus), 3.5 µg/kg/hour CRI.
  - Xylazine (0.5–1 mg/kg IV bolus), 1 mg/kg/hour CRI.
- Xylazine, detomidine and romifidine carry an equine label. Dexmedetomidine and medetomidine are drugs with a small-animal label that can also be used in the equine.
- In general, the more alpha-2 specific agents like detomidine, medetomidine and dexmedetomidine can be predicted to have longer and stronger effects.
- Can contribute to ataxia in recovery.

6.7.4 Lidocaine

- Local anesthetic.
- When used intravenously, it has the following effects:
  - MAC sparing.
  - Antinociceptive.
  - Improves gastrointestinal function postoperatively.
  - Negative inotropy.
- Bolus dose + CRI (1.5 mg/kg IV + 30 µg/kg/min).
- Can contribute to ataxia in recovery, so recommend discontinue CRI 30 minutes prior to recovery.

6.7.5 Combinations with the Addition of Guaifenesin or a Benzodiazepine

- "Triple drip" or GG/xylazine/ketamine.
  - Made by adding 500 mg (5 ml of 100 mg/ml) xylazine and 1 gram (10 ml of 100 mg/ml) ketamine to a liter of GG (**Figure 6.9**).

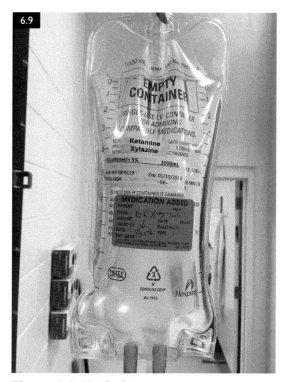

Figure 6.9 Triple drip

- Can be used to supplement inhalant anesthesia for surgeries that are particularly painful.
- Infusion rate is approximately 1–2 ml/kg/hour.

6.8 CASE EXAMPLES

6.8.1 Relatively Healthy Horse (450 Kg) Undergoing Colic Surgery

- The horse needs to be induced for abdominal surgery after intravascular volume replacement of fluid deficits. A sample protocol might include:
  - Xylazine 100–300 mg IV, depending on the condition of the horse and the amount of alpha-2 agents given during the preoperative workup period.

- Butorphanol 10 mg IV.
- 5% GG: given to effect, especially useful when a lower dose of xylazine is being used due to the condition of the horse. The horse is induced when showing sufficient signs of sedation such as knee buckling and swaying.
- Induction: 1000 mg ketamine + 25 mg diazepam mixed together.
- The horse is positioned in dorsal recumbency on a padded table.
- Anesthesia is maintained with isoflurane in circle system and mechanical ventilation.
- Lidocaine is given 1.5 mg/kg IV plus 30 µg/kg/min CRI started. This is discontinued approximately 30 minutes prior to moving to the recovery area.
- Additional butorphanol may be given as intermittent boluses every 30 minutes to 1 hour or a CRI started.
- Care is taken to ensure that mean arterial pressure is maintained above 70 mmHg with fluid therapy and inotropic support.

6.8.2 A Young Racehorse (450 Kg) Undergoing Sesamoid Fracture Repair

- The horse will be positioned in left lateral recumbency on a padded table.
- Detomidine 5 mg IV.
- Butorphanol 10 mg IV.
- Induction with 1000 mg ketamine mixed with 50 mg of midazolam.
- The horse is positioned with the dependent leg pulled forward to relieve pressure on the brachial plexus.
- "Triple drip" is used to provide additional analgesia and reduce MAC. The rate used is 0.5 ml/kg/hour.
- The horse is maintained on isoflurane in a circle system and a mechanical ventilator used.

FURTHER READING

Gozalo-Marcilla M, Gasthuys F, Schauvliege S (2014) Partial intravenous anaesthesia in the horse: A review of intravenous agents used to supplement equine inhalation anaesthesia. Part 1: Lidocaine and ketamine. *Vet Anes Analesia* **41**:335–345.

Gozalo-Marcilla M, Gasthuys F, Schauvliege S (2015) Partial intravenous anaesthesia in the horse: A review of intravenous agents used to supplement equine inhalation anaesthesia. Part 2: Opioids and alpha-2 adrenoceptor agonists. *Vet Anes Analesia* **42**:1–16.

Nannarone S, Spadavecchia C (2012) Evaluation of the clinical efficacy of two partial intravenous anesthetic protocols, compared with isoflurane alone, to maintain general anesthesia in horses. *Am J Vet Res* **73**:959–967.

Steffey E (2009) Inhalation anesthetics and gases. In: *Equine Anesthesia Monitoring and Emergency Therapy*, 2nd edn. (eds Muir WW, Hubbell JAE), Saunders Elsevier, St. Louis, pp. 288–314.

ANESTHESIA MONITORING AND MANAGEMENT

Jane Quandt

7.1 INTRODUCTION

Monitoring is necessary to ensure the safe outcome of an anesthetic episode and to recognize potential complications and institute treatment in a timely fashion. Monitoring guidelines for horses undergoing general anesthesia are available on the American College of Veterinary Anesthesia and Analgesia website (www.acvaa.org/docs/Equine).

Anesthetic depth is generally assessed by:
* Eye activity.
* Movement.
* Physiologic parameters.
* End tidal concentration of exhaled inhalant agents.

Monitoring of the cardiovascular system should consist of:
* Digital pulse palpation.
* Capillary refill time.
* Mucous membrane color.
* Electrocardiogram if indicated.
* Arterial blood pressure if indicated, especially if inhalant anesthesia is used.

The respiratory system is monitored by:
* Observation and respiratory rate and rhythm.
* Pulse oximetry if indicated.
* Capnometry if indicated.
* Arterial blood gas analysis if indicated.

7.2 ANESTHETIC DEPTH

* In equine anesthesia, it is imperative that the anesthetist constantly monitor anesthetic depth.
* An equine patient that inadvertently enters a light plane of an anesthesia during a procedure poses a risk to both itself and the personnel involved with the procedure.
* Conversely, too deep a plane of anesthesia can cause compromised oxygen delivery to vital organs and can result in cardiovascular collapse.
* Diligent monitoring of anesthetic depth allows the anesthetist to titrate the anesthetic agents being used to maintain a surgical plane of anesthesia that is safe for both the patient and the personnel.

7.2.1 Eye Signs
* The eye rotates ventrally and medially in the early stages of anesthesia but becomes central with deep levels of anesthesia (**Figure 7.1**).
* Lateral nystagmus is seen in the very early stages of anesthesia or if the patient becomes light during anesthesia. Nystagmus should not be present when a surgical plane of anesthesia is achieved.
* Lacrimation is noted during a light surgical plane of anesthesia and disappears at deeper levels (**Figure 7.2**).
* The palpebral reflex, closure of the lids when the cilia are stimulated, becomes progressively depressed as anesthesia

DOI: 10.1201/9780429190940-7

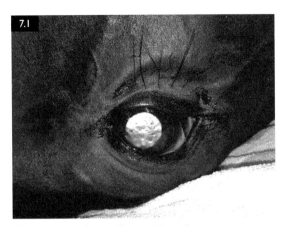

Figure 7.1 Centrally positioned eye

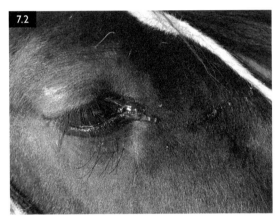

Figure 7.2 Lacrimating eye

deepens. It may be slow and sluggish at a surgical plane of anesthesia.

- The corneal reflex, closure of the lids when pressure is applied to the cornea, should be present during anesthesia; its absence indicates excessive anesthetic depth.
- Be aware that repeated stimulation of the eye reflexes may result in reflex depression. The effects of the dissociative anesthetics, such as ketamine and tiletamine, may limit the value of eye reflexes as these drugs may cause spontaneous blinking, nystagmus, central eye position, and lacrimation.

7.2.2 Movement

- Movement of head and limbs and tensing of neck muscles are indicative of a light plane of anesthesia.
- Anal tone may be useful when access to the head is limited. Stimulation of the anus should result in reflex contraction of the anal sphincter. The absence of anal tone indicates that the level of anesthesia is too deep.

7.2.3 Physiologic Parameters

- Heart rate (HR).
  - In horses tends to remain stable. Resting HR in the awake horse is 24–40 beats/minute.
  - The HR of the anesthetized horse will vary between 35–45 beats/minute, with the HR of foals going as high as 60 beats/minute.
  - An increase in HR may not accompany a light plane of anesthesia, and therefore a normal HR is not necessarily an indication of adequate anesthesia.
  - A decrease in HR could indicate too deep a plane of anesthesia or impending cardiac arrest.
- Respiratory rate (RR).
  - In the awake horse 15 breaths/minute with a tidal volume of 10 ml/kg.
  - The RR during spontaneous ventilation is 6–20 breaths/minute.
  - Inhalant anesthetics depress ventilation and therefore intermittent positive pressure ventilation (IPPV) should be provided if the patient is unable to maintain a normal end-tidal carbon dioxide ($ETCO_2$).
- Blood pressure.
  - Hypotension is commonly encountered even at adequate anesthetic planes.
  - Inhalant anesthetics cause a decrease in inotropy and systemic vascular resistance.
  - Positive inotropic agents are commonly administered to equine patients under

inhalational anesthesia. However, an increase in blood pressure may be indicative of a lightening plane of anesthesia.

- In general, physiologic parameters decrease as the plane of anesthesia deepens. A simultaneous decrease in HR, RR, and blood pressure could indicate impending disaster.

7.2.4 End-Tidal Inhalant Concentration

- The end-tidal (expired) concentrations of inhaled anesthetics at equilibrium reflect the amount of anesthetic in the blood and also in the brain. Therefore, the end-tidal agent concentrations provide a real-time indication of the depth of anesthesia (**Figure 7.3**).
- The minimum alveolar concentration (MAC) of an inhalant is the minimum amount that prevents 50% of the population from responding to a noxious stimulus, when no other drugs, such as sedatives and analgesics, are administered.

- Movement response to a noxious stimulus, such as surgery, may occur at 1 MAC.
- MAC is decreased by multiple factors including injectable anesthetic agents in partial intravenous anesthesia (PIVA) (Chapter 6).
- MAC is a measurement of the potency of inhaled agents, and it is species-specific (**Table 7.1**)

7.3 CARDIOVASCULAR SYSTEM

- Cardiovascular depression results in decreased oxygen delivery to vital organs in addition to the large muscle bellies of the equine patient.
- Cardiovascular collapse is cited in some studies as the leading cause of mortality in equine anesthetic patients.
- Catastrophic injury in recovery is also sometimes cited as the leading cause of mortality. A contributing factor to catastrophic injury is myopathy due to compromised perfusion during the anesthetic event. The incidence of myopathy is increased in patients that suffer prolonged hypotension under anesthesia.
- The anesthetist should monitor the cardiovascular system diligently in order to ensure continued oxygen delivery to vital organs and muscle tissue.

7.3.1 Subjective Monitoring

- Capillary refill time (CRT) is a visual indication of perfusion. Normally, it should be less than 2.5 seconds; a prolonged CRT (> 3 seconds) is indicative of poor perfusion and low cardiac output.

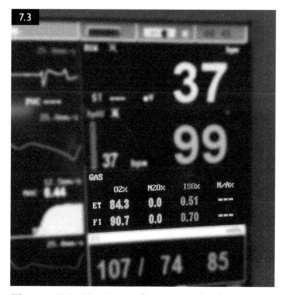

Figure 7.3 Monitor indicating end-tidal agent

Table 7.1 **Minimum alveolar concentration of different inhalant agents in horses**

DESFLURANE	HALOTHANE	ISOFLURANE	SEVOFLURANE
7.02–8.06%	0.88–1.05%	1.31–1.64%	2.31–2.84%

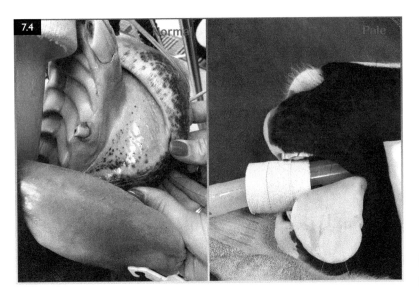

Figure 7.4 Pink versus pale mucous membranes

- The color of mucous membranes is an indicator of respiratory and cardiovascular status (**Figure 7.4**).
  - Pale mucous membranes indicate peripheral vasoconstriction and/or decreased circulating red cells.
  - Brick red mucous membranes and a prolonged CRT indicate poor gas exchange and blood sludging in the capillaries.
- Digital palpation of an arterial pulse is reliable for rough assessment of cardiac output, rate, and rhythm (**Figure 7.5**).

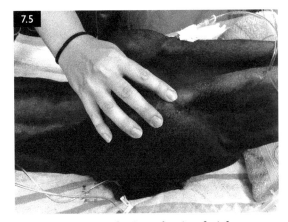

Figure 7.5 Anesthetist palpating facial artery

7.3.2 Electrocardiography (ECG)
- Used to monitor HR and rhythm via a visual representation of the electrical activity in the heart.
- A base-apex lead is used in order to augment the p-wave (**Figure 7.6**).
- Base-apex lead description:
  - The right arm electrode is clipped to the neck in the right jugular furrow.
  - The left arm electrode is passed between the front legs and clipped at the apex of the heart over the left intercostal space.
- The left leg electrode is clipped to the neck or shoulder.
- Lead I will give a negative R wave, and a bifid P wave is common due to the size of the equine atria (**Figure 7.7**).
- A normal ECG does not indicate normal hemodynamics or normal cardiac contraction; it only gives information on electrical activity.
- Use of an ECG is requisite for definitive diagnosis of arrhythmias.
  - AV block is normal in horses and may be observed while under anesthesia,

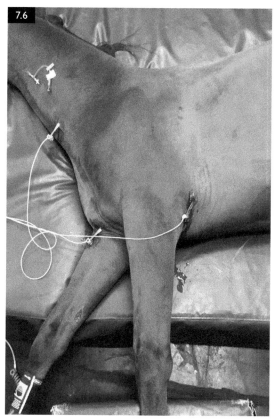

Figure 7.6 Base-apex lead setup

especially in the presence of alpha-2 agonists (**Figure 7.8**).

- The most common pathologic arrhythmia observed in horses is atrial fibrillation and is commonly identified peri-anesthetically.
- Ventricular premature complexes (VPCs) are sometimes seen in systemically ill patients.
- Supraventricular premature complexes are occasionally seen in anesthetized horses, and they may precede atrial fibrillation.
- Foals with uroabdomen suffering from hyperkalemia may exhibit bradycardia, VPCs, sinus arrest, asystole, and/or ventricular fibrillation.

7.3.3 Blood Pressure

- Arterial blood pressure is directly correlated with cardiac output. Blood pressure can be measured indirectly (noninvasively) using Doppler or oscillometric methods or directly (invasively) by arterial catheterization.

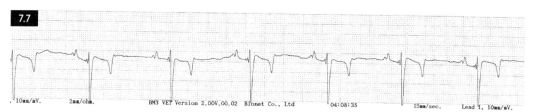

Figure 7.7 Normal equine ECG
Courtesy of Dr. Michelle Barton

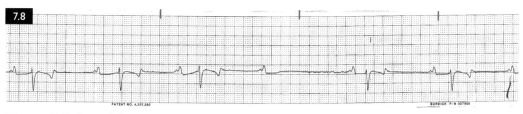

Figure 7.8 Second degree atrioventricular (AV) block
Courtesy of Dr. Michelle Barton

- Doppler ultrasonic flow detector (Doppler) (**Figure 7.9**)
  - It detects blood flow through an artery when pressure is released from an occlusive cuff.
  - It provides an estimation of the systolic blood pressure.
  - The Doppler transducer is placed distal to the cuff that is attached to a sphygmomanometer. The placement is either on the tail or a limb.
  - The width of the cuff is 20 to 40% the circumference of the tail.
- Automatic oscillometric technique
  - It uses an air-filled cuff placed around the tail or leg (**Figure 7.10**).
  - Good equivalence for mean arterial pressure was found between oscillometric technique and invasive measurements when the cuff width-to-tail circumference ratio was 0.25 and the cuff was placed on the tail.
  - The cuff is inflated to a pressure in excess of systolic blood pressure, then slowly released. Arterial pressure pulsations cause pressure oscillations within the cuff as the pressure falls. These oscillations are superimposed over a declining pressure curve. Systolic pressure is where the fluctuations begin to increase in size and MAP is where the fluctuations are the largest.
  - These devices are automatic and give a digital readout.
  - They become less accurate when the MAP is < 65 mmHg.
- Arterial catheterization (**Figure 7.11**).
  - This represents the most accurate method for assessing blood pressure.

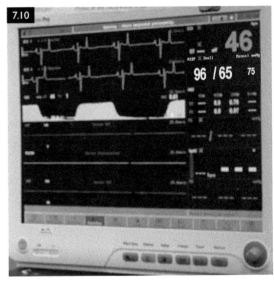

Figure 7.10 Oscillometric blood pressure

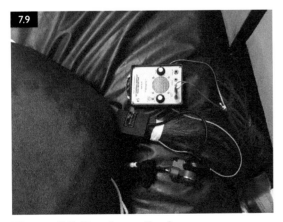

Figure 7.9 Doppler, cuff, sphygmomanometer

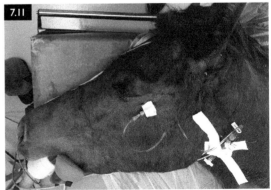

Figure 7.11 Arterial catheter placed in transverse facial artery

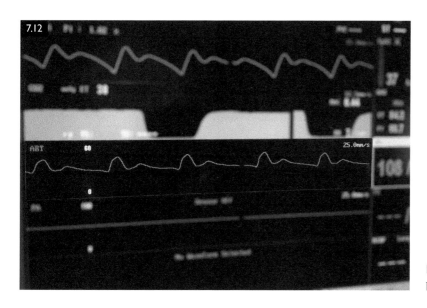

Figure 7.12 Arterial blood pressure waveform

- The catheter is attached to a pressure transducer to give direct arterial blood pressure readings (**Figure 7.12**).
- A 20- or 22-gauge catheter is most commonly used.
- It allows for beat-to-beat determination of heart rate, blood pressure, and arterial waveform configuration.
- The arteries accessible for catheterization in the equine include the lateral nasal, facial, transverse facial, and metatarsal.
- Complications are rare if there is asepsis during catheter insertion, use of sterile solutions for flushing, and appropriate pressure on the artery after catheter removal.
- The transducer is flushed with sterile saline and zeroed to room air at the level of the right atrium where it is placed.
- Systolic pressure variation, pulse pressure variation, or "cycling" caused by controlled ventilation is an indication of hypovolemia and may respond to IV fluid therapy.

- Mean arterial blood pressure of 70 mmHg is desirable to maintain adequate muscle perfusion in horses weighing less than 500 kg.
- Maintaining MAP of 80 mmHg is recommended for horses greater than 500 kg.
- Every effort should be made by the anesthetist to maintain blood pressure above these thresholds.

7.4   RESPIRATORY SYSTEM

- General anesthesia and recumbency in horses lead to significant derangements in gas exchange and respiratory function. Monitoring of respiration is done to ensure adequate oxygenation and ventilation are maintained.
- Monitoring parameters are RR, pulse oximetry, capnometry, arterial blood gas analysis, mucous membrane color, thoracic wall compliance, movement of the re-breathing bag, and tidal volume.
- When the horse is breathing spontaneously, RR less than 5 breaths per minute is likely to result in hypoventilation and increased

$PaCO_2$, which can lead to hypoxemia (low PaO_2).

- Intermittent positive pressure ventilation (IPPV) is used to manage hypoventilation when undergoing inhalant anesthesia. Respiratory rate of 6 to 8 breaths per minute is adequate for the adult horse. Higher RR, up to 10 to 12 breaths per minute, may be used in foals.
- The tidal volume for each breath should be 10 to 15 ml/kg. The peak airway pressure with a normal tidal volume should be 15 to 25 cmH_2O in the healthy adult horse.
- Horses with abdominal distension (i.e. colic surgery) may require potentially harmful peak airway pressures (up to 40 to 45 cmH_2O) to deliver an adequate tidal volume due to the severe compression of the enlarged gastrointestinal tract against the diaphragm.
  - These high pressures will lead to a decrease in venous return and subsequently decreased cardiac output.
  - These horses need rapid surgical intervention and decompression of the gastrointestinal tract to reduce the peak inspiratory pressure necessary to generate an adequate tidal volume.

7.4.1 Capnography

- Ventilation is assessed by monitoring the carbon dioxide (CO_2) via an arterial blood gas ($PaCO_2$) or $ETCO_2$. Normal $ETCO_2$ is 35–45 mmHg, with less than 35 mmHg defining hyperventilation and greater than 45 mmHg defining hypoventilation.
- Capnographs utilize infrared technology to measure the amount of CO_2 within the gas sample.
- The capnograph is a non-invasive device with an adaptor that connects between the endotracheal tube and the Y-piece, or samples directly from the endotracheal tube.
  - Sidestream sampling: exhaled gas is aspirated from the adapter between the endotracheal tube and the Y-piece and delivered to the capnometer (**Figure 7.13**).
  - Mainstream sampling: the measuring device itself is placed between the endotracheal tube and the Y-piece (**Figure 7.14**).
- The amount of CO_2 in the last part of the exhaled breath, $ETCO_2$, equals the amount of CO_2 in the alveoli and closely matches $PaCO_2$.
- The $ETCO_2$ usually underestimates the $PaCO_2$.
  - Normal $PaCO_2$-to-$ETCO_2$ gradient in the awake horse is 5 to 10 mmHg.
  - This gradient will increase under anesthesia due to atelectasis, decreased cardiac output, and increased dead space ventilation.
  - The $ETCO_2$ in healthy horses under anesthesia tends to be 10 to 15 mmHg lower than the $PaCO_2$.
  - Up to 20 mmHg difference is commonly observed in the distended horse undergoing colic surgery.
  - This gradient is expected to be larger in horses in dorsal recumbency versus lateral recumbency.
- The $ETCO_2$ waveform, the capnogram (**Figure 7.15**), is useful to help identify potential complications.
  - Unexpectedly low $ETCO_2$ may be due to cardiac arrest, a significant decrease in cardiac output, hypotension, air embolism, pulmonary embolism, disconnected or broken sampling line, leaking/deflated endotracheal tube cuff, or small/inadequate tidal volume.
  - Absent $ETCO_2$ can be noticed with apnea, disconnection of the endotracheal tube from the Y-piece, airway obstruction, or esophageal intubation.
  - Re-breathing CO_2 is seen when the waveform does not go back to zero (baseline) during inspiration. This

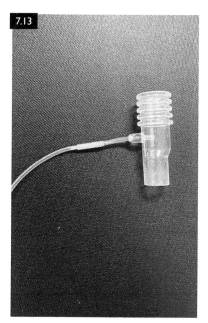

A. Sidestream capnograph connection for standard 15mm circuit connection.

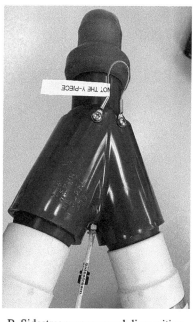

B. Sidestream capnograph line exiting Y-piece of large animal circuit.

Figure 7.13 Sidestream gas analyzer sampling lines

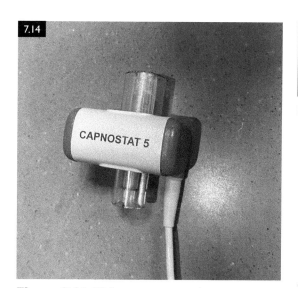

Figure 7.14 Mainstream gas analyzer

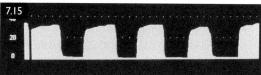

Figure 7.15 Capnogram

- A prolonged inspiratory or expiratory slope may be due to a gas sampling rate that is too low, a partial airway obstruction, a leak around the endotracheal tube cuff, bronchoconstriction, or an obstruction or crack in the sampling line.

7.4.2 Arterial Blood Gas

- Arterial blood gases may be obtained from an arterial catheter or with direct insertion of a blood gas needle/syringe in the artery (**Figure 7.16**). The blood gas should be analyzed immediately after sampling for the best results.
- Blood gas values will give accurate information on ventilation, oxygenation,

could be due to large dead space of the apparatus, incompetence of the expiratory valve of the circle system (if valve is stuck open or closed), exhaustion of CO_2 absorbent, or rapid and shallow breathing.

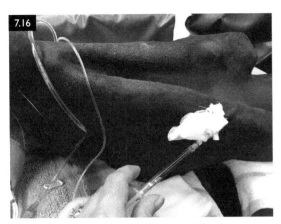

Figure 7.16 Sampling of arterial blood

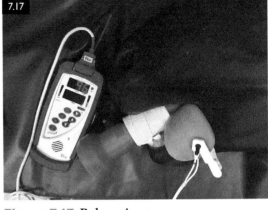

Figure 7.17 Pulse oximetry

as well as the acid-base status. This is especially important for the critically ill equine patient. The normal values are:

- pH 7.38 to 7.41.
- $PaCO_2$ 36–46 mmHg.
- PaO_2 on room air at sea level should be approximately 100 mmHg in healthy subjects.
  - On 100% oxygen, as with anesthesia, PaO_2 values should exceed 200 mmHg (can be as high as 5 x inspired oxygen concentration, approximately 500 mmHg).
- An increased $PaCO_2$ (hypoventilation) with values of 60 mmHg or higher are indicative of severe respiratory depression.
- A PaO_2 value of less than 60 mmHg constitutes severe hypoxemia. This is commonly due to atelectasis (lung collapse) during prolonged recumbency and ventilation/perfusion mismatch.

7.4.3 Pulse Oximetry

- The pulse oximeter (**Figure 7.17**) is a non-invasive device that provides the SpO_2, which is an estimate of the percentage of arterial blood hemoglobin that is saturated with oxygen (SaO_2).
- This monitor works by flashing red and infrared light through tissue and measuring

the absorbance of light. Oxygenated and deoxygenated hemoglobin absorb light at different wavelengths, with deoxygenated absorbing more red light and oxyhemoglobin absorbing more infrared light. Arterial blood is differentiated from venous blood by analyzing only pulsatile absorbance.

- The oximeter also detects the pulse rate. This pulse rate must correspond to the rate obtained by palpation or the ECG with the sensor in place for at least 30 seconds for the oximeter value to be considered accurate.
- A reading may be difficult to obtain with severe vasoconstriction and dark pigmented skin or mucous membranes.
- The pulse oximeter can detect desaturation before it may be clinically apparent. Hypoxemia is defined as a PaO_2 of 60 mmHg or less and this corresponds to a SpO_2 of 92%. A low value indicates corrective action needs to be taken such as oxygen supplementation, intermittent positive pressure ventilation, or assisted ventilation.
- Sites for probe placement include the tongue, lip, nostril, prepuce, and vulva.

7.5   SUMMARY

- The astute anesthetist should utilize all of the above modalities in monitoring the equine anesthetic patient.
- There is no single monitor that can provide all necessary information, and only the integration of data from multiple monitoring modalities will provide a comprehensive picture of the condition of the patient.
- All actions of the anesthetist in maintaining a stable and adequate anesthetic plane should be guided by thorough and diligent monitoring.

7.6   CLINICAL CASE EXAMPLES

7.6.1 12-Year-Old Quarter Horse to Be Anesthetized for Stifle Arthroscopy

- Physical exam and pre-operative blood work within normal limits.
- Monitoring used:
  - Visual inspection of eye position, palpebral reflex, mucous membrane color, capillary refill time (CRT), heart rate (HR), and respiratory rate (RR).
  - Multiparameter monitor for capnography, pulse oximetry, ECG, and invasive blood pressure.
- One hour into procedure.
  - No eye movement, normal mucous membrane color and CRT.
  - RR 5 breaths/minute.
  - $EtCO_2$ 55 mmHg.
  - SpO_2 95%.
  - Normal sinus rhythm, HR 32 beats/minutes.
  - Blood pressure 120/55 (80) mmHg.
  - This patient is currently hypoventilating, and this could be what has caused the saturation to be low.

- The anesthetist increases the tidal volume to achieve a peak inspiratory pressure of 25 cmH$_2$O and increases the RR from 5 to 8 breaths/minute.
- Five minutes later.
  - No eye movement, normal mucous membrane color and CRT.
  - $EtCO_2$ 45 mmHg.
  - SpO_2 98%.
  - Normal sinus rhythm, HR 32 beats/minute.
  - Blood pressure 120/55 (80) mmHg.

7.6.2   1-Year-Old Male Arabian to Be Castrated in the Field

- Physical exam within normal limits.
- Monitoring used: visual inspection of eye position, palpebral reflex, mucous membrane color and CRT, and handheld pulse oximetry.
- Ten minutes into the procedure.
  - Rapid nystagmus, swift palpebral, and spontaneous blinking.
  - SpO_2 97%, HR 40 beats/minute.
  - This patient's plane of anesthesia is too light.
- The anesthetist administers a bolus of ketamine and xylazine to deepen the anesthetic plane.
- Five minutes later.
  - No nystagmus, slow palpebral.
  - SpO_2 97%, HR 35 beats/minute.

FURTHER READING

Hubbell JAE, Muir WW (2009) Monitoring anesthesia. In: *Equine Anesthesia Monitoring and Emergency Therapy*, 2nd edn. (eds Muir WW, Hubbell JAE), Saunders Elsevier St. Louis, pp. 149–170.

Murrell JC (2006) Monitoring the anesthetized horse, monitoring the central nervous system. In: *Manual of Equine Anesthesia & Analgesia* (eds Doherty T, Valverde A), Blackwell Publishing Ames, pp. 186–191.

Trim CM, Clarke KW (2014) Patient monitoring and clinical measurement. In: *Veterinary Anaesthesia*, 11th edn. (eds Clarke KW, Trim CM, Hall LW), Saunders Elsevier, St. Louis, pp. 19–63.

Wilson DV (2006) Monitoring the anesthetized horse, monitoring the respiratory system. In: *Manual of Equine Anesthesia & Analgesia* (eds Doherty T, Valverde A), Blackwell Publishing, Ames, pp. 191–199.

CHAPTER 8

FLUID THERAPY

Jarred Williams and Elizabeth Hodge

8.1 INTRODUCTION

This chapter describes catheter placement as well as different types of intravenous fluids available for administration to anesthetized patients, including crystalloids, colloids, and blood products. Fluid selection and indications for fluid therapy in a variety of clinical conditions will be discussed.

8.2 INTRAVENOUS CATHETERS

8.2.1 Jugular Vein Catheters

- The jugular vein is most commonly used for venous access in adult horses and foals (**Figure 8.1**).
- 14-gauge 5.25-inch over-the-needle (OTN) or over-the-wire (OTW) catheters are typically used; 10- or 12-gauge OTN can be used when more rapid fluid resuscitation is required. 16- or 14-gauge OTW catheters are appropriate for use in foals.
- Teflon catheters should not be left in place for more than 3 days due to their thrombogenic effect as compared to polyurethane or silicone catheters, which can be left in for 3–4 weeks.
- To place a jugular vein catheter:
  - An area in the cranial one third of the neck of the jugular furrow should be aseptically prepared and 1–2 ml of 2% lidocaine, for local anesthesia during placement, can be injected subcutaneously at the desired insertion site prior to catheter placement using sterile technique (**Figure 8.2**).
- The vein is distended by holding off with the knuckles of the nondominant hand in the distal jugular groove. The catheter is held in the dominant hand with the thumb and middle finger holding the stylet and the catheter hub together (**Figure 8.3**).
- The index finger can be held over the stylet but must be lifted when checking for blood to indicate appropriate placement (**Figure 8.4**).
- With the catheter parallel to the jugular groove, directed towards the heart, it is advanced through the skin and into the jugular vein at a 30-degree angle until venous blood is seen in the stylet when the index finger is lifted.
- The angle is then decreased and the catheter advanced several centimeters prior to using the nondominant hand to hold the stylet (**Figure 8.5**).
- The dominant hand is then used to feed the catheter off the stylet into the vein (**Figure 8.6**).
- The stylet is then removed and the vein occluded once again to confirm venous blood flow (**Figure 8.7**).
- A catheter injection cap or T-port with cap should be secured onto the catheter and sutured in place with 2–0 nonabsorbable suture in a manner that holds the catheter in the jugular groove (**Figure 8.8**).

DOI: 10.1201/9780429190940-8

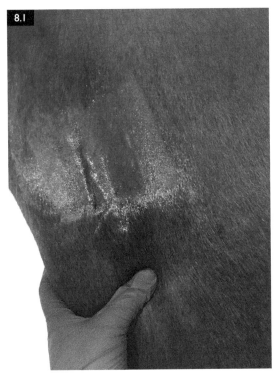

Figure 8.1 Jugular vein

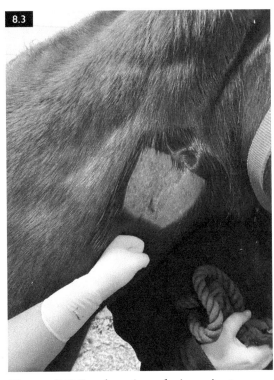

Figure 8.3 Jugular vein occlusion prior to catheter placement

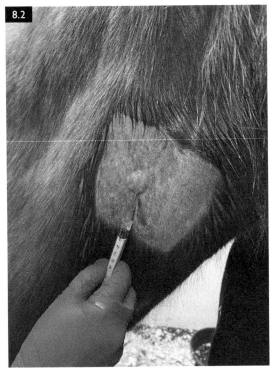

Figure 8.2 Lidocaine bleb prior to catheter placement

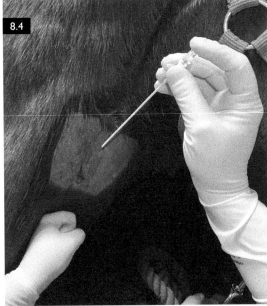

Figure 8.4 Index finger over end of catheter

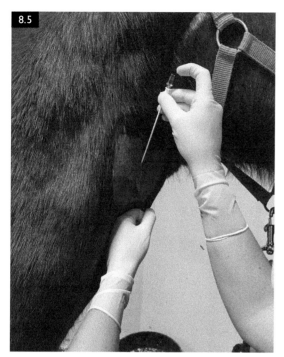

Figure 8.5 Advancing stylet

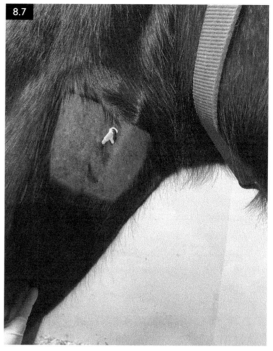

Figure 8.7 Stylet removed, occluding jugular, blood coming out of catheter

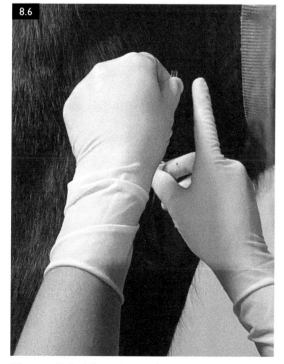

Figure 8.6 Advancing catheter

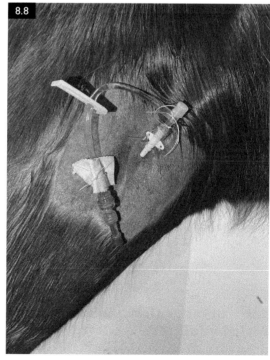

Figure 8.8 Secured catheter with T port

8.2.2 Saphenous Vein Catheters

- The saphenous vein can be used in adult horses undergoing advanced imaging or when surgery of the head and neck precludes use of the jugular vein.
- Following induction of anesthesia with the horse in lateral or dorsal recumbency, or in the standing, sedated patient, the saphenous vein can be identified in the medial aspect of the proximal hind limb.
- The vein may need to be held off for 1 minute or longer to distend the most proximal aspect.
- A 16- or 14-gauge 2–5.25-inch OTN catheter is placed and secured similarly to jugular vein catheterization. An OTW catheter can also be used.

8.2.3 Superficial Lateral Thoracic Vein Catheters

- The lateral thoracic vein can be catheterized using a 16- or 14-gauge OTW catheter in the standing sedated horse or recumbent foal.
- The lateral thoracic vein can be palpated running horizontally between the external abdominal oblique and ascending pectoralis (pectoralis profundus) muscles at the level of the elbow.
- Placement is similar to placing an OTW in the jugular vein; 2% lidocaine should be used at the desired insertion point, then a 14-gauge 1–1.5 inch needle or short catheter should be seated into the vein.
- Blood should flow from the needle prior to feeding the wire.
- Horses may kick while the catheter is being inserted and sutured in place.
- A catheter wrap may be required.

8.3 PRINCIPLES

8.3.1 Composition and Fluid Distribution within Animals

- An adult horse's total body water is approximately 60% of the body weight.

Blood volume is approximately 8% of the body weight.
- A foal's total body water is approximately 75% of the body weight. Blood volume is approximately 9% of the body weight.
- Body fluid compartments can be divided into intracellular (ICF) and extracellular (ECF) compartments.
- The ECF compartment is composed of the intravascular and interstitial fluid.
- In adults the ECF to ICF compartment ratio is 1:2.
- In foals the ECF to ICF compartment ratio is 1:1.

Electrolytes are chemical particles that dissociate in solution to form electrically charged particles or ions.
- Sodium is the primary extracellular cation, and bicarbonate and chloride are the predominant extracellular anions. Potassium is the primary intracellular cation.
- Water will move to follow sodium.
- Proteins do not readily diffuse through the capillary membrane and thereby maintain intravascular volume by exerting colloid oncotic pressure (COP).
- The majority of COP, 70%, comes from albumin, globulins, and fibrinogen.
- Starling's law describes the forces that move fluid between the interstitial and vascular space.

8.3.2 Four Main Forces that Determine Fluid Distribution across Capillaries

- COP of the plasma is the primary force keeping fluid in the vessels.
- COP of the interstitium opposes that of the plasma.
- Intravascular hydrostatic pressure is the primary force pushing fluid out of the vessels.

- Interstitial hydrostatic pressure opposes that of the intravascular space.

8.3.3 Indications for Fluid Therapy under General Anesthesia

- Fluid therapy is a vital tool to help provide cardiovascular support and maintain appropriate perfusion during anesthesia by optimizing cardiac preload.
- 5–10 ml/kg/hour intravenous fluids is an appropriate rate for a normally hydrated, healthy horse.
- Preoperative fasting in addition to ongoing losses from urination may result in hypotension, which can be combated with high volumes of intravenous fluids for a short period of time following induction of anesthesia, referred to as fluid loading. A starting bolus can range from 2 to 5 ml/kg, depending on the dehydration of the patient. This dose can be repeated if necessary.
- Packed cell volume (PCV) and total solids (TS) are a relatively quick and simple method to gauge hydration in addition to physical exam findings. Normal PCV can range from 30%-45% and TP from 6–7.5 mg/dl.
- Morbidity and mortality associated with general anesthesia are higher in horses than other species.
- Inhaled anesthetic agents cause a dose-dependent vasodilation of the peripheral vessels and reduction in cardiac output resulting in hypotension.
- Hypotension (mean arterial pressure less than 65–70 mmHg) greatly increases the risk of myopathies and anesthetic recovery complications.

8.4   TYPES AND RATES OF FLUID THERAPY

8.4.1 Fluid Classification

- Careful evaluation of each patient preoperatively will help establish the proper course of fluids required during the anesthetic period.
- Fluids are administered intravenously for replacement needs, but they may also be delivered intraosseously in foals.
- Fluids administered during general anesthesia are predominantly classified as crystalloid, colloid, or blood products.

1) Crystalloids
   - Normal saline (**Figure 8.9**), hypertonic saline (**Figure 8.10**), Lactated Ringer's

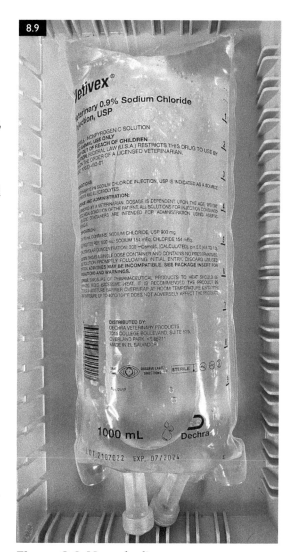

Figure 8.9 Normal saline

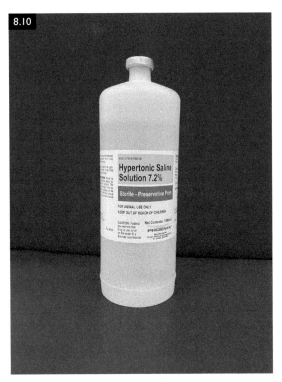

Figure 8.10 Hypertonic saline

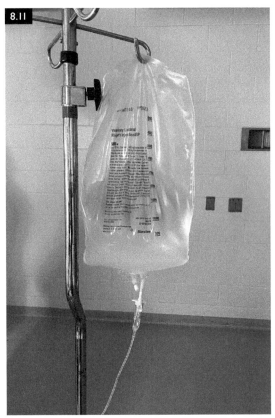

Figure 8.11 Lactated Ringer's solution

solution (LRS) (**Figure 8.11**), and Plasma-Lyte A are all crystalloid fluids.

- They contain small particles that are osmotically active and can pass through capillary membranes.
- Crystalloids disseminate throughout the body fluid spaces, while colloids tend to remain within the intravascular spaces.
- Based on tonicity, crystalloids can be further divided into hypotonic, isotonic, and hypertonic fluids. Tonicity of a fluid compares the osmolality (concentration of solute per unit of solvent) of the fluid with the intracellular osmolality.
- Based on their usage, crystalloid fluids can also be classified as maintenance or replacement fluids, and these differ in their electrolyte concentration.
- Maintenance fluids are usually hypotonic, containing lower sodium and higher potassium concentrations.

- Replacement fluids are usually isotonic and are considered balanced, as they have similar electrolyte composition and tonicity to plasma. They are suitable for rapid volume restoration.
- Replacement fluids, such as Plasma-Lyte A, are most commonly used during general anesthesia, because they are isotonic and can be given rapidly intravenously to expand the intravascular compartment.

Types of crystalloid fluids and their clinical indications

a) Lactated Ringer's solution and Plasma-Lyte A
- These are balanced isotonic fluids.
- They contain acetate, lactate, or gluconate, which serve as

alkalinizing agents to maintain acid-base balance.

- Commonly used as replacement solutions under general anesthesia at a rate of 5–10 ml/kg/hour.
- Fluids with additional potassium chloride supplementation should be used with caution during general anesthesia in case large volumes must be administered rapidly. Life-threatening hyperkalemia may occur with bolus administration of potassium greater than 0.5 mEq/kg/hour.

b) Hypertonic saline
- Hypertonic saline has an osmolality of 2,400 mOsm/l, approximately 8 times the tonicity of plasma, which classifies it as hypertonic.
- It is commercially available as 3.0–7.5% solutions of sodium chloride; 7–7.5% is most commonly used in horses.
- It is used primarily to treat hypovolemic shock at 2–4 ml/kg intravenously once as a bolus in adult horses.
- It exerts beneficial effects primarily through improvement in intravascular volume and reduction in afterload as the solute load draws fluid from both the extracellular and intracellular compartments. Vital organ blood flow is, therefore, improved.
- The effects of hypertonic saline are transient with distribution to the interstitium within 30 minutes. Regular isotonic crystalloid solutions must be used in order to replace the body water lost.
- One liter of hypertonic saline expands the plasma volume 3–4 liters.
- Contraindicated in patients with hypernatremia, risk of volume overload, or renal insufficiency. Neonatal kidneys may not be able to excrete additional sodium and can develop severe hypernatremia.

c) Dextrose added to fluids
- Dextrose can be added to crystalloid solutions at a variety of concentrations, with 2.5% and 5% being the most commonly used.
- Dextrose 5% in water is considered isotonic, but the glucose is rapidly metabolized by cells such that the remaining free water is hypotonic, resulting in electrolyte abnormalities in the extracellular fluid if large volumes are bolused rapidly.
- 5% dextrose contains 170 kcal/l.
- 50% dextrose must be diluted prior to administration as it is hypertonic and can cause phlebitis. It is given slowly intravenously in a large vein to minimize venous irritation.
- If dextrose administration is desired, dextrose can be added to LRS or Plasma-Lyte A, resulting in an initially hypertonic solution. When the dextrose is metabolized, the solution will be isotonic.
- For example, to make 2.5% dextrose in LRS, 50 ml of LRS is removed from a 1-liter bag and replaced with 50 ml of 50% dextrose. $C1V1 = C2V2$ (50% dextrose)(x ml) = (2.5% dextrose)(1000 ml) x= 50 ml.
- Indications for adding dextrose to crystalloid fluids:
  - Pediatric patients.
  - Patients with severe liver dysfunction.
  - Over-conditioned, off-feed, and/or hypertriglyceridemic patients.

d) Normal saline/0.9% NaCl.
- Does not contain any bicarbonate precursors.
- Considered an acidifying solution.
- Large volumes administered rapidly will dilute plasma bicarbonate, causing a dilutional acidemia.
- Indications for use of normal saline:

- Patients with metabolic alkalosis.
- Patients with hyperkalemia, such as horses with hyperkalemic periodic paralysis (HYPP) or uroabdomen.

Advantages of Crystalloid Fluids
- Can be used for volume replacement for normal patients undergoing general anesthesia.
- Can be administered at high rates for patients in hypovolemic shock. Approximately 1 blood volume (8% of body weight = 36 liters in a 450 kg horse) could be delivered per hour: 60–80 ml/kg/hour in adult horses with the use of a large-bore catheter.
- Cost-effective.
- Rapid onset of effect.
- Long shelf life.
- Easily obtained and available.

Disadvantages of Crystalloid Fluids
- Dilution of plasma proteins.
- Need 3 times the equivalent volume to replace lost blood and replenish oxygen-carrying capability and clotting factors.
- Relatively short duration of effect. Only 25% of administered volume remains in the intravascular space after 1 hour.

2) Colloids.
- Colloid fluids may be naturally occurring (plasma, whole blood) or synthetic (dextrans, hydroxyethyl starch, gelatins).
- Colloid solutions are aqueous solutions containing particles with large molecular weights.
- Some of these particles can diffuse through capillary membranes, but many cannot and remain within the intravascular space. This tends

to increase intravascular oncotic pressure, which retains fluid within the intravascular space and also draws some fluid in from the interstitial space.
- If colloids are used with crystalloids, the amount of crystalloids should be reduced by 40 to 50% to avoid volume overload.

Indications for Colloid Fluid Therapy
- Rapid volume replacement with less redistribution to interstitial space.
- Low plasma proteins.
- Increased capillary permeability (e.g. systemic inflammatory response syndrome).
- Hypovolemia with cerebral or pulmonary edema.
- Patients with third-space losses.

Adverse Reactions and Contraindications for Colloid Fluid Therapy
- Potential for volume overload, as the fluid stays primarily within the intravascular space.
- Potential for coagulopathies with synthetic colloids.
- Potential for hypersensitivity reactions with natural colloids.
- Should be avoided in patients with existing renal disease, septicemia, or coagulopathy.
- More costly to administer than crystalloids.

Type of Colloid Fluid—Hetastarch
- Hetastarch (**Figure 8.12**) is a synthetic polysaccharide, with starch molecules of varying molecular weights.
- Long-lasting vascular expansion (up to 24 hours).

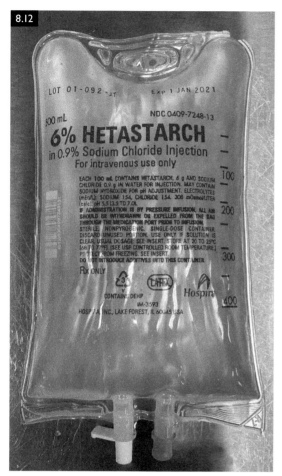

Figure 8.12 Hetastarch

- Store at room temperature.
- Dose is 2–10 ml/kg/day.
- Under general anesthesia the fluid can be administered as a bolus or a constant rate infusion (CRI).

3) Blood products
   - Blood products can be natural or synthetic.
   - Natural blood products include fresh or stored whole blood and frozen plasma.
   - Synthetic products in veterinary medicine are limited to Oxyglobin®, which is not currently available.

Patients Requiring Blood Products before General Anesthesia
- Patients with severe blood loss or with anemia (PCV < 0.2 l/l [20%]) or an anticipated blood loss of < 30% of blood volume. Blood volume in horses is 80–90 ml/kg.
- Hypoproteinemic patients with TP < 35 g/l (3.5 g/dl) or albumin < 20 g/l (2 g/dl).
- Patients with bleeding disorders (e.g. coagulopathies or thrombocytopenia).
- Whole blood is the best replacement for acute blood loss when both PCV and TP levels are low.
- Administration of 30–40 ml/kg intravenous crystalloids prior to onset of blood loss assists in maintaining intravascular volume and dilutes PCV/TP, reducing the amount of red cells lost per unit volume.
- Plasma is used to treat sepsis/endotoxemia or protein loss when red blood cells remain adequate; however, the amount of plasma required to raise the total protein by 1 g/dl is expensive (ranges from 3–10 liters of plasma in a 450-kg horse).

Cautions When Administering Natural Blood Products
- A filtered blood administration set should be used when administering blood or blood products.
- Blood products should be slowly warmed to body temperature prior to administration.
- Horses should be cross-matched if time allows.

Dose Rates of Whole Blood
- 10–22 ml/kg/hour.
- 25–50% of total blood loss should be replaced in acute hemorrhage.

- 2.2 ml of whole blood per kg body weight (or 1 ml of whole blood per lb body weight) raises PCV by 0.01 l/l (1%), provided the donor's PCV is approximately 0.4 l/l (40%).
- Administer slowly initially (0.3 ml/kg over 10–20 minutes; monitor for transfusion reaction). Then increase rate as needed up to 20–40 ml/kg/hour.

Signs of Transfusion Reaction (under General Anesthesia)
- Tachycardia.
- Tachypnea or dyspnea.
- Increased body temperature.
- Hypotension.
- Urticaria.
- Edema.

8.5   CLINICAL CASE EXAMPLES

- A healthy horse undergoing general anesthesia for an elective procedure should receive LRS or Plasm-Lyte A at 5–10 ml/kg/hour IV.

- A foal with a ruptured urinary bladder presenting for bladder repair with a mild hyperkalemia should receive 0.9% NaCl or LRS at 10 to 20 ml/kg/hour IV.

- A horse with colitis, with total solids of 3 g/dl, undergoing abdominal explore

under general anesthesia, should receive a balanced, isotonic replacement fluid such as LRS or Plasma-Lyte A at 10 ml/kg/hour. Hetastarch at 0.4 ml/kg/hour can be added.

FURTHER READING

Cruz JF, Peatling JE (2010) How to utilize saphenous vein catheterization during general anesthesia for selected surgical and diagnostic procedures. *Proceedings of the 56th Annual Convention of the American Association of Equine Practitioners*, Baltimore, pp. 41–43.

Fielding CL, Magdesian KG (2015) *Equine Fluid Therapy*, Wiley Blackwell, Ames.

Hart KA (2014) Review of fluid and electrolyte therapy in neonatal foals. *Proceedings of the 60th Annual Convention of the American Association of Equine Practitioners*, Baltimore, pp. 93–97.

Nolen-Walston RD (2012) Flow rates of large animal fluid delivery systems used for high-volume crystalloid resuscitation. *J Vet Emerg Crit Care* **22**:661–665.

Orsini JA, Divers TJ (2014) *Equine Emergencies: Treatment and Procedures*, 4th edn., Elsevier Saunders, St. Louis.

Snyder LB, Wendt-Hornickle E (2013) General anesthesia in horses on fluid and electrolyte therapy. *Vet Clin North Am Equine Pract* **29**: 169–178.

Wagner AE (2008) Complications in equine anesthesia. *Vet Clin North Am Equine Pract* **24**:735–752.

CHAPTER 9

ANESTHETIC RECOVERY

Philip Kiefer, Jane Quandt and Michele Barletta **125**

9.1 INTRODUCTION

Among all the procedures commonly performed in veterinary medicine, recovery of equine patients from general anesthesia can be among the most precarious.

- The risk of complications and catastrophic injury during recovery from even routine procedures is markedly higher than in most other domestic species.
- Modern studies show that orthopedic injuries compose the bulk of major complications.
- Substantial risks exist to not only the recovering patient, but also the personnel involved in the recovery.
- Careful preparation, planning and experienced personnel are essential to maximize positive patient outcomes.

9.2 RECOVERY MODALITIES

- Selection of a recovery method is dictated by numerous variables.
  - Available facilities.
  - Patient temperament and status.
  - Reason for anesthesia.
  - Availability and experience of personnel.
- Little information exists in the literature examining the effect of recovery methods on patient outcome.

9.2.1 Free Recovery
- The patient is allowed to recover without intervention (**Figure 9.1**).

- A true free recovery is usually conducted in a padded recovery stall, although this method is occasionally used in a normal stall, paddock, round pen or similar areas. (True free recoveries are relatively uncommon.)
- Free recoveries may be elected for:
  - Young, healthy patients recovering from elective procedures.
  - Horses of temperaments unsuitable to other methods.
  - Animals anesthetized for short period of time.
  - When injectable anesthesia is used.
  - Field anesthesia.
- The patient may be placed on a mattress in the recovery location to provide padding.

9.2.2 Hand-Assisted
- The patient is guided while attempting to stand (**Figure 9.2**).
- This usually consists of one person guiding the patient via a hand on the patient's halter or lead rope, and one person providing traction on the tail.
- Additional personnel may be added to either the head or the tail, or they may stabilize the patient from either side.
- In adult horses, those assisting usually provide only guidance and stability, as enough force cannot be generated to lift the patient.
- Foals may be lifted by hand if they are small enough.
- This method is commonly used in the field for patients of all sizes and in a hospital setting for smaller patients.

DOI: 10.1201/9780429190940-9

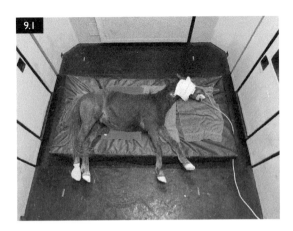

Figure 9.1 Horse in recovery with no ropes

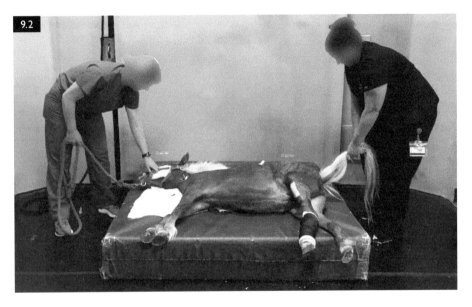

Figure 9.2
Hand-assisted
recovery

9.2.3　Rope-Assisted

- Leverage and stabilization are provided to the patient via long ropes attached to the halter and tied to the tail (**Figure 9.3**), which are then run through rings on the wall.
- Rope recovery requires a recovery stall.
- Ropes should be inspected before every use and cleaned after every use.
- Ropes may be run through the rings to outside the stall, where recovery can be directed and observed from relative safety, or may be run through the rings to the inside of the stall, where more control can be exerted over the patient.

9.2.4　Sling-Assisted

- During entry to the recovery stall, the patient is placed into a sling (**Figure 9.4**).
- The patient is encouraged to recover quietly until they are judged capable of standing.

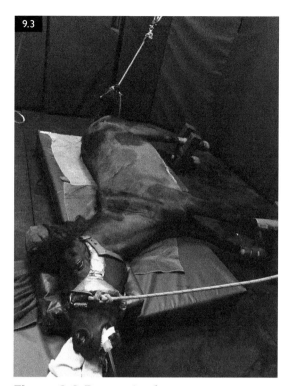

Figure 9.3 Rope-assisted recovery

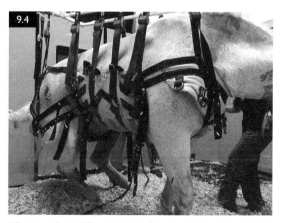

Figure 9.4 Sling-assisted recovery

- Once this stage has been reached, the sling is used to raise the patient, and the horse is allowed to gain its feet.
- The sling may then be removed, or it may be left in place to support the patient.

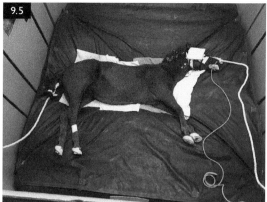

Figure 9.5 Horse on air mattress

- Sling recoveries are relatively rare due to their complicated nature and inherent effort.
- Suitable horses are those with significant musculoskeletal injuries, neurologic issues, or large size who cannot be otherwise assisted.
- Assistance from a sling may also be used for patients that have been unable to recover via other means and require additional assistance.

9.2.5 Inflatable Air Mattress
- This technique involves using an air compressor to inflate a mattress under the anesthetized horse (**Figure 9.5**).
- The mattress provides some padding to the patient and, while it is inflated, theoretically keeps the horse from attempting to stand.
- Once the horse is judged to be awake, the air compressor is shut off, the mattress deflates, and the patient is allowed to attempt to stand.
- The patient may or may not be assisted by ropes.

9.2.6 Pool Recoveries
- A rare form of recovery due to the expensive equipment and advanced training and experience necessary to successfully utilize this technique (**Figure 9.6**).

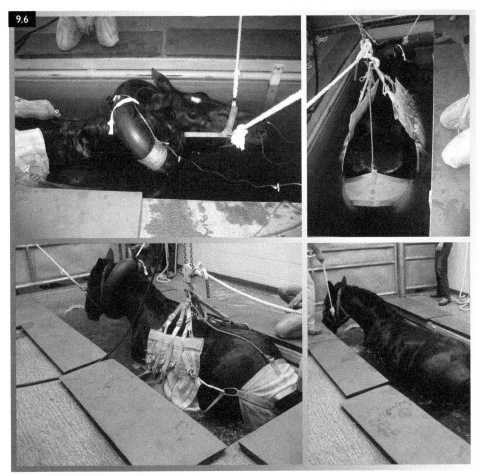

Figure 9.6 Pool recovery
Courtesy of Dr. Tamara Grubb

- It is usually reserved for patients undergoing orthopedic surgery.
- Two major variations exist:
  1) The first involves a rectangular pool with a floor attached to a scissor lift.
     - The horse is placed in a sling and lowered into the pool with the scissor lift in the down position.
     - Once the horse is awake, the floor is raised under the horse simultaneously with the sling, until the horse and the floor are level with the surrounding surface.

2) The second variation is the pool raft recovery system.
   - It lowers the slung, anesthetized horse into a rubber raft floating in a large pool.
   - The horse is allowed to recover suspended in the raft.
   - Once the horse is awake, it is blindfolded and lifted out of the raft via the sling and into a recovery stall, where it is placed on its feet.
- Water entering the surgical site is a concern, and plastic bags and waterproof

adhesive tape are used to attempt to protect this area.
- This is less of a concern in the raft recovery system as the raft provides some protection from direct contact with the water.

9.2.7 Tilt Table
- Another rare form of recovery.
- Usually reserved for significant orthopedic repair.
- After sedation, the horse is secured to a rotating table, starting in a horizontal position.
- Once the horse awakens, the table is rotated to a vertical position, and the restraints are removed.

9.3 RECOVERY ENVIRONMENT

9.3.1 Field Anesthesia
- Patients with short general anesthetic procedures such as those typically undertaken on the farm (routine castrations, simple laceration repair, etc.) can be successfully recovered where they are anesthetized.
- This is usually a grassy area in a field or near the barn, an arena, a round pen or the like (**Figure 9.7**).
- For younger, flightier, or less well-broke horses, some sort of confinement like a round pen, paddock or indoor area may be desired. Ideally, this area should be clean and dry, with good footing.
- A halter and lead rope can be used to control the animal during recovery.
- A soft surface that provides some cushioning is preferable.
- The area should be free of rocks, sticks and other debris that might injure the patient or the practitioner.
- Lighting should be appropriate and the environment as calm and quiet as possible.

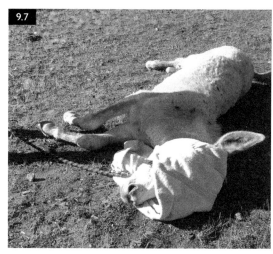

Figure 9.7 Horse recovering in a field

- A towel should be placed under the dependent eye to protect it from dirt and grass.
- Another towel should be placed on the other eye to protect it from the sunlight.
- Avoid areas with a slope and near water.

9.3.2 Hospital Setting
- When general anesthesia is to be performed regularly, construction of a specific recovery stall is advisable (**Figure 9.8**).
- This stall also frequently serves as the induction stall.
- This should be a separate room from the operating room.
- There are many variations, but the design should reflect the prevailing desired recovery method.
- The construction should be sturdy, with padded walls of adequate height.
- The flooring should have good footing and may consist of rubber or synthetic construct, sand or similar type of footing.
- The stall should be easy to clean between patients.
- Well-anchored rings for recovery ropes and a hoist system for placing the patient on

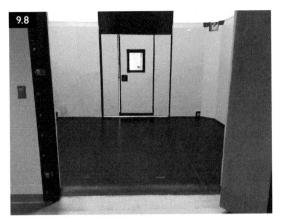

Figure 9.8 Recovery stall

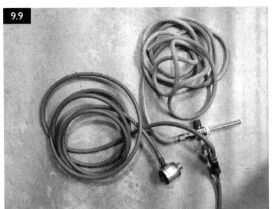

Figure 9.9 Oxygen drop with demand valve

the surgical table and for slings should be included in the design.

- Multiple electrical outlets are desirable and should be installed in areas not accessible to the horse.
- A fluid hanging system should also be placed for unstable patients or those experiencing a poor recovery.
- An oxygen drop with demand valve should be easily accessible (**Figure 9.9**).
- Doors should be sturdy, with good hinges and secure locking capability.
- The stalls should be inspected for any protuberances, corners or sharp edges that a patient may injure themselves on. Lighting in the stall should be easily controllable.

9.4   RECOVERY DRUGS

- Horses anesthetized using inhalants commonly have poor recoveries if they attempt to stand prior to eliminating a significant amount of the agent.
- In order to encourage the patient to lie in recovery longer and eliminate more of the anesthetic agent, additional sedation is often administered at this time.

- Alpha-2 agonists including xylazine (0.2–0.8 mg/kg) and romifidine (0.02–0.08 mg/kg) are commonly administered.
  - The dose administered is based on the patient's anesthetic depth at the time of arrival in recovery.
  - If the patient seems quite deep, then only a small dose may be given, whereas if the patient already has rapid nystagmus, spontaneous movement or other indication of a very light plane of anesthesia, then a larger dose may be given.
- A small amount of acepromazine (1–3 mg total dose per adult horse) can be used based on health status and demeanor of the patient.
- Opioids are commonly administered at the recovery period in patients that underwent painful surgical procedures. This has been shown to improve the quality of recovery in addition to providing analgesia during the recovery period.

9.5   COMPLICATIONS

9.5.1 Airway Obstruction
- Airway obstruction can occur in the recovery period.

- Most commonly due to edema in the nasal cavity preventing nasal breathing after extubation.
- Other causes include blood clots or foreign bodies obstructing the airway.
- Phenylephrine (**Figure 9.10**) can be administered intranasally prior to recovery in order to reduce any nasal edema.
  - The dose used is 15 mg of phenylephrine per adult horse diluted in 10 ml of 0.9% normal saline. Half of this volume (5 ml) is administered per each nostril using a canula.
- Further precaution can be taken by placing nasopharyngeal tubes to maintain a patent upper airway throughout recovery.
- If the anesthetist is concerned about airway obstruction, an orotracheal tube can be maintained throughout recovery in order to ensure a patent airway.

- The tube is generally secured to the patient's mandible with tape.
- Any time that there is a possibility of airway obstruction, the anesthetist should have a tracheostomy kit available in order to facilitate provision of an emergency airway.

9.5.2 Myopathy

- Compromised oxygen delivery to the equine musculature during anesthesia can result in myopathy (**Figure 9.11**).
- Myopathy is more likely to occur in patients that:
  - Suffered from hypotension during the anesthetic event.
  - Underwent a prolonged anesthesia event.
  - Are not adequately padded.
  - Are incorrectly positioned.
  - Are very large (i.e. draft horses).
- Clinical signs of myopathy:
  - Difficulty standing in recovery.
  - Swollen firm muscle mass, generally on the dependent side.
  - Patients generally appear painful.
  - Red/brown urine due to myoglobinuria.

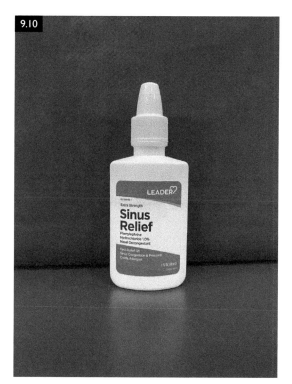

Figure 9.10 Intranasal phenylephrine

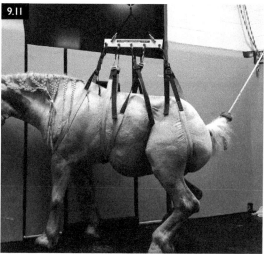

Figure 9.11 Myopathy

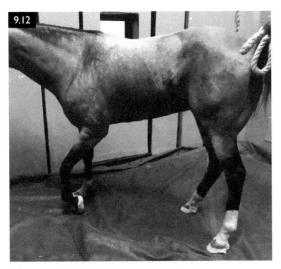

Figure 9.12 **Radial nerve paralysis**

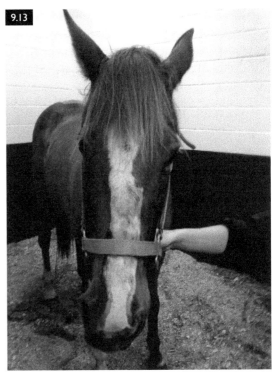

Figure 9.13 **Facial nerve paralysis**
Courtesy of Dr. Kelsey Hart

- Myoglobin will be released from damaged myocytes and eliminated via the kidneys.
- Large amounts of myoglobin can result in acute renal failure.
- Diagnostics:
  - Patients with myopathy will have an increased creatine kinase (CK).
  - A normal CK will rule out myopathy.
- Therapy:
  - NSAIDs for pain (flunixin meglumine, phenylbutazone).
  - Intravenous fluids to support clearance of the myoglobin and renal function.

9.5.3 Neuropathy
- Damage to nerves can occur in equine patients under anesthesia.
- Similar to myopathy, this is more likely to occur in patients that suffered from hypotension, underwent a prolonged anesthesia, were not adequately padded, were incorrectly positioned or are very large.
- The radial nerve (**Figure 9.12**) and facial nerve (**Figure 9.13**) are most commonly affected.

- The radial nerve can often be protected from injury by properly padding the equine patient and pulling the dependent forelimb forward in order to relieve direct pressure over the dependent radial nerve.
- The facial nerve should be carefully padded to avoid compression.
  - Halters should be removed, and the space beneath the horse's head should be free of firm objects.

9.5.4 Catastrophic Injury
- One of the leading causes of anesthetic-associated mortality in horses is catastrophic injury in recovery.
- Fractures and dislocations are often a death sentence to the equine patient (**Figure 9.14**).
- Older mares that may suffer from osteoporosis and patients that already are

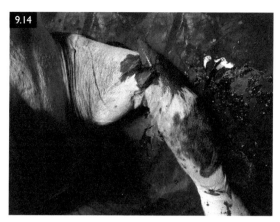

Figure 9.14 **Horse with fracture**
Courtesy of Dr. Valerie Moorman

suffering from myopathy or neuropathy are at increased risk for fracture in recovery.
- In the event that a patient does suffer catastrophic injury in recovery, the patient should be quickly re-anesthetized to provide analgesia and prevent further injury.
- Once anesthetized, it is safe to investigate the extent of the injury and contact the owner to determine their wishes.

9.6 RECOVERY TIMELINE

9.6.1 Preanesthesia
- Assess patient.
  - Temperament, signalment, American Society of Anesthesiologists (ASA) status.
- Designate recovery area.
  - Clean, dry footing.
  - Adequate space.
  - Sufficient lighting.
- Assemble recovery essentials.
  - Well-maintained, sturdy halter, with appropriate padding.
  - Towels.
  - Ropes.
  - Oro-/nasotracheal tube.
  - White tape/elasticon.
  - Needles, syringes, flush.

- Specific recovery items (i.e. slings, rafts, etc.).
- Cuff syringe (oro/nasotracheal tube).
- Oxygen and lines (if available).
- Tracheostomy kit (if indicated).
  - Scalpel #10/15 blade, disposable or with #3 blade handle.
  - Kelly hemostat.
  - 2% lidocaine.
  - Syringes/needles.
  - Sterile 4x4 gauze.
  - Self-retaining tracheostomy tube(s) of appropriate size.
- Calculate recovery and emergency drug doses.
- Assemble recovery and emergency drugs.
- Evaluate patient's feet and shoes.
  - Remove shoes if necessary (poorly fitting/ loose, caulks, heel/toe grabs, MRI).
  - Cover shoes/feet if warranted (shoes left on, slippery surface, poor hoof condition).
- Position mattresses/other supplies for easy use.
- Plan for recovery emergencies:
  - Tracheostomy.
  - Traumatic event.
  - Immediate re-induction of anesthesia.

9.6.2 During Anesthesia
- Avoid prolonged hypotension.
- Ensure the horse is positioned appropriately and the table/surface is well-padded.
- Discontinue lidocaine and other drugs in a timely manner to allow time for washout prior to recovery (see chapter 6).
- Discontinue ventilation when appropriate to encourage self-ventilation once in recovery stall.
- Ensure sufficient anesthetic depth at the end of the procedure to allow the patient to be safely moved to the recovery area (if necessary).
- If possible, place a urinary catheter and maintain it in place until the horse is in

recovery. Horses under general anesthesia receive alpha-2 agonist drugs (which increase urine production) and IV fluids. A full bladder may cause discomfort during recovery and, once standing, the horse may urinate in the recovery stall, making the floor wet and potentially slippery.
- Ensure the recovery area is set up.

9.6.3 Entering the Recovery Area Immediately after the Procedure
- Evaluate patient status, including anesthetic depth, and communicate with team members to ensure safety.
- Ensure patent airway with sufficient airflow.
  - Secure oro-/nasotracheal tube if being left in place.
- If necessary, supply oxygen via demand valve. Do not over-ventilate patient, as this may delay the return of spontaneous ventilation.
- Monitor position of dependent eye.
- Apply elastic tape to hooves/shoes if desired.
- Ensure down thoracic limb is pulled forward to minimize risk of neuropraxia.
- Place halter with padding.
- Apply head and tail ropes (if being used).
- Administer recovery drugs (see 9.4 "Recovery drugs").

9.6.4 Recovery
- Monitor patient, especially respiratory system.
  - Make sure the horse is breathing regularly.
  - Check the color of mucous membranes.
    - Pulling the tongue out to the non-dependent side of the mouth will allow the anesthetist to monitor the color of the mucous membranes from a distance.
  - If there are concerns about the respiratory pattern or color of mucous membranes, provide ventilatory and oxygen support.

- Use demand valve if the endotracheal tube is still in place. If the animal is not breathing, reintubate and use the demand valve.
- If the color of mucous membranes suggests hypoxia, provide oxygen support. This can be done using an oxygen line attached to a flowmeter and inserted in one nostril or into the endotracheal tube if the animal is still intubated. Oxygen flow should be set at 15 l/min in adult horses.
- Keep recording all the events during this time:
  - Drugs administered.
  - Spontaneous ventilation.
  - Nystagmus (start and end).
  - First movement.
  - Change from lateral to sternal recumbency.
  - Change from sternal recumbency to standing.
  - Complications, if any.
- Monitor anesthetic emergence, and be ready to address concerns if necessary.
- Remain safe and make sure all personnel involved are in a safe place in case of an emergency.

9.6.5 Once Standing
- Assess patient status.
- Provide support with ropes, if used, or by holding the halter.
- Remove tail rope (may cause patient discomfort).
- Assign a score to the recovery.
  - Unfortunately, there is not a universal score system for equine recovery, which can be quite subjective. However, it is recommended that the veterinarian or the institution chooses one scale and uses the same scale for each case (**Table 9.1**).
  - Using a score system will maintain a record of recovery events and can help decide for a different approach (i.e.

Table 9.1 Example of adult equine recovery score

SCORE	DESCRIPTION
1	Excellent. The horse stood at the first attempt with no complications or struggle. No to minimal ataxia after standing.
2	Good. The horse stood at the second attempt without complications. Some struggle noticed. Mild ataxia after standing.
3	Fair. Less than 4 attempts were made before standing. Minor complications were observed without real danger. Mild to moderate ataxia after standing.
4	Poor. Rough recovery with struggle (pedaling, rolling from side to side) and several uncoordinated attempts (more than 4). Potential danger of injury (i.e. fractures). The horse may not be able to stand. If standing, moderate to severe ataxia.
1 R	Excellent with ropes. The horse stood at the first attempt with no complications or struggle. No to minimal ataxia after standing.
2 R	Good with ropes. The horse stood at the second attempt without complications. Some struggle noticed. Mild ataxia after standing.
3 R	Fair with ropes. Less than 4 attempts were made before standing. Minor complications were observed without real danger. Mild to moderate ataxia after standing.
4 R	Poor with ropes. Rough recovery with struggle (pedaling, rolling from side to side) and several uncoordinated attempts (more than 4). Potential danger of injury (i.e. fractures). The horse may not be able to stand. If standing, moderate to severe ataxia.

ropes versus no ropes, different drugs in recovery) if the same horse needs to be anesthetized and did not have a good recovery the first time.

FURTHER READING

Bettschart-Wolfensberger R (2015) Horses. In: *Veterinary Anesthesia and Analgesia: The Fifth Edition of Lumb and Jones*, 5th edn. (eds Grimm KA, Lamont LA, Tranquilli WJ et al), Wiley Blackwell, Ames, pp. 857–866.

Driessen B (2006) Assisted recovery. In: *Manual of Equine Anesthesia & Analgesia* (eds Doherty T, Valverde A) Blackwell Publishing, Ames, pp. 338–351.

Elmas CR, Cruz AM, Kerr C (2007) Tilt table recovery of horses after orthopedic surgery: Fifty four cases (1994–2005). *Vet Surg* **36**:252–258.

Hubbell JAE, Muir WW (2009) Considerations for induction, maintenance and recovery. In: *Equine Anesthesia Monitoring and Emergency Therapy*, 2nd edn. (eds Muir WW, Hubbell JAE), Saunders Elsevier, St. Louis, pp. 381–396.

Lukasik VM, Gleed RD, Scarlett JM et al (1997) Intranasal phenylephrine reduces post anesthetic upper airway obstruction in horses. *Equine Vet J* **29**:236–238.

Sullivan EK, Klein LV, Richardson DW et al (2002) Use of a pool-raft system for recovery of horses from general anesthesia: 393 horses (1984–2000). *J Am Vet Med Assoc* **221**:1014–1018.

CHAPTER 10

COMPLICATIONS OF EQUINE ANESTHESIA

Ann Weil

10.1 INTRODUCTION

Complications develop commonly in anesthesia of equine patients. These complications can begin prior to initiation of the anesthetic episode and extend into the post-anesthetic period. Complications can be mild, moderate, or severe, even resulting in death of the patient. Prevention and rapid management of these complications will reduce the incidence of poor outcomes.

10.2 PRIOR TO ANESTHESIA

10.2.1 Hypovolemia

- Horses should not be deprived of water prior to general anesthesia. Equine patients should be assessed for adequacy of hydration prior to administering general anesthetics. Horses at risk for hypovolemia include:
  - Those presenting with signs of colic.
  - Animals who have exercised heavily prior to anesthesia (traumatic injury).
  - Mares with dystocia.
  - Horses with traumatic blood loss.
- Every effort should be made to restore fluid losses prior to anesthetizing the horse.
- Rapid rehydration is necessary when horses are painful and in need of colic surgery.
- Caution should be used with sedative/analgesic drugs when hypovolemia is present.
- Fluid choices include (see Chapter 8):
  - Isotonic-balanced crystalloid solutions in large volumes.
  - Hypertonic saline in conjunction with isotonic solutions.
  - Colloids.
  - Blood products if hemorrhage has occurred.
- Performing necessary fluid resuscitation prior to general anesthesia will help offset the detrimental cardiovascular effects of the anesthetic drugs.
- Complete fluid resuscitation may not be possible before it is necessary to induce the horse, depending on the emergent nature of the situation.

10.2.2 Electrolyte Imbalance

- Most common electrolyte imbalances in horses presented for general anesthesia include:
  - Hypokalemia.
    - May be common in horses with colic presented for anesthesia and surgery.
    - Caution must be used if potassium-supplemented fluids are used during general anesthesia due to the risk of administering too much potassium too quickly if rapid bolus administration of fluids occurs.
    - Normal serum concentration ranges depend on the laboratory reference values used, but an example would be 3.3–4.3 mmol/l (mEq/l).
  - Hyperkalemia.
    - Serum potassium should be checked if there is any indication of hyperthermia or elevated CO_2 in the anesthetized horse, as it may be a sign of increased

DOI: 10.1201/9780429190940-10

metabolism as a result of a genetic muscle disorder.

- Foals with a ruptured urinary bladder may also have hyperkalemia.
- Hyperkalemia is a life-threatening disorder, especially in the context of general anesthesia, and should be addressed immediately.
- Every effort should be made to lower serum potassium to as normal a level as possible prior to general anesthesia.
- ECG signs of hyperkalemia include:
  - Bradycardia.
  - Peaked T waves.
  - Small or missing P waves.
  - Widened QRS complexes.
  - Prolonged P-R intervals.
- Treatment of hyperkalemia includes:
  - 0.9 % NaCl at 5–20 ml/kg/hour IV.
  - 5% dextrose at 5 ml/kg/hour IV.
  - 23% calcium gluconate (**Figure 10.1**) in 5% dextrose, 0.2–0.4 ml/kg IV.
    - Alternatively, administer IV 0.2 mg/kg calcium chloride or 100–200 mg/kg calcium borogluconate.
  - Regular insulin at 0.05–0.1 IU/kg.
  - Control of CO_2. Hypercapnia should be eliminated and the mechanical ventilator set to normalize CO_2 levels if possible.
  - If pH is less than 7.2, consider $NaHCO_3$ at 1–2 mEq/kg IV over 15 minutes.
- Hypocalcemia.
  - Hypocalcemia is common in horses presented for emergency abdominal surgery. Ionized calcium can be measured quickly with the point-of-care monitors in common use (i-STAT, IRMA, EPOC, etc.) (**Figure 10.2**). Reference ranges vary, but normal ionized calcium can range from 1.45–1.75 mmol/l (~50% of

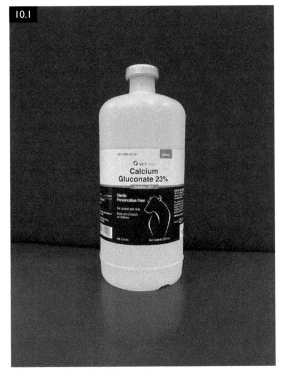

Figure 10.1   Calcium gluconate

total calcium). Ionized calcium will also depend on the serum albumin concentration.

- Hypocalcemia can be associated with reduced cardiac output in the anesthetized horse.
  - Calcium supplementation was very common in horses anesthetized with halothane, due to its pronounced cardiovascular depressant effects.
- Calcium gluconate solution (0.1–0.5 ml/kg) can be added to a 5-liter bag of balanced isotonic crystalloid fluids and given at anesthesia fluid rates.
- Ionized calcium should be rechecked if exogenous calcium is being administered.
- Hypomagnesemia.
  - Also reported in horses with surgical intestinal colic due to ileus, endotoxemia, and sepsis.

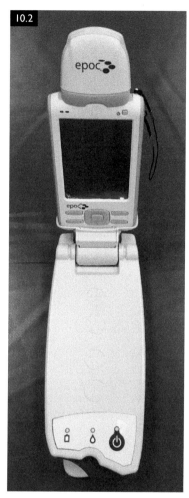

Figure 10.2 Point-of-care monitor (EPOC)

- Like hypocalcemia, hypomagnesemia may contribute to hypotension or cardiac arrhythmias in the anesthetized horse.

10.2.3 Blood Loss
- Anticipate hypovolemia from blood loss if the horse has presented with a laceration.
- Look for mentation changes in horses that have lost blood. Sometimes the owner will not be able to provide historical information that helps estimate the severity of the trauma.
- The ability of the equine spleen to contract may make it difficult to assess blood loss based on the PCV alone. A low total protein may be a clue to hemorrhage.
- PCV should be at least 20% prior to anesthetizing the horse.
- Crystalloid fluids +/- colloid fluids may be used to restore volume status. The ratio of volume replacement is roughly 3:1 (crystalloid fluid volume:blood volume lost).

10.2.4 Shock
- Shock can generally be defined as a lack of oxygenation to tissues. Horses, like other animals, can go into shock when the circulatory system does not meet the body's need for oxygen.
- Some conditions that can incite shock in the horse include:
  - Blood loss from trauma (hypovolemic shock).
  - Pain and infection from colic (septic or toxic shock).
  - Heart failure (cardiogenic shock).
  - Allergic reaction (anaphylactic shock).
  - Dehydration (hypovolemic shock).
  - Trauma to the nervous system, e.g. head trauma (neurogenic shock).
- Most horses have an extraordinary ability to be in severe shock and remain standing. However, some horses in shock will certainly become recumbent.
- Signs of shock in the horse include:
  - Rapid heart rate.
  - Weak pulse.
  - Rapid respiratory rate.
  - Pale, tacky mucous membranes.
  - Cool skin and extremities.
  - Ataxia.
- Any horse suffering from signs of shock will most certainly require significant intravenous fluid therapy treatment (except for cardiogenic shock) as well as treatment for the inciting cause of the shock.
- General anesthesia should be avoided if possible until the animal can be stabilized.

10.2.5 Severe Lameness

- Horses that are very lame (ambulating primarily on three legs) are at risk during the induction process as they may not be able to handle the ataxia produced by preanesthetic doses of alpha-2 agents.
- Most horses do not become recumbent with high doses of xylazine or detomidine, but a severely lame horse may fall before the onset of anesthetic unconsciousness.
- It is helpful to have the animal positioned in the induction area prior to sedative administration if possible. Every effort should be made to induce the animal smoothly and quickly once signs of ataxia are observed.

10.2.6 Failure to Sedate

- One good adage to live by when anesthetizing horses is "Never induce an unsedated horse."
- An intravenous catheter is almost always a good idea to avoid an inadvertent perivascular injection and subsequent failure to induce anesthesia.
- Always check the catheter for patency (and ability to aspirate blood) prior to use for anesthesia.
- Excited horses may be more difficult to sedate with "normal" doses of pre-anesthetic sedatives.
- Temperament and athletic condition of the horse should be taken into account when selecting preanesthetic sedatives and doses.
- Stallions are not necessarily difficult to sedate.

10.2.7 Intra-Arterial Injections

- Inadvertent intra-arterial injections are not uncommon in sedating horses.
- Every effort should be made to determine that the needle or catheter is in the jugular vein, not the carotid artery.
- Signs of arterial sticks include bright red blood color and arterial spurting of blood from the needle or catheter.

- A needle of sufficient diameter (18–20 gauge) to show arterial spurting should be used.
- Xylazine is one of the more frequent medications accidentally administered in this manner.
- Horses will appear to "drop off the needle" and often flip over backwards, potentially striking their head.
- Seizures may be the result of an intra-arterial injection.
- If seizures occur, intravenous diazepam (0.05–0.1 mg/kg IV) should be given once it is safe for personnel to approach the horse.
- Once the horse is recumbent, supportive care may be necessary. If the horse is breathing and has a steady heart rate, it is this author's opinion that the horse should be allowed to remain recumbent until it is ready to stand on its own. This usually takes between 30 and 60 minutes.

10.2.8 Catheter Management

- Always check the catheter by aspirating blood prior to anesthesia to ensure catheter patency.
- Catheters that are questionable in terms of patency should be replaced prior to use.
- It is important to check that all injection caps and extension fastenings are tight so that air aspiration cannot occur.
- If a horse is found with an open jugular catheter, air aspiration may have occurred. Auscultate the heart for the presence of air, which may sound turbulent.
- Other signs of air embolism include:
  - Collapse/seizure.
  - Anxiety.
  - Malaise.
  - Tachycardia.
  - Tachypnea.
  - Muscle fasciculations.
  - Agitation with abnormal behavior including kicking and flank biting.
  - Cyanosis.

10.2.9 Inability to Intubate

- Most horses are intubated blindly (the larynx is not visible). Pulling the tongue forward and ensuring that the endotracheal tube is not caught against the edges of the teeth will help the process.
- In an adult horse that is anesthetized and recumbent, it is difficult to place the endotracheal tube inadvertently into the esophagus. Most of the time it will go into the trachea or nowhere. Regardless, placement of the tube into the trachea should be ascertained by feeling breath expiring through the tube or using a capnometer.
- In contrast to the adult horse, it is very easy to place an endotracheal tube in the esophagus of a foal. The anesthetist must take care to make sure that the animal is appropriately intubated.
- Horses with recurrent laryngeal nerve paralysis may be more difficult to intubate blindly. A smaller diameter endotracheal tube may be helpful during this time. A smaller tube such as a stomach tube may be used as a stylet to facilitate placement of the endotracheal tube (**Figure 10.3**).

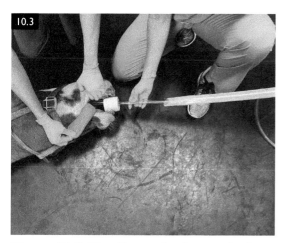

Figure 10.3 Use of stomach tube as stylet for endotracheal intubation

- An endoscope may be very helpful to assist with intubation in horses that are difficult to blindly intubate (**Figure 10.4**).
- Many horses that are anesthetized for colic surgery may become significantly bloated as soon as they are induced to anesthesia and recumbent. Intubation must be accomplished quickly so that assisted ventilation can begin.
- If a stomach tube is desired, it should be placed while the horse is still standing. It is relatively difficult to place a stomach tube in an anesthetized, recumbent horse.

10.3   DURING ANESTHESIA

10.3.1 Respiratory Complications

- Hypoventilation
  - Hypoventilation is a very common consequence of general anesthesia. Every patient that is anesthetized is likely to experience respiratory depression as a normal sequelae to the anesthesia process. The anesthetized central nervous system may not respond to higher blood levels of carbon dioxide as well as the non-anesthetized brain. General anesthesia will also negatively affect respiratory muscle function.
- $PaCO_2$ between 35 and 45 mmHg is considered to be "normal."
- All injectable and inhalant anesthetics cause hypoventilation and a resultant increase in $PaCO_2$.
- Adjunctive drugs like xylazine or butorphanol will contribute to respiratory depression.
- It is common to see a reduced size of breath and reduced respiratory rate in the spontaneously breathing anesthetized horse.
- Horses anesthetized with ketamine will exhibit an apneustic or breath-holding respiratory pattern.

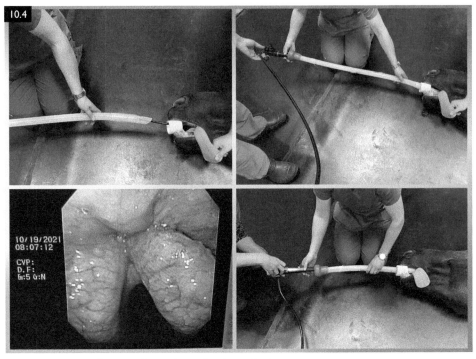

Figure 10.4 **Use of endoscope for endotracheal intubation**

- The large body mass of adult horses also contributes to respiratory depression as functional residual capacity is reduced with general anesthesia and recumbency.
- Atelectasis of the dependent lung occurs over time. This contributes to impaired gas exchange.
- Dorsal recumbency tends to have the most negative effect on respiratory function.
- Abdominal enlargement can greatly compromise ventilation in the horse. Fasting improves the ability of the horse to ventilate as abdominal fill is smaller, thus reducing the abdominal pressure against the diaphragm.
- The horse is an obligate nasal breather, and recumbency increases the work of breathing in the anesthetized horse.
- Intubating horses, regardless of whether they will be maintained on inhalant anesthetic, may help reduce the work of breathing.
- Mechanical ventilation can improve the respiratory function in the anesthetized horse.
- It is this author's preference to initiate mechanical ventilation at the start of the anesthetic procedure, especially if the horse is in dorsal recumbency.
- Some permissive hypercarbia may be desirable in the anesthetized horse. $PaCO_2$ of 60 mmHg helps improve cardiac function, increasing cardiac output and improving blood pressure.
- Excessive hypercarbia may be a sign of increased and aberrant muscle metabolism or a problem with the anesthetic equipment that allows rebreathing of CO_2. Very elevated $PaCO_2$ levels contribute to arrhythmia, narcosis, and myocardial depression leading to death.

- Machine or equipment problems that may show up as hypercarbia include:
  - One-way valve stuck in the open position (usually due to excessive moisture within the machine).
  - Exhausted chemical CO_2 absorbent. The chemical absorbent should be evaluated by the anesthesia provider at the start of every anesthetic episode.
  - Capnography can be very helpful in showing an inspiratory baseline of CO_2, indicative of rebreathing CO_2. The inspiratory baseline should be zero.
- Mechanical ventilator settings:
  - 7–8 breaths/minute is helpful to get an adequate minute volume in the anesthetized adult horse.
  - Tidal volume should be approximately 10 ml/kg.
  - Peak airway pressure should be 20 cmH_2O or less ideally, but many patients in dorsal recumbency undergoing abdominal surgery may require a higher airway pressure than that. Many horses presented for colic surgery will have significant abdominal distension upon being anesthetized and recumbent. Time is of the essence to get the abdomen open and help relieve abdominal pressure so that an appropriate amount of tidal volume can be delivered without excessive airway pressure.
- Hypoxemia
  - $PaO_2 < 60$ mmHg is considered to be severe hypoxemia and a cause for concern in the anesthetized horse.
  - Low arterial oxygen tension is more common in the anesthetized horse than in any other commonly anesthetized domestic species.
  - When hypoxemia is identified (via pulse oximetry or by blood gas analysis), it is helpful to consider the 5 classic causes of hypoxemia:
    - Hypoventilation.
    - Decreased FiO_2.
    - Ventilation/perfusion (V/Q) mismatch.
    - Barriers to diffusion.
    - Right to left shunting (physiologic and anatomic).
  - Hypoventilation (hypercarbia) can be improved by the use of mechanical ventilation.
  - Decreased FiO_2 may be produced by:
    - Oxygen source failure.
    - Too low an oxygen flow rate.
    - Occluded or kinked endotracheal tube.
  - Ventilation/perfusion mismatch occurs frequently in the adult horse:
    - Gas exchange requires the close proximity of blood from pulmonary circulation and air from ventilation in the lung.
    - Lung pathology as well as general anesthesia can alter both ventilation and circulation through the lung.
    - Ideal ventilation/perfusion ratio is approximately 0.8.
  - Right to left shunt (venous admixture).
    - Physiologic.
      - Can be considered the ultimate V/Q mismatch!
      - Most common when the horse is positioned in dorsal recumbency but may occur in lateral recumbency.
      - Often a result of blood flow to regions of the lung that are not ventilated.
    - Anatomic.
      - Includes congenital cardiac abnormalities, such as ventricular septal defect and patent ductus arteriosus.
  - Barriers to diffusion

- This is a relatively rare problem in the normal anesthetized horse.
- It is not advisable to anesthetize a horse with pneumonia or pleuritis unless absolutely necessary.
- Pulmonary edema may be a result of airway obstruction or stressed recovery experience in the horse.
- Treatment of pulmonary edema in the horse includes oxygen therapy with 100% oxygen via nasal cannula or endotracheal tube and furosemide (1.0 mg/kg IV).
- Heavy alpha-2 agonist administration in an already excited horse may exacerbate potential for pulmonary edema due to an increase in pulmonary vascular pressures.
- Treatment of low oxygen tensions in the anesthetized horse may include:
  - Increased oxygen flow rate if too low a flow is present.
  - Increased ventilation if significant hypercarbia is present.
  - The use of positive end expiratory pressure (PEEP) may be helpful to improve oxygenation in the anesthetized horse (10 cmH$_2$O). This helps reduce the opening pressure needed within the alveoli.
  - Recruitment maneuvers at higher airway pressure may be attempted.
  - Reduced anesthesia duration and a return to sternal recumbency and/or standing as soon as practically possible.
  - Administration of bronchodilating agents:
    - Aminophylline (5–12 mg/kg IV).
    - Isoproterenol (0.1–0.2 mg/kg).
    - Albuterol (2 mcg/kg administered via atomizer via endotracheal tube).
- Horses that are hypoxemic should be administered supplementary oxygen in recovery until it is no longer possible to do so.

- 15 l/min of oxygen flow is necessary to influence oxygen tensions in an adult horse.

10.3.2 Bradycardia

- Bradycardia is defined in the anesthetized horse as heart rate < 25 beats/minute.
- Several of the drugs used in an anesthesia protocol may contribute to bradycardia, especially alpha-2 agents like xylazine or detomidine.
- Some individuals may have particularly high vagal tone with low resting heart rates.
- Hypertension may also cause bradycardia in some individuals.
- When bradycardia is identified:
  - Is dobutamine running? If so, check rate and blood pressure. If blood pressure is high, slow down the infusion.
  - Is the horse hypotensive and bradycardic? This is an indication for anticholinergic therapy. Atropine at 0.01 mg/kg IV is this author's preference due to its rapid onset and short duration of action. It is important to note that it takes only a low dose to influence the heart rate in the horse. Do not administer a small-animal dose to an equine.
  - Epinephrine 5–10 µg/kg IV bolus may also be administered in a horse that has a very low heart rate and hypotension.

10.3.3 Hypotension

- Reliable and accurate blood pressure monitoring is very important in horses that are anesthetized with inhalant anesthetics.
- Arterial catheterization should be considered for monitoring blood pressure in procedures that are anticipated to be greater than 45 minutes.
- The facial artery (**Figure 10.5**), transverse facial artery (**Figure 10.6**), or greater metatarsal artery (**Figure 10.7**) may be easily cannulated to monitor blood pressure.

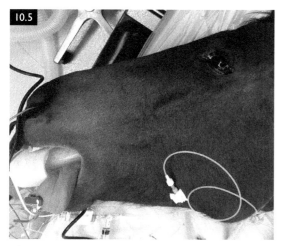

Figure 10.5 Catheter in facial artery

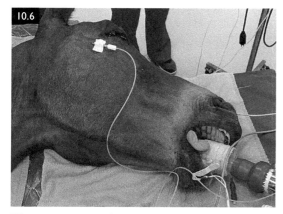

Figure 10.6 Catheter in transverse facial artery

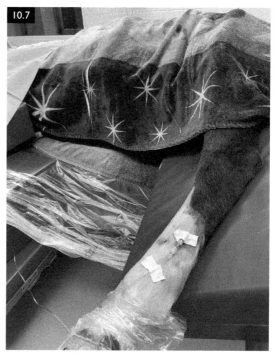

Figure 10.7 Catheter in great metatarsal artery

It is also convenient to have an arterial catheter in place for blood gas sampling.

- Indirect blood pressure monitoring can be used for short duration procedures.
- Horses that are anesthetized with injectable anesthetics are not as likely to be hypotensive due to the vasoconstriction produced by alpha-2 agents and the increased cardiac output produced by dissociative anesthetics.
- Inhaled anesthetics reduce blood pressure by:
  - Reduction in cardiac output.
  - Vasodilation.
- Modern inhaled anesthetics like isoflurane, sevoflurane, and desflurane have less impact on cardiac output than halothane (see Chapter 6). They are, however, very potent vasodilators.
- There are two factors known to impact the likelihood of postanesthetic myopathy (a potentially life-threatening complication of general anesthesia) in the horse:
  - Hypotension.
  - Duration of general anesthesia.
- Every effort should be taken to ensure that arterial blood pressure is preserved throughout the anesthetic process. It is this author's opinion that hypotension should be corrected as soon as it is identified, rather than waiting for vasoconstriction from surgical pain and stimulation to raise the measured pressures.
- Mean arterial blood pressure (MAP) is the best estimate of tissue perfusion pressure.

- MAP should be maintained greater than 70 mmHg in the anesthetized horse.
- The anesthetist may be in the uncomfortable position of having a very light horse in terms of anesthetic depth with significant hypotension. It is incumbent on the anesthetist to improve blood pressure without further reducing anesthetic depth.
- Methods of correcting hypotension include:
  - Improving peripheral vascular volume.
    - Use of 10 ml/kg/hour crystalloid fluids.
    - Inclusion of colloids (Vetstarch) or plasma if necessary.
  - Reducing anesthetic depth if possible.
    - Lower vaporizer settings can greatly improve blood pressure.
    - Use of anesthetic-sparing drugs like alpha-2 agonists can have an inhalant-sparing effect.
  - Use of positive inotropes (increase contractility).
    - Horses have more reduction in cardiac output under equipotent anesthetic levels than other common domestic species. In other words, their cardiac output is affected more by inhalant anesthetics, and it is common to require inotropic support while undergoing anesthesia.
    - Dobutamine, a synthetic catecholamine, is a common choice to increase contractility, thus increasing stroke volume and cardiac output with a resultant rise in blood pressure. Dobutamine is often administered "to effect" or about 1–5 µg/kg/min.
    - Horses are typically more "sensitive" to both endogenous and exogenously administered sympathomimetic drugs. When dobutamine is administered at appropriate rates, it is typical to see a reduction in heart rate in the anesthetized horse. This occurs because dobutamine has more inotropic effect than chronotropic effect at the β-1 receptor. The horse's baroreceptors will sense the rise in blood pressure, and the parasympathetic nervous system (via a vagally mediated reflex) will slow the heart rate. Slowing the dobutamine infusion rate should be done if significant bradycardia occurs.
    - If the horse becomes significantly tachycardic (high heart rate), then the dobutamine infusion should be slowed or stopped.
    - Horses that are volume-depleted will not have a beneficial response to dobutamine therapy, as they will not be able to increase the stroke volume as contractility increases. Hypovolemia must be corrected in order for inotropic therapy to have its maximum effect.
    - Dopamine, a naturally occurring catecholamine, is another option for inotropy.
  - Vasopressor therapy.
    - Vasopressor therapy is warranted when the initial steps to control hypotension have been unsuccessful.
    - Sympathomimetic drugs include phenylephrine, ephedrine, vasopressin, and norepinephrine (**Table 10.1**).
    - Most are administered as a constant rate infusion, but ephedrine may be given as a bolus.
    - Blood pressure and heart rate must be monitored carefully when these drugs are given. They are best "titrated" to a desired end-point, such as MAP greater than 70 mmHg. Heart rate may go down as these drugs are given.
    - Mucous membranes may become pale as these drugs are administered.

Table 10.1 **Inotropic and vasoactive agents used for support of blood pressure in anesthetized horses**

AGENT	DOSE	MECHANISM OF ACTION	COMMENTS
Dobutamine	0.5–5 µg/kg/min	Beta receptor agonism.	Most commonly used inotrope in horses.
Dopamine	1–5 µg/kg/min	Alpha and beta receptor agonism.	
Ephedrine	0.03–0.06 mg/kg	Alpha and beta receptor agonism.	Longer duration of action (20–30 min); tachyphylaxis may develop with repeated dosing.
Norepinephrine	0.1–1 µg/kg/min	Alpha and beta receptor agonism.	Useful in refractory hypotension.
Phenylephrine	0.5–1 µg/kg/min	Alpha receptor agonism.	Possible reflex bradycardia.
Vasopressin	0.1–1 mU/kg/min	Vasopressin (V1) receptor agonism.	Useful in refractory hypotension, acidemia. Possible reflex bradycardia.

10.3.4 Arrhythmias

- Arrhythmias of ventricular origin are relatively uncommon in the anesthetized horse.
- It is helpful to evaluate an ECG on a horse prior to anesthesia to help identify issues like atrial fibrillation or excessive vagal tone (i.e. bradycardia, second-degree AV block).
- If bradyarrhythmias are present in the horse prior to anesthesia, that may be an indication to reduce the dose of alpha-2 agent used as a premed. Most of the time, the sympathomimetic action of ketamine will produce an increase in heart rate, but not always. Horses with pre-existing bradycardia may be more at risk when anesthetized (see 10.3.2, Bradycardia, for treatment).
- Atrial premature contractions (APCs) (**Figure 10.8**) are arguably the most common arrhythmia seen in the anesthetized horse. They have a pulse wave associated with them, but the following pulse will have a smaller waveform as there is less blood in the ventricle at the time the heart contracts.
- It is important to note and record the presence of APCs as they can be a sign of increased sympathetic tone. Dobutamine infusions may increase the number of APCs,

so if it is possible to slow the rate of infusion and maintain desired blood pressure, consider doing so.
- APCs rarely cause a large drop in blood pressure, and most horses are able to maintain sufficient blood pressure and cardiac output to continue the procedure, although keeping the duration of anesthesia as short as possible is always a good idea.
- Atrial fibrillation is a relatively rare rhythm disturbance (**Figure 10.9**). Horses often are able to maintain adequate blood pressure during the procedure, but it may be prudent to discontinue the anesthesia as quickly as is feasible.
- Treatment of atrial fibrillation includes:
  - Lidocaine: 2 mg/kg IV bolus, 50 µg/kg/min CRI.
  - Quinidine: 1 mg/kg slow IV (over 10 minutes) repeated up to a total of 4 mg/kg.
  - Electrocardioconversion; more likely to be successful if patient has not been in atrial fibrillation for a long period of time.

10.3.5 Inadequate Depth of Anesthesia

- Dealing with an inadequately anesthetized horse is always problematic.

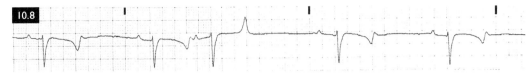

Figure 10.8 Atrial premature complex
Courtesy of Michelle Barton

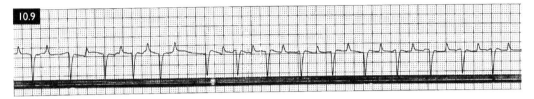

Figure 10.9 Atrial fibrillation
Courtesy of Dr. Michelle Barton

- Small doses of injectable anesthetic (most commonly ketamine) can be used to help reduce movement of the horse.
- Usually 100–300 mg (1–3 ml) of ketamine is sufficient to stop movement, unless the horse is completely awake.
- One should always double check that there is not an equipment issue leading to the problem, such as:
  - Empty inhalant level in the vaporizer.
  - Machine is not properly put together.
  - Inadequate oxygen flow rate is used.
  - Leaks in the circuit or endotracheal cuff.
- If high vaporizer levels and repeated boluses of injectable anesthetic are required to keep a horse "down" for the procedure, a continuous rate infusion of adjunctive drugs may be necessary to produce analgesia and an improvement in anesthetic conditions (see Chapter 6).

10.3.6 Hypothermia
- Many horses will cool down during long duration of anesthesia, especially when a body cavity is open, such as in colic surgery.

- Smaller-sized patients, such as foals, can become significantly hypothermic quite quickly. External heating devices should be used for foals during surgery.
  - Circulating water blankets.
  - Forced air warmers (**Figure 10.10**).
- Prolonged recovery can occur as the horse cannot be adequately rewarmed.
- Blankets and external warming devices should be used in recovery until it is no longer safe to do so.

10.3.7 Hyperthermia
- Horses may experience malignant hyperthermia-type syndromes while undergoing general anesthesia.
- True malignant hyperthermia is a genetic disease that is triggered by stress, inhalants, and succinylcholine.
- Hyperkalemic periodic paralysis (HYPP) is a genetic disease of American Quarter Horses that has some similar signs in the anesthetized horse.
- In either case, a rise in end-tidal CO_2 may appear before a rise in body temperature.
- Signs of hyperthermic reactions may include:

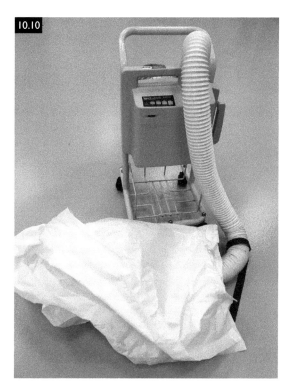

10.10

Figure 10.10 Forced air warming blanket device

- Tachycardia.
- Hypertension.
- Sweating.
- Hard muscles or muscle fasciculations.
- Metabolic and respiratory acidosis.
- Increased serum K.
- Dark-colored urine (myoglobinuria).
- If an individual is identified as having this problem, then symptomatic care needs to be started immediately. This may include:
  - Ending the anesthesia if at all possible.
  - Controlling the end-tidal CO_2.
  - Treatment for hyperkalemia (see 10.2.2, Electrolyte Imbalance).
  - External cooling.
  - Dantrolene (1–2 mg/kg IV) if malignant hyperthermia rather than HYPP is suspected.
  - Many of these horses will have problems with prolonged and weak recovery.

10.4 RECOVERY

- The recovery period is the most difficult period of the anesthesia process to control and have a predictably good outcome.
- Complications during the recovery period are numerous, and the possibility of catastrophic musculoskeletal injury is always present.
- As a general guideline, any horse anesthetized with an injectable anesthetic has less risk of a poor recovery outcome than one anesthetized with inhalant anesthesia. However, some surgeries require a longer duration of anesthesia with control of ventilation and oxygenation, necessitating inhalant anesthesia.
- Care should be taken to avoid excited recoveries and emergence delirium. The use of sedative drugs may be helpful in the recovery period as long as they don't produce excessive ataxia and muscle weakness.
- Most horses will benefit from ventilation and oxygenation assistance in the recovery stall. This can be routinely provided with a demand valve and/or insufflation of 100% oxygen at 15 l/min.
- Occasionally a horse will not wean off the ventilator and resume spontaneous ventilation quickly. It is helpful to supplement 1–2 breaths/min until the horse is breathing on its own. Do not administer alpha-2 agents until the horse has spontaneous ventilation as they depress ventilation. If they are administered in the recovery stall, ventilation must be monitored carefully. Doxapram (0.5 mg/kg, IV) can be given if a demand valve is not available.

10.4.1 Obstructed Airway

- The horse is an obligate nasal breather. When recumbent for any duration of time, the nasal tissues tend to become swollen and edematous.

- Airways may also be obstructed by laryngeal swelling, laryngospasm, and displacement of the soft palate.
- There is a great debate amongst anesthesiologists about whether a horse should be recovered to standing with an oral endotracheal tube in place. Nasal edema is very common in anesthetized horses. Laryngospasm and laryngeal paralysis are relatively uncommon but are an emergency situation if they do occur. If the horse is extubated while still recumbent, then it is somewhat easier to deal with laryngospasm and an obstructed larynx. Signs of an obstructed airway may include:
  - A musical or high-pitched inspiratory sound.
  - Greatly increased respiratory effort.
  - Flaring of nostrils.
  - Increased heart rate.
- Every effort must be made to quickly relieve the obstruction. A nasotracheal tube of sufficient length can be placed so the end of the tube is past the area of obstruction, or a tracheostomy can be performed. These tend to be more difficult if a dyspneic horse is already standing.
- Any horse with nasal edema should have a nasopharyngeal (**Figure 10.11**) or nasotracheal tube placed at the time of oral endotracheal tube extubation to ease the burden of breathing. Oxygen may be insufflated through the tube if needed.
- Phenylephrine may be used in the nasal passage to relieve edema, but a nasopharyngeal/nasotracheal tube is required most of the time.
  - The intranasal phenylephrine dose used is 15 mg of phenylephrine per adult horse diluted in 10 ml of 0.9% normal saline. Half of this volume (5 ml) is administered per each nostril using a canula (**Figure 10.12**).
- Dorsal recumbency tends to produce the most nasal edema, and more nasal edema will be present with increased duration of anesthesia.

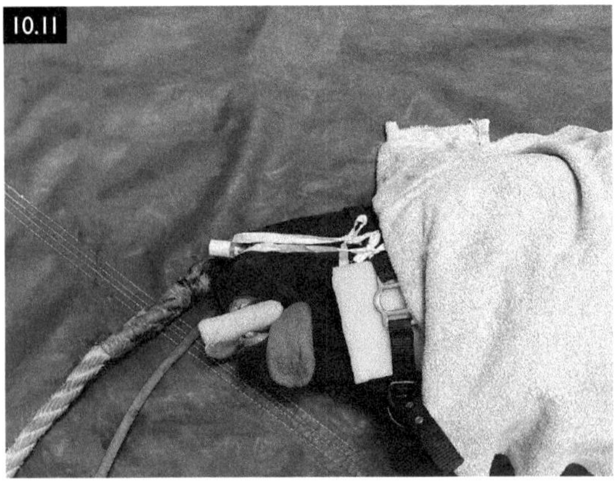

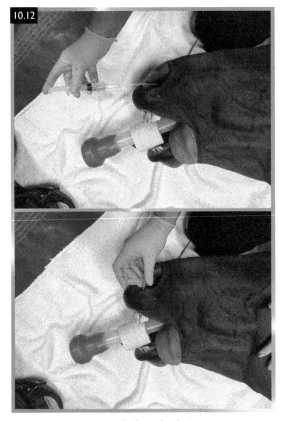

Figure 10.12 Nasal phenylephrine administration

Figure 10.11 Nasopharyngeal tube

- Horses should be able to swallow when extubated. Swallowing enables the horse to replace the position of the epiglottis to its normal relationship with the soft palate. "Bumping" the larynx gently with a nasotracheal tube may elicit a swallow and relieve a displaced palate.

10.4.2 Myositis

- Careful monitoring and attention to detail during the maintenance phase of the anesthetic period will greatly decrease the amount of myositis seen in the recovery stall.
- Every effort should be made to keep anesthesia duration as short as possible. Efficiency is an essential component to excellent equine anesthesia.
- It is this author's opinion that we do not see as much myositis with isoflurane or sevoflurane anesthesia as when we used a lot of halothane. Perhaps the increased vasodilation produced by the more modern inhalant anesthetics assists with improved muscle blood flow.
- Nonetheless, padding is critical to protect muscles from pressure points and damage.
- Meticulous blood pressure management remains a key component to avoiding myositis. Fluids and inotropes should be used to maintain MAP above 70 mmHg.
- Heavy muscled horses and draft breeds should have a MAP above 75–80 mmHg if at all possible.
- Signs of myositis in the recovery stall include:
  - Prolonged recovery.
  - Hard, swollen, and painful muscles.
  - Excited or "rough" recovery.
  - Myoglobinuria.
- Treatment of myositis includes:
  - Fluid administration (balanced isotonic crystalloid).
  - Pain relief (NSAIDs).
  - Sedation if necessary.

10.4.3 Nerve Paralysis

- All the principles of good muscle care apply to the nervous system as well.
- Nerve damage in recovery is often a positioning problem.
- Care should be taken to use padding whenever possible.
- The down forelimb should be pulled forward as much as possible to avoid injury to the brachial plexus.
- The hind limbs should be supported in a neutral position, neither abducted nor adducted.
- Care should be taken to avoid facial nerve damage from halters or hard surfaces.
- The non-dependent limbs are also vulnerable to nerve damage, so care should be taken not to tie them in abnormal positions.
- Nerve damage in the recovery stall is often manifested as a reluctance to stand or prolonged recovery. The animal may require assistance or a splint in order to remain standing. These problems may correct in time, so nerve damage is not always permanent.

10.4.4 Violent Recovery

- The old anesthesiologist's adage is a horse will get up as it goes down; of course, that is not always true.
- However, horses that tend to be excitable and are weak from a long duration of anesthesia may be predicted to be more at risk for difficult recovery than other horses.
- Some anesthesiologists may elect to transition a horse to injectable anesthetic if a difficult recovery is predicted. Others may use a recovery pool or some other method of assisting recovery. Nonetheless, sedation may be necessary to help control emergence delirium.
- It is crucial to avoid excessive noise and stimulation when recovering horses.

10.4.5 Pulmonary Edema

- Pulmonary edema in recovery may result from:
  - Fluid overload during prolonged procedures (relatively uncommon).
  - Obstructed airway.
  - Excessive excitement during recovery.
  - Recovering horses in water.
- Treatment for pulmonary edema consists primarily of:
  - Furosemide (1 mg/kg IV).
  - Oxygen therapy. It can be useful to place a nasotracheal tube in the standing horse, so that high flows of oxygen can be administered without disturbing the horse. Nasopharyngeal tubes can be placed bilaterally and oxygen insufflated on both sides if necessary. 15 l/min O_2 flow can be administered.

FURTHER READING

Muir WW, Hubbell JAE (2008) Anesthetic-associated complications. In: *Equine Anesthesia, Monitoring and Emergency Therapy*, 2nd edn. (eds Muir WW, Hubbell JAE), Saunders Elsevier, St Louis, pp. 397–417.

CHAPTER 11

SPECIFIC DISEASES AND PROCEDURES

Cynthia Trim

11.1 INTRODUCTION

The information in this chapter addresses horses with specific disease conditions that require medical or surgical procedures and provides directions for anesthetic management that may be important to achieve a successful outcome. Where more in-depth, detailed explanations of specific points and anesthetic drug combinations are needed, the reader is directed to look elsewhere in this book or to the suggested further reading.

This chapter is organized according to body areas: head and neck, thorax, abdomen, and limbs. Within these sections, the conditions are titled alphabetically (**Table 11.1**).

11.2 OVERVIEW OF STANDING SEDATION, INTRAVENOUS ANESTHESIA, INHALATION ANESTHESIA

- Many procedures can be performed on horses that are sedated but standing. The feasibility of this approach depends on the temperament of the animal, the environment, the drugs and personnel available, and the anatomical location of the procedure.
  - Sudden, unexpected movements of the horse may result in damage to nearby equipment and people or may compromise the success of the procedure.
  - Nonetheless, standing sedation is frequently employed for such procedures

as diagnostic imaging and endoscopy, ophthalmologic procedures, dental surgery, castration, and laparoscopy, to name a few. Short-duration procedures may be accomplished after administration of a combination of agents, with one or two supplemental injections (see Chapter 3).
- Intravenous continuous rate infusion (CRI) of agent(s) will provide more consistent sedation for longer-duration procedures of 2–3 hours. Furthermore, the addition of local analgesia is preferable whenever applicable to the procedure.
- General anesthesia, whether provided by injectable agents or an inhalation agent, has the inherent risks of injury or mortality for the animal, requiring the veterinarian to obtain specific training.
  - The essentials of monitoring equipment, oxygen supply, and an anesthetic delivery system substantially increase the cost of this approach over sedation alone. However, general anesthesia may be advisable or necessary for some animals and some procedures.
- The preanesthetic evaluation, comprising assessment of health status, behavior, available facilities, and clinical aims, is used when planning anesthetic management.
- Routine general management, such as washing out the mouth before anesthesia, combinations of anesthetic agents, and precautions for recovery, has been covered in previous chapters and may not be mentioned for all conditions in this chapter.

DOI: 10.1201/9780429190940-11

Table 11.1 **Chapter organization**

SECTION	PROCEDURES
Head and neck	Cerebrospinal fluid collection
	Ear surgery
	Esophageal obstruction (choke)
	Dentistry
	Guttural pouch disease
	Laryngeal surgery
	Myelography
	Ophthalmology
	Sinuses
Thorax	Diaphragmatic rupture
	Thoroscopy
Abdomen	Colic
	Dystocia and Caesarian hysterotomy
	Laparoscopy
	Ovariectomy
	Urinary bladder rupture in foals
Limbs	Arthroscopy
	Feet
	Orthopedic surgery

11.3   HEAD AND NECK

- Monitoring depth of anesthesia in horses, during inhalation anesthesia in particular, is greatly assisted by observation of the position of the eye and the direction of rotation of the globe within the orbit, character and presence/absence of nystagmus, and the strength of the palpebral reflex. Access to the eye may be limited for some procedures around the head and neck.
- The anesthetist should take every opportunity to see the eye(s) during breaks in the surgical procedure.
- In anticipation of not being able to see the eye, the animal should be taken to the desired plane of anesthesia before the surgical procedure begins.
- Administration of a sedative or analgesic, such as lidocaine, an alpha-2 agonist, or an opioid, as a CRI may avoid large swings in the depth of anesthesia.

- A local anesthesia nerve block should be administered whenever possible. By providing constant analgesia, the animal is less likely to respond to changes in intensity of surgical stimulus.
- In a hospital where the surgical caseload involving general anesthesia is high, strong consideration should be given to the purchase of an anesthetic gas analyzer (**Figure 11.1**). Since the large-animal circle anesthetic concentration is generally very different from the vaporizer setting, monitoring inspiratory and end-tidal isoflurane or sevoflurane concentrations significantly contributes to maintaining a constant depth of anesthesia and avoiding inhalant anesthetic overdose.

11.3.1   Cerebrospinal Fluid (CSF) Collection

- General anesthesia is required for cervical collection of CSF (**Figure 11.2**). Total intravenous anesthesia (TIVA) or inhalation anesthesia may be used whether CSF collection only is required or if other procedures, e.g. diagnostic imaging, will follow.
- When the horse is ataxic, sedatives will increase the severity of ataxia, and the horse may fall over before induction of anesthesia or be unable to stand after anesthesia.
- The horse may react adversely to the increase in ataxia; the response depends on the horse's temperament.
  - One option is to administer a fraction of the calculated premedication drugs, enough to provide mild sedation without exacerbating ataxia, and then to inject the remainder immediately before the induction agents.
- When the horse is already recumbent and unable to stand, induction and recovery will take place in the animal's stall.
- If endotracheal intubation is planned, the horse will have to be propped up with the pharynx higher than the nose to encourage

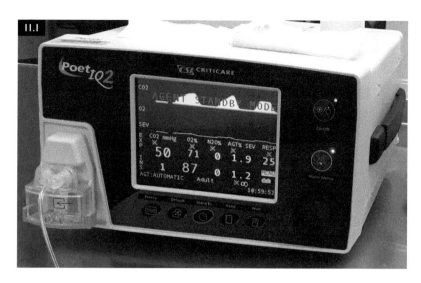

Figure 11.1 Anesthetic gas analyzer

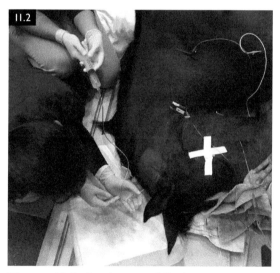

Figure 11.2 Cerebrospinal fluid (CSF) collection

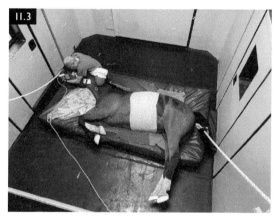

Figure 11.3 Kneeling on a horse's neck in recovery

drainage when flushing the mouth with water to clean it before anesthesia.

- Induction of anesthesia should be routine. TIVA is administered for collection of CSF or for transportation to radiology.
- The anesthetist should have a plan of action for recovery to manage a horse making repeated attempts to rise.
  - Options for recovery from anesthesia could be physical restraint, e.g., kneeling on the horse's neck and holding the head and neck in extension (**Figure 11.3**), or additional administration of sedatives. The floor and walls should be padded and sharp/protruding edges covered to protect the horse and personnel. When a horse can stand before anesthesia but with difficulty, recovery could be facilitated by use of a sling, if available.
- Increased intracranial pressure (ICP) may already be suspected in some animals. In others, an increase in ICP will have an adverse effect on outcome.

- Protocol design should include an alpha-2 agonist sedative (xylazine, detomidine, romifidine) for premedication to help to prevent increased ICP. Thiopental and guaifenesin, if available, will also decrease ICP.
- Lowering the head below heart level will increase ICP, and this should be avoided. The head must be supported level with the spine in a standing animal while sedated or during transportation while anesthetized (**Figure 11.4**).
- Increased arterial carbon dioxide ($PaCO_2$) from hypoventilation will increase ICP.
- Controlled ventilation is advisable to keep $PaCO_2$ within a normal range (approximate mean value 40 mmHg, 5.3 kPa).
- Capnography can be used to monitor adequacy of ventilation, but note that the arterial CO_2 will be approximately 4–6 mmHg (0.5–0.8 kPa) higher than the capnography value when the horse is artificially ventilated. Capnography values may not be reliable estimates of arterial CO_2 during spontaneous breathing because the lungs progressively collapse, creating discrepancies between arterial and alveolar CO_2.

11.3.2 Ear Surgery

- Examination, laser, or cryosurgery procedures.
- The ear is sensitive to manipulation even when the horse is heavily sedated or anesthetized with TIVA.
- Ring block with local anesthetic solution is often unsatisfactory analgesia.
- Proximity to the parotid gland and guttural pouch decreases safety of injections for local anesthesia.
- A recent study in cadaver horses describes a two-injection technique that may be useful for providing local anesthesia of the ear, while avoiding inadvertent injection of the parotid gland that may lead to inflammation (Cerasoli et al. 2017).
  - The great auricular nerve can be located by digital palpation at the cranial edge of the wing of the atlas (**Figure 11.5**). This nerve arises from the second cervical vertebral nerve and passes superficially toward the base of the ear, dividing into a variable number of branches to innervate

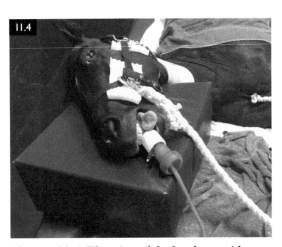

Figure 11.4 Elevation of the head to avoid increased intracranial pressure (ICP)

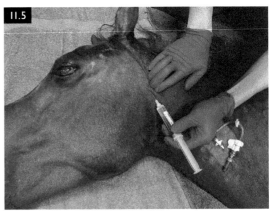

Figure 11.5 Palpation of the great auricular nerve at the cranial edge of the wing of the atlas

both external and internal surfaces of the pinna. This study identified success using dissections and imaging after subcutaneous injection of 2 ml of solution.

- The second injection was made with the pinna facing rostrally. The parotid gland was palpated and a 21-gauge needle was inserted between the parotid gland and the base of the ear, to a depth of about 2 cm (Warmblood breed) and 10 ml of solution injected (**Figure 11.6**).

11.3.3 Esophageal Obstruction (Choke)

- Initially, sedative drugs may be administered to either sedate the horse or relax the esophagus. Then an endotracheal tube is inserted through the ventral nasal meatus and into the trachea (nasotracheal intubation) (**Figure 11.7**). The cuff of the endotracheal tube is inflated to minimize the risk of pulmonary aspiration when the esophagus is lavaged to dislodge the esophageal foreign body.
- In the event that general anesthesia becomes necessary, the animal must be evaluated for presence of fluid aspiration into the lungs and for dehydration as a result of interrupted water intake.

- Adjust drug dosages for anesthesia when there is residual sedation from a standing procedure.
- During lavage in the standing horse, fluid may accumulate in the esophagus proximal to the obstruction. Drain this fluid (lower the horse's head) because remaining fluid may reflux into the pharynx during

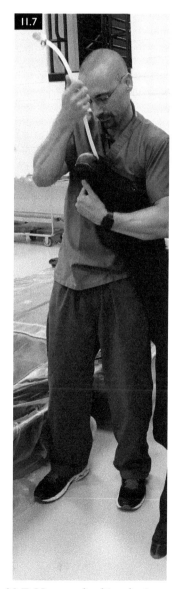

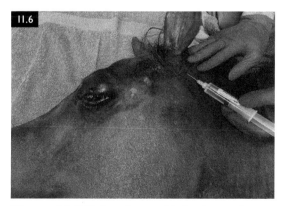

Figure 11.6 Point of second injection at the base of the ear

Figure 11.7 Nasotracheal intubation

induction of anesthesia and be carried into the trachea during oral insertion of the endotracheal tube.

- At the time of induction of anesthesia, consider holding the horse in sternal position with the head up until the endotracheal tube is inserted and the cuff inflated (**Figure 11.8**).
- When the horse is under general anesthesia, the animal's neck, and particularly the area of the obstruction, should be positioned higher than the head so that fluid and debris freely drain.
- Nasal congestion may develop when the head is dependent during anesthesia, resulting in airway obstruction after extubation.
- Leave the endotracheal tube in place for recovery from anesthesia (**Figure 11.9**). Position the tube so it exits the mouth at the interdental space, and wrap white porous tape around the tube and around the animal's muzzle or poll to hold the tube in place. Leave the cuff inflated if blood or fluid is in the pharynx or upper part of the trachea. Only remove the tube when the horse is standing, finger palpation of the nasal mucosa cannot

detect swelling, and the horse's head is lowered.

- To detect mucosal edema and swelling:
  - Insert a finger as far as possible into a ventral nasal meatus.
  - Palpate the medial wall of the meatus with your finger.
  - Normal mucosa is closely adhered to the nasal bone.
  - It is abnormal if your finger touches the mucosa and then the tissue must be depressed before the bone can be touched, as if there is a space between the mucosa and the bone.
  - Remember that even though no swelling is detected near the nostril, mucosal congestion can be present at the caudal end of the meatus and obstruct airflow after extubation.
- Maintain continuous observation of the animal with an orotracheal or nasotracheal tube during the entire recovery from anesthesia.
  - Hazards of endotracheal tubes left in place during recovery from anesthesia:
  - The tube can be kinked, limiting or obstructing breathing when:
  - The horse is in sternal position with muzzle resting on the floor.

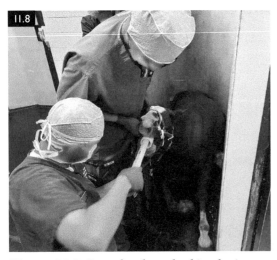

Figure 11.8 Sternal endotracheal intubation

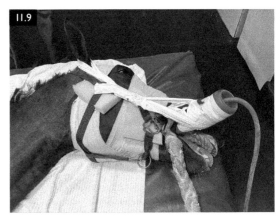

Figure 11.9 Recovery with endotracheal tube in place

- The horse is standing with the muzzle pressed against a padded wall.
- The horse is standing with the head pressing with extreme head/neck flexion.
- Tube is repositioned between clenched incisor teeth.
- The tube can be become obstructed with blood clots.
- Tracheal abrasions can occur from movement of the tube.
- Vasoconstrictor spray, such as phenylephrine 0.15% solution, into the nose may speed elimination of the congestion.
- Occasionally hemorrhage occurs during extraction of an esophageal foreign body. Attempt to remove the clots with a flow of water into the pharynx through a tube inserted through the mouth until the tip is in the pharynx. Leave the orotracheal tube in place during recovery, and remove when the horse is standing, head lowered, and can cough or sneeze out remaining clots.

11.3.4 Dentistry

- Many dental procedures can be completed in the standing sedated horse using local anesthesia nerve blocks (**Figure 11.10**).
- Detomidine is frequently part of the sedation protocol, sometimes as a continuous infusion and often combined with an opioid, such as butorphanol.
- Jerky movements and tremors of the head that interfere with the procedure may be features of sedation induced by single injections of xylazine and butorphanol.
- Nerve blocks provide analgesia and improve surgical conditions (e.g., mental nerve block for the incisors; infraorbital block for the upper canines; maxillary and mandibular nerve blocks for the incisors, premolars, and molars) (see Chapter 12).
- General anesthesia may be necessary for repair of fractures of maxilla or mandible or extraction of molar teeth.
  - Include regional anesthesia block in the anesthetic protocol.
  - Perform endotracheal intubation and inflate the cuff to an airtight seal to avoid

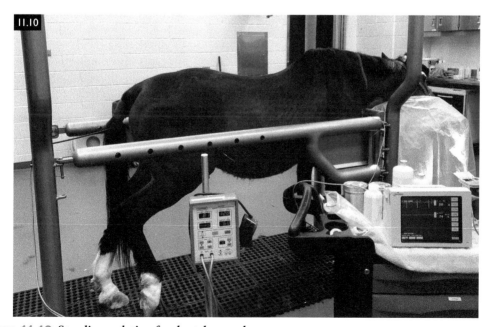

Figure 11.10 Standing sedation for dental procedure

pulmonary aspiration of blood. Risk of aspiration is present even for repair of a fracture close behind the incisors because the surgeon may elevate the nose to assess the repair and alignment, allowing blood to flow from that site into the pharynx.

- Consider nasotracheal intubation or intubation through a tracheotomy for bilateral mandibular fracture repair, which will require complete closure of the mandible during anesthesia to achieve an accurate alignment. Both procedures for intubation can be performed after the horse is anesthetized but before the start of surgery.

- A mouth gag will be needed to hold the jaws apart. Various gag designs are available (**Figure 11.11**). To provide best exposure for the procedure, choice of gag design and position will depend on where in the mouth the procedure is to be performed.

- Position the head with the nose dependent to promote blood draining from the mouth and not into the trachea (**Figure 11.12**).

- Anticipate and prepare to treat moderate or severe hemorrhage (steps also apply to other surgeries, e.g. guttural pouch, ethmoid tumors):
  - A large catheter should be pre-placed in the jugular vein and bags of balanced electrolyte fluid immediately available.
  - Keep a running tab of blood loss. To facilitate accurate measurement, take an empty white bucket and add water liter by liter. Mark the fluid level using a permanent marker pen after each liter, and when full, empty the bucket and add numbers for 5, 10, and 15 L. Place this bucket on the floor under the surgical site.
  - A second and third IV catheters are sometimes essential for rapid fluid infusion. These can be inserted into the other jugular vein (depending on whether the horse is in dorsal or lateral recumbency), into a saphenous vein, into a median vein, and/or into the internal thoracic vein.
  - For cases with a high risk for major blood loss, invasive monitoring of

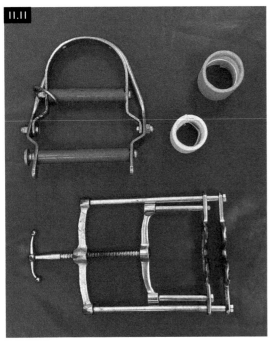

Figure 11.11 Various mouth gags

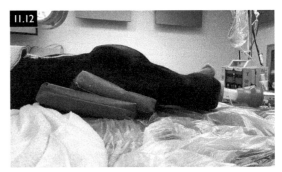

Figure 11.12 Positioning the head with nose dependent to allow drainage out of the mouth during dental procedures

arterial blood pressure is recommended so that failure to keep pace with blood loss can be recognized by decreasing pulse pressure and/or arterial pressure (see Chapters 7 and 10).

- Infuse IV-acetated or lactated Ringer's solution at 2x volume of blood lost up to 20 ml/kg. Add hypertonic 7.5% saline, 2–4 ml/kg, in addition to crystalloid fluid during severe hemorrhage to maintain mean arterial pressure (MAP) > 70 mmHg.

- Airway management for recovery from anesthesia is similar to the description in the section on choke.

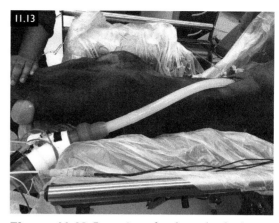

Figure 11.13 Insertion of endotracheal tube through tracheotomy site

11.3.5 Guttural Pouch Disease

- Diseases of the guttural pouch may be diagnosed in the standing animal using radiography, endoscopy, and computerized tomography (CT). Medical management and some surgical procedures can be performed in the standing horse. General anesthesia may be employed for more complex surgeries.

- When distension of the guttural pouch is causing partial airway obstruction and difficulty breathing before anesthesia, decide before anesthesia on the method to obtain a patent airway.

- Performing a tracheotomy in the standing animal under local anesthesia before induction of anesthesia may be advisable. The endotracheal tube can be inserted through the tracheotomy after induction of anesthesia (**Figure 11.13**).

- Alternatively, ensure that a flexible endoscope is available in the induction area to facilitate orotracheal intubation. Check that when the endoscope is inserted inside the endotracheal tube it is long enough to reach the end of the tube and provide an adequate view during insertion.

- Manual manipulation and guiding the endotracheal tube into the larynx (as in

cattle) are rarely possible because of the narrow space of the equine pharynx. An exception may be a large horse and a person with a small hand.

- Depending on the surgical procedure performed, hemorrhage may be a problem.

11.3.6 Laryngeal Surgery

- Intubation may be difficult in a horse with laryngeal paralysis. Consider using an endotracheal tube with an internal diameter (ID) one size smaller than the usual size for that horse, e.g., use a 24 mm ID endotracheal tube for a 450–500 kg horse.

- Pull gently at the time of withdrawal of the endotracheal tube in case the tube has been inadvertently sutured to the larynx.

- Change in body position and intraoperative extubation:
  - Have injectable drugs available to maintain anesthesia after the inhalant is discontinued when the endotracheal tube must be withdrawn for intralaryngeal surgery.
  - If the horse has been in lateral recumbency for the surgery and must be turned to dorsal recumbency for a laryngotomy, maintain inhalation

anesthesia until the surgeon is ready to make a laryngeal incision, briefly disconnecting the endotracheal tube from the circle circuit during repositioning.
- Check for a decrease in MAP after the horse is on its back.
- Deflate the cuff before moving the tube. Attach a 60-ml syringe to the pilot balloon, aspirate air from the cuff, and, leaving the syringe connected to the tube, then inject the same amount of air into the endotracheal cuff for reinflation.
- Reinsertion of the tube for recovery probably will require assistance from the surgeon to guide the tube into the trachea.

11.3.7   Myelography

- Commonly, the animal is anesthetized in a designated induction stall and transported by hoist, cart, or forklift to the radiology room, and the process is reversed for recovery from anesthesia.
- Considerations listed for CSF collection may apply to an animal scheduled for a cervical myelogram for neurologic disease.
- Use mechanical ventilation to maintain $PaCO_2$ within normal limits and avoid increased ICP.

- Administer IV fluid therapy 5–10 ml/kg/h to promote diuresis and excretion of the contrast agent.
- One person should be dedicated to preventing the endotracheal tube from moving within the trachea, monitoring for kinking of the endotracheal tube, and disconnections from the anesthesia and/ or oxygen delivery system when the head and neck are flexed or extended for imaging (**Figure 11.14**).
- The head should be elevated during injection of contrast to encourage caudal flow of contrast agent, decreasing rostral flow that might predispose to seizures.
- An acute decrease in arterial pressure may occur after injection of contrast agent. Decrease anesthetic administration, and deliver an IV fluid challenge of balanced electrolyte 5–10 ml/kg.
- Assisted recovery will probably be necessary since ataxia is likely to be increased after anesthesia.
- Twitches and tremors may develop during recovery and at any time during several hours after anesthesia. Decreasing environmental noise (ear plugs) and administration of a small dose of xylazine (0.1–0.2 mg/kg) intravenously to sedate and to promote contrast elimination may be effective treatment.

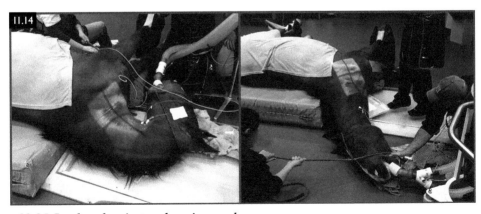

Figure 11.14 Intubated patient undergoing myelogram

11.3.8 Ophthalmology

- Many ophthalmic procedures can be performed in the standing sedated horse with adjunct local nerve blocks.
  - Administer 2% lidocaine for the nerve blocks, and provide topical local anesthesia of the cornea with proparacaine or tetracaine.
  - The auriculopalpebral block will block motor control of the eyelids but provides no analgesia.
  - Blocking the supraorbital, the lacrimal, the infratrochlear, and the zygomatic nerves will desensitize the eyelids.
- General anesthesia must provide immobility of the eyelids or globe, avoid increased intraocular pressure (IOP), for some procedures ensure that the globe is in a central position within the orbit, and analgesia.
  - Note that TIVA with an alpha-2 agonist sedative and ketamine, with or without guaifenesin, is accompanied by varying degrees of nystagmus that may interfere with the surgical procedure.
  - The presence of rapid globe movement during TIVA is a common reason for choosing inhalation anesthesia for ophthalmologic procedures. Nystagmus will be absent, but the eye may slowly rotate during a light-moderate plane of inhalation anesthesia.
  - Blinking can be prevented by an auriculopalpebral nerve block, but this block provides no analgesia.
- Several anesthetic factors impact IOP:
  - IOP is not increased during induction of anesthesia with ketamine in horses if the horse is premedicated with an alpha-2 agonist sedative (xylazine, detomidine, romifidine), which decreases IOP.
  - When the horse is lifted by hoist from the induction stall to an operating table, IOP will be increased if the head is positioned below the level of the horse's heart. Ensure head is held up during transportation (**Figure 11.15**).
  - The head should be elevated above the level of the spine, usually with foam pads or on a table headboard with an elevated angle, when the horse is positioned on the operating table (**Figure 11.16**)
- Hold the animal's head securely during induction of anesthesia when the cornea is fragile, e.g., deep ulcer. If the halter shifts to compress the eye or the head thumps on the ground, the cornea may rupture.
- It is normal for the horse's eye to rotate rostroventrally in the orbit during inhalation anesthesia. The optimal globe position for a keratectomy or conjunctival flap will depend on the location of the surgery.
- A peribulbar nerve block can be performed as a 3 or 4-point injection around the globe (avoiding the medial canthus) to paralyze the extraocular muscles but is generally recommended only for enucleation because of the risk of tissue damage.
- When the use of stay sutures to stabilize the position of the globe may compromise the surgical outcome, a central eye position can be achieved by intravenous administration

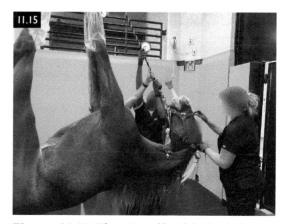

Figure 11.15 Elevation of head during hoisting to avoid increase in intraocular pressure (IOP)

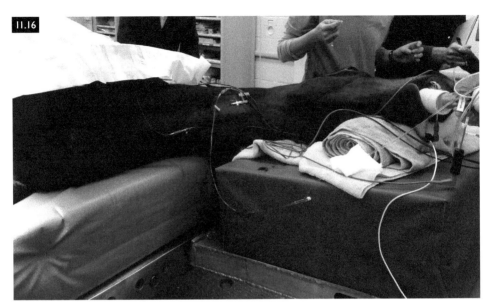

Figure 11.16 Elevation of head on the table in lateral recumbency

of a neuromuscular blocking agent (NMBA) such as atracurium or vecuronium. Note that the NMBA will paralyze all skeletal muscles, including the respiratory muscles.

- Training in the use of NMBAs is essential.
- An NMBA causes paralysis so that an animal cannot indicate if it gains consciousness or is experiencing pain.
- Respiratory muscles are paralyzed so mechanical ventilation is necessary.
- The animal should be adequately anesthetized before an NMBA is administered. The anesthetist must know how to differentiate between signs indicating inadequate anesthesia and signs of inadequate neuromuscular blockade.
- The cardiovascular system is monitored using invasive arterial pressure, heart rate, gum color, and capillary refill time (CRT). A decrease in MAP and prolongation of CRT may be a warning of anesthetic overdose.
- A peripheral nerve stimulator will provide an approximate measure of the

degree of neuromuscular blockade.
- Needles inserted over the common peroneal nerve are stimulated, and the foot twitches.
- Administration of atracurium (0.1 mg/kg IV) will block neuromuscular transmission (several-minute onset) so that no twitches will occur when the nerve is stimulated.
- A sequence of four electrical stimulations (train-of-four feature, or TOF) is used to evaluate the intensity of neuromuscular block (**Figure 11.17**). Full blockade is present when, after administration of the NMBA, none of the four peripheral nerve stimulations elicits foot twitches. Common use is to administer the NMBA just until the twitches are absent or until only one twitch is present. When a second twitch is observed, a supplemental dose of NMBA is administered to maintain neuromuscular block for surgery.

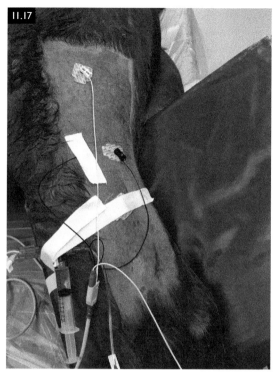

Figure 11.17 Use of train-of-four (TOF) on common peroneal nerve

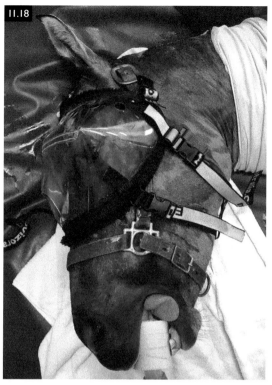

Figure 11.18 Horse with eye protector on for recovery

- When the surgical procedure is completed, the action of the NMBA is reversed by administration of an anticholinesterase inhibitor. This is usually neostigmine. Historically, edrophonium was the preferred agent for use in horses. However, this drug was recently discontinued. Return of neuromuscular transmission (four full-strength twitches) may take 10 minutes after administration of reversal. Complete reversal is essential for horses to ensure strong limbs for standing in recovery from anesthesia.
- Rotation of the eyeball into a rostroventral position is evidence of returned neuromuscular transmission since the eye muscles return to normal function later than limb muscles.
- Acceleromyography is a more

complete method for monitoring neuromuscular transmission. Quantitating the degree of neuromuscular block is more accurate than a visual assessment of the strength of foot twitch and because even a small degree of block that cannot be detected visually may impair muscular function in recovery.
- A commercially available eye protector, a hood with a left or right eyecup, should be placed over the head to protect the operative eye during induction and recovery from anesthesia (**Figure 11.18**).
  - It is important to be meticulous when securing the protector in place so that the edge cannot slide over the eye when the horse is active in attaining sternal and standing positions in recovery.

- Attentive care should be used when securing a protective thick foam hood with cutout holes for the eyes and ears, making sure that the adjustable straps are sufficiently tight when the head and neck are flexed and extended.
- Do not attach tubing from a subpalpebral lavage to the halter for recovery from anesthesia to avoid possible breakage or a dislodged catheter when the halter moves or twists during the horse's efforts to stand. Braid a lock of mane close to the poll and secure the tube to the proximal part of the braid near the skin.
- Enucleation is often performed during general anesthesia but can be done in a standing sedated horse. Enucleation appears to be excessively painful because the procedure may elicit movement in an animal assessed as adequately anesthetized.
  - Recovery from anesthesia has been documented as poorer quality after enucleation when compared with other types of ophthalmic or peripheral limb surgery.
  - Retrobulbar/peribulbar nerve block is recommended (20 ml 2% lidocaine for a 450-kg horse) with the lidocaine injected during anesthesia but 5–10 minutes before start of surgery.
  - Parenteral administration of analgesic agents, such as butorphanol or another opioid, or CRIs of lidocaine or an alpha-2 agonist sedative.
  - Traction on the eye may induce bradycardia or asystole via a vagus nerve reflex. Use of a retrobulbar nerve block prevents vagal stimulation. In the past, atropine has been administered before enucleation surgery to block the vagal effect; however, atropine may have a significantly long duration (days) on intestinal motility in horses. If

administered, to avoid colic, intestinal sounds must be auscultated before feeding the horse after surgery.

11.3.9   Sinuses

- General anesthesia in combination with nerve blocks for analgesia.
- Hemorrhage can be severe; therefore, volume of blood loss must be monitored (see 11.3.4, Dentistry).
- Plan for airway obstruction from blood clots and nasal congestion during recovery from anesthesia. Management may include recovery with endotracheal tube present (see 11.3.3, Esophageal Obstruction [Choke]).

11.4   THORAX

11.4.1 Diaphragmatic Rupture

- Diagnosis of diaphragmatic rupture in a horse is difficult before anesthesia as the clinical signs resemble colic. The condition can be present in foals.
- When identified during an abdominal exploratory surgery, the area of rupture may be exposed to air, resulting in pneumothorax. Hypoxemia and a tension pneumothorax may complicate anesthetic management.
  - Inspired gas should be increased to > 90% and IPPV instituted, if it has not already been done.
  - Insertion of a chest tube on the side of the rupture may facilitate aspiration of air.
  - Continuous positive airway pressure (CPAP) or an alveolar recruitment maneuver (ARM) with positive end-expiratory pressure (PEEP) may partially counteract the lung collapse associated with pneumothorax.
  - The surgery table may have to be tilted 'head-up', in reverse Trendelenburg position, to improve surgical exposure of the diaphragm (**Figure 11.19**).

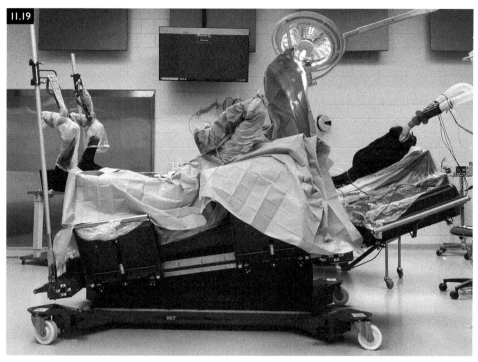

Figure 11.19 Reverse-Trendelenburg, dorsal recumbency

- The position of the arterial pressure transducer must be adjusted to heart level to maintain accurate measurement.
- A possible consequence of this position is increased pressure on the gluteal muscles and gluteal ischemia, with swelling, myositis, and lameness in recovery.

11.4.2 Thoracoscopy

- Can be performed in the standing horse because of the anatomical separation between the left and right lungs.
  - Sedation is achieved by administration of an alpha-2 agonist with or without an opioid.
  - Local infiltration with lidocaine, mepivacaine, or another local anesthetic provides analgesia for insertion of the scope.

- Thoracoscopy may be performed with the horse under general anesthesia and in dorsal recumbency.
  - Unlike laparoscopy, insufflation of the thorax with carbon dioxide is not recommended as an increase in intrathoracic pressure to > 2 mmHg will significantly decrease cardiac output and oxygenation.
  - Furthermore, the lung collapse will not immediately reverse when the gas is aspirated from the thorax at the end of the procedure.

11.5 ABDOMEN

- A variety of intra-abdominal surgical procedures can be performed in the standing horse using drug combinations for sedation as previously described (Chapter 3).

- Depending on the anticipated duration of surgery, administration of a sedative as a CRI may be advisable.
- Local analgesia utilizing infiltration of the abdominal wall with local anesthetic solution, paravertebral nerve blocks, or epidural injections of one or more agents (local anesthetic, alpha-2 agonist, morphine) may provide supplemental analgesia.
- A ventral midline abdominal celiotomy will be performed with the horse under general anesthesia (TIVA, inhalation anesthesia, or a combination of the two [partial IV anesthesia, PIVA]) and most commonly in dorsal recumbency.
  - Cardiopulmonary monitoring is very important for general anesthesia because these agents and dorsal recumbency will result in decreased cardiovascular function and impaired breathing.

11.5.1 Colic

- Horses with colic that require general anesthesia for surgery may be relatively healthy or have cardiopulmonary compromise, uremia, and endotoxemia.
- All these horses are subject to the adverse effects of anesthetic agents and the impact of dorsal recumbency and celiotomy with increased risk for hypoventilation, hypoxemia, hypotension, injury during recovery from anesthesia, and postanesthetic myopathy/neuropathy.
- Animals that are hypovolemic, acidotic, endotoxemic, with electrolyte imbalance, abdominal distension, and exhaustion are at increased anesthetic risk for death during or in the week following anesthesia.
- Animals with colic may have significantly decreased requirement for anesthetic agents from usual dose rates for healthy animals.

- Guidelines for colic patients include:
  - Perform a thorough preanesthetic evaluation to identify abnormalities, including seeking the patient history, assessment of the animal's mental status, physical examination particularly of the cardiovascular and respiratory systems, results of laboratory hematologic and biochemical tests, information from the rectal examination and abdominal fluid analysis, and volume of gastric reflux (**Table 11.2**).
  - Hypovolemia, hypocalcemia, and hypoxemia in all animals, and hypoglycemia in foals, should be corrected before induction of anesthesia.
  - Anesthetic agents and dose rates are chosen based on results of the preanesthetic evaluation.
  - Be prepared: use checklists to ensure all equipment is ready and available; make plans for likely complications.
  - Physiologic variables must be maintained within normal limits during anesthesia for the greatest outcome success.
- Before induction of anesthesia
  - See checklist (Table 11.2)
  - Administer IV antibiotics ≥ 30 minutes before induction of anesthesia. Many antibiotics decrease myocardial contraction and cause hypotension lasting about 45 minutes. When administered intraoperatively, the antibiotic should be injected at a very slow rate while simultaneously monitoring for decreased MAP.
  - Preoperative plans must include management of inadequate depth of anesthesia, gastric reflux flowing around the nasogastric (NG) tube, decreased MAP < 70 mmHg, abrupt severe hypotension (MAP < 60 mmHg), bradycardia (rate < 20 beats/min), and hypoxemia (PaO_2 < 60 mmHg, 8.0 kPa).

Table 11.2 Colic anesthesia checklist before anesthesia

OBSERVATION	SIGNIFICANCE	ACTION
Recent drug administration.	Evaluate behavior in relation to administration.	• Anticipate animal response to chosen drug protocol. • Adjust dose rates of chosen protocol based on previous drug administration and response.
Current behavior.	Calm but not depressed, accepting of new environment and people interaction. Excited, resistant to intensive care manipulations. Anxious eye, shivering/tremors.	• May respond well to routine anesthesia protocol. • Design premedication to achieve sedation, anticipate hyperactivity during recovery. • May have a reduced requirement for anesthetic drugs.
Large volume of gastric reflux.	Risk of pulmonary aspiration during induction of anesthesia. Gastric distension may impair ventilation during anesthesia.	• Attempt removal of reflux immediately before induction of anesthesia.
Extreme abdominal distension and labored breathing.	Hypoxemia and hypotension even before anesthesia. If intestinal centesis is not effective, immediate induction of anesthesia may be necessary; risk of death imminent.	• Minimize time lapse from premedication to induction. • Decrease dose rates for anesthetic agents from usual by up to 50%. • Administer oxygen by nasal insufflation. • Administer low dose dobutamine IV. • Induce into sternal position for endotracheal intubation. Start artificial ventilation with a demand valve immediately. • Rapid transfer to surgery table and rapid onset of surgery for abdominal decompression.
Signs of impaired circulation: mucous membranes bright red or purple or pale, CRT very fast or ≥2 seconds, bounding peripheral pulse or weak pulse strength, tachycardia, auscultation of mitral murmur, irregular cardiac rhythm.	Abnormally bright red membranes, rapid CRT, bounding pulse: Indicative of hyperdynamic cardiovascular function (sepsis or endotoxemia). Abnormally slow CRT, pale membranes, weak pulse: Possible causes are hypovolemia, decreased cardiac output, and/or hypotension. Tachycardia: Associated with pain, anxiety, hypotension, hypercarbia, hypoxemia, endotoxemia, gastric distension. Irregular rhythm: May contribute to decreased cardiac function during anesthesia, atrial fibrillation may be accompanied by normal or fast heart rate, premature ventricular depolarizations may be associated with endotoxemia.	• Patient with hyperdynamic circulation may require higher drug doses for induction of anesthesia but will soon change during anesthesia (30 minutes) to decreased requirement and depressed cardiovascular function. • Evaluate for low blood volume; expand with fluids if assessment indicates fluid deficit. • Measure arterial blood pressure; use pressure with CRT for evaluation of response to volume expansion. • Evaluate an ECG. Anticipate hypotension during anesthesia if atrial fibrillation.

(Continued)

Table 11.2 (Continued)

OBSERVATION	SIGNIFICANCE	ACTION
Abnormal laboratory tests.	PCV is commonly elevated in horses with colic and may not indicate hypovolemia. Hypocalcemia will be associated with hypotension during anesthesia. Hyperglycemia is common and is a reflection of administration of alpha-2 sedatives and sympathetic stimulation. Azotemia may reflect decreased fluid intake and be associated with hypovolemia. Will contribute to CNS depression, pH, blood gas, and base excess abnormalities.	• Recommend fluid volume expansion when PCV > 45%. • Administer calcium (approximately 0.5 ml/kg 23% calcium borogluconate IV, based on sequential determinations of iCa^{++}). • No action. • Requires fluid administration; may decrease anesthetic requirement. • Identify cause of hypoxemia before anesthesia. Moderate or severe metabolic acidosis (base excess 15 to—20 mmol/L) should be partially corrected by slow infusion of sodium bicarbonate, but administration of balanced electrolyte to improve circulation will begin to correct the acidosis in many patients.
Preparation.	Although several people are involved in preparation for surgery, ideally the responsibilities should be evenly distributed and the same duties assigned to the same people for every horse, so that the necessary procedures are performed quickly, efficiently, and as a team. The anesthesia equipment should always be assembled (without oxygen and electrical connections) to facilitate response to emergency situations.	• Patient: one or two IV catheters, volume expansion, calcium-containing fluid if indicated, IV antibiotic administration at least 30 minutes before induction, nasogastric reflux immediately before induction. • Equipment: Connect oxygen, and compressed air if used, to the anesthesia machine, check delivery system for leaks, select endotracheal tubes and check cuffs for leaks, connect electrical equipment, prepare pressure transducer and gas analyzer for use, calculate and prepare adjunct drugs (dobutamine, ephedrine, lidocaine, any alpha-2 agonist or opioid you plan to administer), and insert syringes or bags in syringe pumps or fluid pumps.

CRT, capillary refill time; ECG, electrocardiogram; PCV, packed cell volume; CNS, central nervous system

- At induction of anesthesia the animal is at risk for aspiration of gastric fluid, hypotension, hypoxemia, and cardiac arrest.
  - Premedication and induction drugs are often combinations of xylazine or romifidine, with or without a small dose of detomidine, followed by ketamine with either diazepam or midazolam or propofol. It is important to assess, based on the preanesthetic evaluation, how much the doses of the alpha-2 agonist and ketamine can be reduced (0–50%) from the doses used for healthy animals.
- Immediately before induction, the NG tube must be lavaged to remove as much gastric fluid as possible.
  - This author prefers that the NG tube should remain in place during induction of anesthesia so that gastric fluid may drain during anesthesia; it is almost impossible to insert an NG tube in an anesthetized horse.

- Insert a stopper (plastic syringe case) in the external end of the NG tube during induction. This has advantages and disadvantages. Gastric fluid may drain continuously in the absence of a stopper, but it will puddle on the floor, risking contact with the horse's eye and resulting in corneal damage. By contrast, blocking flow from the NG tube during induction may prevent fluid on the floor and further draining (room contamination) while the horse is being transported to the operating table, but because the tube may maintain the cardia partially open, reflux into the pharynx can still occur.
  - Reflux around the NG tube and into the pharynx may occur with or without a stopper in place.
- Gastric fluid entering the pharynx during induction of anesthesia may enter the trachea before an endotracheal tube can be inserted. Maintain the animal in sternal recumbency with the head elevated during induction and until the endotracheal tube is inserted and the cuff inflated. This potentially may prevent aspiration. After cuff inflation, the horse is allowed to assume lateral recumbency.
- Horses with pre-existing central nervous system (CNS) depression, low blood volume, hypoxemia, metabolic acidosis, and excessive abdominal distension will become hypotensive after induction of anesthesia.
  - Rolling or turning the horse into dorsal recumbency results in decreased arterial pressure, even in healthy animals.
  - Horses with pre-existing low blood pressure or increased risk for hypotension may benefit from a continuous infusion of dobutamine (1–5 µg/kg/min) throughout the induction period.
- Arterial oxygenation will decrease when a horse is turned from lateral to dorsal recumbency.

- Administer 6–8 positive pressure breaths/min with oxygen using a demand valve between induction of anesthesia and beginning transportation to the surgical table. This should be routine practice in all adult horses in a hospital environment.
- Horses with purple or blue/white mucous membranes, with excessive abdominal distension impairing breathing, or with confirmed hypoxemia by blood gas analysis should be administered oxygen by nasal insufflation (15 L/min for a 450 kg horse) during induction of anesthesia. After endotracheal intubation, artificial ventilation with oxygen is applied using a demand valve.
- Maintenance of anesthesia is provided by injectable agents with an inhalation anesthetic agent. The anesthetist determines the relative proportions of IV and inhalation agents.
- The goals are to provide unconsciousness, muscle relaxation, and analgesia; minimal impact on the circulation; and a smooth, injury-free recovery from anesthesia.
  - Set the initial vaporizer setting at a percentage lower than is routine for a healthy horse. When a measurement of MAP is obtained, initiate treatment if the animal is hypotensive. If the animal is not hypotensive, then the vaporizer can be increased if the depth of anesthesia is too light.
  - Immediately initiate controlled ventilation with the ventilator delivering 10 breaths/min (this author's preference). Peak inspiratory pressure normally is about 22–26 cmH$_2$O (17–20 mmHg). A higher pressure may be necessary with abdominal distension but should not exceed 50 cmH$_2$0 (38 mmHg).
  - The inspired oxygen concentration will be determined by the usual practice at the hospital but may have to be increased

to > 90% if hypoxemia (PaO_2 < 60 mmHg, 8.0 kPa) is present.

- Remove the NG stopper as soon as the horse is on the table, and allow fluid to drain into a bucket dedicated for gastric reflux.
- Electrodes should be attached in a base-apex configuration and the electrocardiogram displayed on Lead 1.
- Insert a catheter into a facial or transverse facial artery for measurement of blood pressure, and place the transducer position level with the thoracic inlet or the point of the shoulder.
- Start IV infusions of balanced electrolyte solution (5–10 ml/kg/h) and a lidocaine infusion (1.5 mg/kg over 15 minutes followed by 0.5 mg/kg/h) as soon as possible.

- Position the animal's head at least as high as the thoracic inlet to minimize development of nasal mucosa congestion, without overextending the head and neck.

- If gastric reflux appears around the NG tube, then the head must be lowered to promote drainage. Then specific steps must be taken in recovery to ensure a patent airway (see 11.3.3, Esophageal Obstruction [Choke]).
- If available, a hot air blanket should be positioned over the animal's neck and thorax to slow heat loss. A body temperature < 35.6 °C (< 96.0 °F) at the end of anesthesia is associated with increased ataxia in recovery.
- Intensive monitoring is vital to providing essential information for appropriate administration of anesthetics and supportive treatment. The goal is for the monitored variables to be close to or within normal limits.
- Aim for end-tidal carbon dioxide (capnography) ≤ 40 mmHg (5.3 kPa) or $PaCO_2$ < 50 mmHg (6.6 kPa), SpO_2 (pulse oximetry) > 90%, PaO_2 > 60 mmHg (8.0 kPa), heart rate 26–55 beats/min, MAP ≥ 70 mmHg, CRT < 2 seconds. Use of an anesthetic record in chart form is an immediate visual aid of the anesthesia progress (**Figure 11.20**).

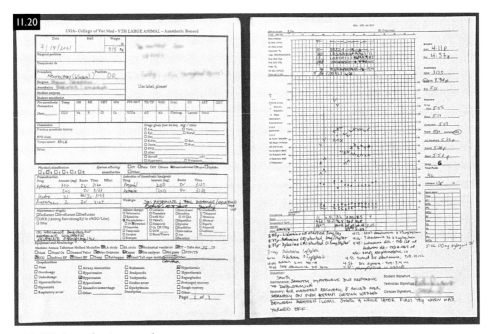

Figure 11.20 Anesthetic record

- Blood glucose should be monitored every 30 minutes in foals and maintained > 100 mg/dl (> 5.5 mmol/L). Infuse 5% dextrose in water at 3 ml/kg/h, adjusting the rate in response to the latest glucose measurement, together with a balanced electrolyte solution at 3–10 ml/kg/h.
- When an anesthetic gas analyzer is used to monitor depth of inhalation anesthesia, the target concentration is usually 0.5–1.2 x minimum alveolar concentration (MAC) for the agent used.
  - Approximate MAC values in horses are for isoflurane 1.3%, for sevoflurane 2.3%, and for desflurane 8%.
  - The anesthetic concentration for each animal depends on the proportion of injectable drugs to inhalation agent administered and the anesthetic requirement of the patient (sick animals need less anesthetic).
  - Thus, a higher inhalant concentration will be necessary when injectable drugs are limited to premedication and induction agents with a lidocaine infusion than when a continuous infusion of a sedative, opioid, or ketamine is administered.
- Management of intraoperative complications is covered in Chapter 10. Inadequate circulation, indicated by hypotension (MAP < 70 mmHg), CRT > 2 seconds, pale or dark mucous membrane color, and dark blood or decreased bleeding at the operative site, is a common complication. Acute hypotension may develop after ischemic bowel is handled or untwisted. Difficulty achieving adequate ventilation may be a problem, indicated by higher than normal $PaCO_2$ or end-tidal concentration and high inspiratory pressure needed to deliver an adequate volume per breath. Some animals may develop hypoxemia despite high inspired oxygen concentration and apparently adequate mechanical ventilation.

- Delivery of an IV fluid challenge, 10 ml/kg of crystalloid in < 15 minutes, may identify the need for blood volume expansion. Improvement is indicated by an increase in MAP and pulse pressure (systolic arterial pressure minus diastolic arterial pressure) and a decrease in amplitude of the pulse pressure variation that cycles with the mechanical ventilator. If these improvements are observed but subsequently the MAP gradually decreases, a second fluid challenge may be delivered.
- Further blood volume expansion can be achieved by IV administration of hypertonic 7.5% saline at initially 2 ml/kg over 15 minutes, up to a further 2 ml/kg. Hetastarch (5 ml/kg) or plasma can also be administered for blood volume expansion.
- Any of several vasoactive drugs may be infused intravenously to promote increased myocardial contractility and/or vasoconstriction, such as dobutamine (0.5–5.0 µg/kg/min) alone or with ephedrine (bolus 0.03–0.06 mg/kg or CRI 0.02 mg/kg/min to effect). Other agents are available for use when these are not effective.
- Oxygenation may improve after the abdominal incision releases the intra-abdominal pressure. Hypoxemia may be responsive to the administration of a bronchodilator, such as albuterol (salbutamol), through the endotracheal tube or application of continuous positive airway pressure (CPAP) or an alveolar recruitment maneuver (ARM) followed by positive end-expiratory pressure (PEEP).

11.5.2 Dystocia and Caesarian Hysterotomy

- Choose doses of anesthetic agents based on individual evaluation because mares with dystocia vary from healthy to exhausted and dehydrated.

- TIVA is most commonly administered for vaginal delivery of the foal. Inhalation anesthesia is commonly administered for hysterotomy.
- Anesthesia setup is urgent and as rapid as possible if the foal is anticipated to be alive.

11.5.2.1 Vaginal Delivery

- Insert a catheter in a jugular vein for drug administration.
- Consider what the mare or jenny would weigh if not pregnant and base doses on that weight. The volume of the uterus contributes little to the initial drug effect in the dam during induction of anesthesia.
- Anesthetic requirement may be much less than usual for some mares with dystocia. Administration of usual doses may result in hypotension.
- When delivery is expected to be relatively easy, e.g. from a mare with a ruptured prepubic tendon, the combination of xylazine (0.9–1.0 mg/kg) and ketamine (1.7–2.0 mg/kg) intravenously will allow vaginal delivery of a live foal.
- When delivery is interrupted and when the foal's head is accessible, it may be possible to insert an endotracheal tube and administer oxygen during manipulations.
- In some cases of fetal malposition or prolonged dystocia, the mare must be suspended by the hind limbs using a hoist while the shoulders, forelimbs, neck, and head are on the ground (**Figure 11.21**). This position allows the clinician to more easily reposition the foal and perform other manipulations. Breathing is difficult for the mare in this position.
  - Administer oxygen (15 L/min for a 450 kg horse) by insufflation through a tube in the ventral nasal meatus or inside an endotracheal tube. Inspired oxygen concentration is higher if insufflation is through an endotracheal tube.

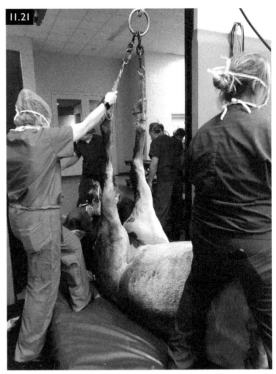

Figure 11.21 **Suspension of mare by hind limbs for vaginal delivery of the foal**

  - Alternatively, insert an endotracheal tube and use a demand valve to either deepen spontaneous breaths or increase the rate of breathing.
- Administration of anesthetic drugs for maintenance of anesthesia is easier using a continuous infusion IV (author's preference is xylazine-guaifenesin-ketamine at 2 ml/kg/h of xylazine 650 mg and ketamine 1300 mg in 1 L of 5% guaifenesin, after induction with xylazine and ketamine) than injection of intermittent boluses. Maintain a light plane of anesthesia.
- Monitoring includes eye position, strength of palpebral reflex, peripheral pulse strength, gum color and CRT, and visual assessment of breathing. Pulse oximetry with a probe on the tongue and a Doppler ultrasound probe on the forelimb can be attempted but may not provide information

as the probes are dislodged by the movements of the animal's body during the attempts to extract the foal.

- Decrease in strength of the arterial pulse, blanching of the mucous membranes (gum color), and CRT > 2 seconds indicate decreased cardiovascular function.
  - Decrease rate of anesthetic administration.
  - Start dobutamine infusion 1.0–2.0 µg/kg/min IV.
  - Administer balanced electrolyte solution (2–5 L for an adult horse) intravenously.
  - Administer hypertonic saline (1 L for an adult horse) intravenously.
  - With the mare in a head-down position, fluid may not flow intravenously rapidly. Bags of fluid can be pressurized to speed delivery, but this probably will stop infusion of anesthetic drugs. A second IV catheter in the opposite jugular vein may be necessary.
- Before recovery, fetal fluids and blood must be cleaned from the floor so that it is not slippery.
- The mare may require assistance to stand. Adductor nerve damage occurs in some mares from pressure of the foal within the pelvis. After the mare is standing, unacceptable ataxia may be reduced by administration of an alpha-2 antagonist, e.g. tolazoline, yohimbine, atipamezole.
- Be prepared for a transition to caesarian hysterotomy in cases where the foal cannot be removed.

11.5.2.2 Caesarian Hysterotomy

- Performed through a ventral midline abdominal incision with the mare in dorsal recumbency.
- Assemble equipment and supplies for resuscitation of the foal (use a previously prepared hospital checklist).
- Most of the anesthetic agents used in horses can be administered to the mare during

caesarian section and result in a live foal. Calculation of anesthetic drugs should be on the estimated non-pregnant weight.

- Guaifenesin is a useful agent for part of the anesthetic protocol. The foal may appear lethargic for about 10 minutes after delivery because guaifenesin crosses the placenta.
- Use a vaporizer setting lower than usual to maintain a light plane of anesthesia. High concentrations of inhalation agents decrease cardiovascular function in the fetus, and metabolic acidosis progressively develops with increased duration of anesthesia.
- Work quickly to achieve a speedy removal of the foal from the mare after induction of anesthesia.
- Administer oxygen and use controlled ventilation for the mare, and attach all routine monitoring. A high inspiratory pressure will be needed until the foal is removed, and then the pressure can be decreased.
- Hypotension after positioning the mare in dorsal recumbency may be *aortocaval syndrome*.
  - Administration of dobutamine only results in tachycardia with no improvement in pressure.
  - The syndrome refers to weight of the uterus compressing the caudal vena cava and aorta and decreasing blood flow to and from the heart.
  - Sometimes tilting the animal to its left is sufficient to change the position of the uterus, restoring blood flow and an adequate arterial pressure; otherwise the surgery must commence immediately to remove the foal.
- The mare may be weak in recovery, and assistance to stand may be needed. Make sure that the floor is not wet and slippery.

11.5.2.3 Resuscitation of the Foal

- Assemble all equipment and supplies before start of anesthesia. A foal resuscitation kit should always be available and checked regularly. Other useful equipment, if available, is a suction device, an anesthesia machine, an ECG monitor, and a capnograph. A printed algorithm for cardiopulmonary resuscitation is helpful.

- A foal resuscitation kit includes:
  - Selection sterile foal naso- and endotracheal tubes 6–12 mm ID.
  - Tube or packets of sterile lubricant and roll gauze.
  - Face mask.
  - Resuscitator (Ambu) bag.
  - Catheters of various sizes and lengths.
  - Pre-drawn syringes containing saline for flushing.
  - 500-ml bags balanced electrolyte and 5% dextrose in water.
  - Administration sets.
  - Selection syringes and needles.
  - Drugs (epinephrine, doxapram, naloxone, atipamezole).
  - Drug dose sheets, preprinted calculations in ml for several foal sizes.
  - Catheter site preparation kit (gauzes, chlorhexidine, alcohol).
  - Clippers, battery-powered, checked (electrical if in clinic).
  - Pulse oximeter, charged.
  - Oxygen supply with regulator and tubing.
- Assessment and appropriate treatment are urgent immediately after the foal is delivered (**Figure 11.22**). If foal is potentially viable, then check for a heartbeat.
  - No heartbeat.
    - Start cardiac massage with foal lying on its right side: 100 compressions/min over the 6th intercostal space, one-third of the distance from the sternum to the back.
    - Make sure compression of the chest is completely released between compressions. Depending on the position of the person applying massage in relation to the foal,

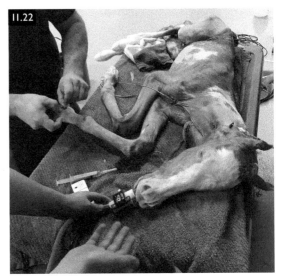

Figure 11.22 **Newborn foal assessment**

stabilizing the foal's body against an immovable object facilitates consistent cardiac compressions.
- A second person can insert an endotracheal tube during cardiac massage to administer oxygen and artificial breaths 8–10 per minute.
- Heartbeat present.
  - Clear fluid from the nasal passages.
  - Remove membranes from the nose, and position head and neck dependent to the body for drainage for 30 seconds.
  - Suction is useful to clear fluid, but apply active suction for no more than 5 seconds at a time because the suction can remove air from the lungs and result in hypoxemia and lung collapse.
  - Supply oxygen between suction periods.
- If the foal is breathing, supply oxygen by face mask.
- If the foal is not breathing or breathing is slow, irregular, gasping, and/or with nasal flaring, insert an endotracheal tube and ventilate.

- Extension of the head and neck into a straight line facilitates insertion of a tube into the trachea.
- Use a tube specifically made for foals so that it is long enough to enter the trachea and not be dislodged by movement of the foal.
- An endotracheal tube provides the best conditions for applied ventilation but eventually will have to be removed. A tube with an internal diameter 2–3 mm smaller than the appropriately sized endotracheal tube is used for nasotracheal intubation, but the smaller lumen may hinder airflow when the cuff is inflated. An advantage is that a nasotracheal tube can be left in position for oxygen administration after the foal starts chewing and lifting its head. Tie the tube to the foal's lower jaw or around the head behind the ears.
- To ventilate the foal, use manual compression (8–10 breaths/min) of a resuscitator bag with air or air/oxygen mix or the reservoir bag on an anesthesia machine system delivering oxygen.
- Measure end-expired carbon dioxide (capnography) by attaching an adapter and the sampling line to the endotracheal tube or by inserting a sampling tube inside the endotracheal tube (IV extension tube with one connector cut off and the other end attached to the sampling tubing). On the monitor, near zero mmHg carbon dioxide indicates either the endotracheal tube is in the esophagus or cardiac arrest; 10–15 mmHg indicates inadequate cardiac output and low to absent arterial pressure; > 20 mmHg indicates presence of peripheral perfusion; and > 45 mmHg indicates hypoventilation.
- Collecting a blood sample to measure pH and blood gases is of no value until circulation has been restored.

- Drugs.
  - Combine with cardiac massage epinephrine 0.01 mg/kg IV.
  - Doxapram is a respiratory stimulant and also will partially antagonize sedation from xylazine or detomidine passed through the placenta from the mare. Inject 0.5 mg/kg, approximately 1.25 ml for a large foal, intravenously.
  - Antagonism of drugs administered to the mare that may have crossed to the foal. Naloxone is an opioid antagonist. Inject 0.01 mg/kg, approximately 1.0 ml (0.4 mg/ml, for a large foal). Atipamezole will antagonize an alpha-2 agonist sedative.
  - Dopamine and dobutamine are cardiovascular stimulants. Dopamine is more effective for resuscitation because it increases heart rate in addition to myocardial contractility. Add 50 mg dopamine (1.25 ml of 40 mg/ml) to 500 ml saline to make a solution of 100 µg/ml. Infuse IV at 7–10 µg/kg/min; for a 50 kg/110 lb foal, 8 µg/kg/min using a 15 drops/ml administration set is one drop/second.
  - Tactile stimulation by rubbing with a towel; tickle inside the nostrils and ears and the perineum.
- Monitoring progress.
  - Bradycardia in a foal is < 60 beats/min. Ensure that the foal is not hypoxemic. Infuse dopamine. Heart rate closer to 100 beats/min is normal.
  - End-expired carbon dioxide value is used to assess adequacy of ventilation and pulmonary perfusion (circulation). Normal value is 35–40 mmHg.
  - Assess strength of peripheral arterial pulse (suggest palpation of metatarsal artery) and use noninvasive pressure monitoring. MAP should be > 60 mmHg and CRT should be one second.
  - Fluid therapy is not immediately necessary unless hemorrhage has

occurred. Measure blood glucose concentration, and if < 80 mg/dl, treat by IV infusion of 5% dextrose in water, starting at 3–5 ml/kg/h.

- Attach a pulse oximeter probe to the tongue. Peripheral hemoglobin oxygen saturation (SpO_2) should be ≥ 93%. Arterial blood will be necessary for blood gas analysis for accurate assessment of oxygenation.
- Measure PCO_2, blood gases, base excess, and glucose once circulation is restored to document adequacy of ventilation and metabolic status. Goal is pH > 7.35 and/ or no base deficit.
- Apply heat to prevent hypothermia.
- Enteral nutrition is essential, and nursing should be encouraged as soon as possible. Watch for regurgitation of milk after the foal has nursed and is lying down, because of the risk of milk aspiration into the lungs.

11.5.3 Laparoscopy
- The horse is under general anesthesia and in dorsal recumbency. The table may be tilted head down (Trendelenburg position) (**Figure 11.23**) for some procedures and even tilted left or right. These positions improve the view through the laparoscope, e.g., undescended testicle, urinary bladder, by shifting the abdominal organs away from the target organs.
- When tilting the table remember the following:
  - Reposition the arterial pressure transducer level with the heart for accurate measurements.
  - Adequate padding to counter increased pressure at contact points with table supports.
  - Ventilation decreased when head down: alter ventilator settings; adjust when assumes horizontal.

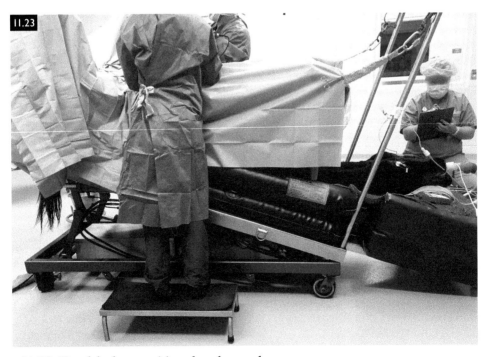

Figure 11.23 Trendelenburg position, dorsal recumbency

- Nasal congestion when head down: prop up head during anesthesia; watch for obstruction of breathing in recovery.
- The abdomen will be insufflated with carbon dioxide to 15 mmHg to facilitate view of organs during laparoscopy. The room lights may be off to improve the view on the monitor, so have a flashlight or small surgery light available for anesthesia monitoring.
- Breathing will be restricted by increased intra-abdominal pressure. Use artificial ventilation to ensure adequate breathing.
- Tilting the table head-down results in the following:
  - Further pressure on the diaphragm, limiting tidal volume.
  - The blood pressure transducer must be repositioned at heart level for arterial pressures to be accurate.

- Avoid congestion of the nasal mucosa when the table is tilted by positioning the head above the level of the heart.
- Check for adequate padding to offset increased pressure on the shoulders or other parts of the body leaning on table supports, thus avoiding local ischemia that can result in myopathy or neuropathy.
- Plan for nasal obstruction from nasal mucosa congestion during recovery from anesthesia (see 11.3.3, Esophageal Obstruction [Choke]).

11.5.4 Ovariectomy

- Ovariectomy may be performed in the standing sedated horse with local infiltration of lidocaine or mepivacaine for either a vaginal or flank approach (**Figure 11.24**).

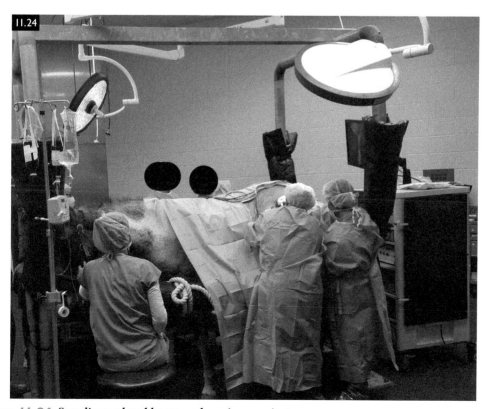

Figure 11.24 Standing sedated horse undergoing ovariectomy

- Alternatively, the horse may be put under general anesthesia for a surgical approach through a flank or ventral midline incision.
  - Use caution when positioning the recumbent horse for a flank incision. Do not pull the upper hind limb caudally because myopathy will result from that position. Secure rope around the fetlock and metatarsus (with padding), and flex and lift the limb perpendicular to the animal's spine, passing the free end of the rope over the hindquarters (adding padding at the contact point) and tying it to the far side of the table or a ring in the wall with a quick-release knot.
  - Removal of a large ovarian tumor may be complicated by excessive blood supply. Surgical attention to these blood vessels may result in extended duration of anesthesia, with implications for myopathy developing in the dependent limbs. A moderate degree of hemorrhage may require more than maintenance fluid administration.

11.5.5 Urinary Bladder Rupture in Foals

- Identify features in these cases that are important to anesthetic management.
- Before anesthesia, measure arterial pressure noninvasively with a cuff around the tail. Measure blood glucose concentration and treat hypoglycemia. Measure serum electrolyte concentrations and treat hyperkalemia > 6.6 mg/dl. Hyperkalemia increases the irritability of the myocardium, leading to dysrhythmias. Uremia causes CNS depression and decreases anesthetic requirement.
- Urine should be drained from the abdomen before induction of anesthesia. If urine is evacuated rapidly during surgery, the loss of abdominal pressure results in an abrupt decrease in MAP.

- To prevent milk reflux into the pharynx, the foal should wear a muzzle to prevent nursing for 30 minutes before anesthesia.
- The foal should remain in proximity to the mare for reassurance until the foal is anesthetized.
- Before the foal is removed, the mare may need to be sedated to prevent self-inflicted injury. A commonly used sedative is acepromazine (0.02 mg/kg) with xylazine (0.3 mg/kg) or detomidine (0.005 mg/kg) IV.
- Anesthesia is frequently induced with diazepam or midazolam and ketamine or propofol or mask induction with sevoflurane or isoflurane, and maintained with sevoflurane or isoflurane. Halothane is more likely to induce cardiac dysrhythmias in these patients compared with other inhalant anesthetics.
  - The dose rates of anesthetic drugs for foals fewer than a few days old are less than those for older foals or adults.
  - Avoid drugs that decrease heart rate, such as alpha-2 agonists, because neonatal foals have high heart rates and cardiac output, and any drug decreasing these functions results in hypotension.
  - Maintenance IV fluids include acetated or lactated balanced electrolyte solution (5 ml/kg/h) with 5% dextrose in water (D5W; 3 ml/kg/min). The D5W infusion rate should be adjusted based on the results of blood glucose measurements performed every 30–60 minutes to maintain blood glucose ≥ 100 mg/dl. A fluid challenge of balanced electrolyte solution (10 ml/kg over 10 minutes) may be necessary to treat low MAP.
- MAP should be kept at 70–80 mmHg during anesthesia. Administration of dobutamine (0.5–1.0 μg/kg/min) or ephedrine (0.03–0.06 mg/kg) intravenously may increase MAP.

- Advanced third-degree atrioventricular heart block is a dysrhythmia that may develop in foals with bladder rupture. Dopamine (7–10 µg/kg/min) is the drug of choice for this complication. Cardiac massage may be required to maintain circulation and delivery of oxygen and drugs to the heart. Atropine (0.02 mg/kg) or ephedrine is administered if additional assistance is needed to increase heart rate.
- Hypothermia easily develops. Prevention includes a hot air blanket over the top of the foal's neck, shoulders, and thorax.
- Recovery from anesthesia should take place in a padded recovery room, where the foal is held in recumbency until judged strong enough to stand. As soon as the foal makes an attempt to stand, one or two people should support it. Try to allow the foal to stand by itself, only limiting forward movement to avoid stumbling; holding the foal up generally results in it abandoning its own efforts to remain standing.
- Carefully supervise introduction of the foal to the mare to avoid the foal being kicked. If the foal is allowed to nurse and then immediately lies down to sleep, regurgitation of milk may occur, seen as flowing out of the foal's mouth. The foal must be immediately woken up to initiate swallowing and prevent pulmonary aspiration.

11.6 LIMBS

11.6.1 Arthroscopy

- Many horses scheduled for this procedure are young and healthy except for joint disease. Therefore, routine anesthetic protocols can be used.
- Analgesia may be systemic administration of an opioid, e.g. butorphanol or morphine, with the inclusion of intra-articular administration of preservative-free morphine (0.1 mg/kg) and/or bupivacaine during closure of the surgical site.

11.6.2 Feet

- Procedures with minimal invasiveness with an expected duration of < 2 hours can be performed with the animal under TIVA with oxygen supplementation.
- Usual anesthetic management is employed. Upper limbs are supported in the horizontal position (**Figure 11.25**). Blood pressure can be monitored noninvasively with an oscillometric monitor. Place towels near the penis or vulva to soak up leaking urine if in an indoor stall.
- Inhalation general anesthesia is used for more involved surgical procedures.
- Add local anesthesia whenever possible whether using TIVA or inhalation anesthesia.
- Intravenous regional analgesia (Bier block) is a useful technique for providing analgesia for extensive debridement.
  - A tourniquet is attached proximal or distal to the carpus or tarsus and 2% lidocaine (20 ml for a large horse) injected intravenously distal to the tourniquet slowly over several minutes.
  - A Butterfly needle directed toward the foot can be easily held in place by hand while the syringe is attached to the extension tubing. The same needle can be used for local IV infusion of an antibiotic, if planned.

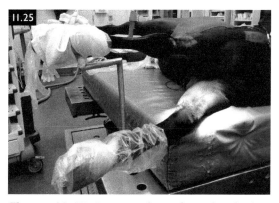

Figure 11.25 Support of non-dependent limbs in lateral recumbency

- Onset of anesthesia is about 10–15 minutes. Note that analgesia disappears within 5–10 minutes after the tourniquet is removed, at which time systemic analgesia must be provided.
- Analgesia is apparent by the decrease in anesthetic agent(s) required and a smooth anesthesia.

11.6.3 Orthopedic Surgery

- Many procedures fall into this category, and they may have different anesthetic requirements, depending on the degree of limb or joint instability and the health and temperament of the patient.
- Fractures of limb bones are repaired during general anesthesia with isoflurane, sevoflurane, or desflurane. The anesthetic protocol will be influenced by the usual protocols used in each clinic, the anesthetic agents available, and the training of the anesthetist.
- Considerations for anesthetic management include estimates of duration, provision of analgesia, and assistance required in recovery. A major concern is preventing the horse from destroying the surgical repair or refracturing the limb during recovery from anesthesia. This may be associated with multiple attempts to stand but can occur even with a quiet recovery and at first attempt when full weight is borne on the repaired limb. The temperament of the patient and its ability to recognize the handicap contribute to the outcome.
- Surgery may be long, requiring attention to adequate padding and positioning to minimize the risk of myopathy or neuropathy.
- Analgesia must be provided. Options include:
  - An opioid, e.g. morphine, hydromorphone, or methadone.
  - An alpha-2 agonist sedative for premedication and a CRI, e.g.

dexmedetomidine, is frequently added.
- Lidocaine CRI.
- Local anesthesia nerve blocks may not be useful if they persist into the recovery period and compromise limb strength and function. A soaker catheter may be inserted in or near a fracture site with the external end emerging at a point distant from the repair (or cast) for instillation of bupivacaine after recovery from anesthesia.
- Recovery must be assisted. Difficulty rising will depend on the location of the fracture. Ropes are attached to the halter and tail to prevent the horse from moving around the recovery area and stumbling or falling. The ropes cannot lift the horse; that effort must be supplied by the animal, but they can stabilize once standing. Lifting can be accomplished using a sling with a fast hoist or a pool arrangement, when available.

11.7 CASE EXAMPLES

11.7.1 A 16-Year-Old 545-Kg Thoroughbred Mare Anesthetized for Deep Debridement and Lavage of the Right Forefoot

- After premedication with detomidine and butorphanol, topped up with xylazine, anesthesia was induced with diazepam and ketamine and maintained with isoflurane in oxygen.
- A Bier Block was planned. After inflation of a tourniquet and intravenous injection of 15 ml 2% lidocaine (Bier block), mean arterial pressure decreased and stabilized around 73 mmHg and heart rate at 26 beats/min for 45 minutes.
- At that time oxygen inflow was 3 L/min, the vaporizer was 2.5%, and the end-tidal isoflurane was 1.3%.
- A butorphanol supplement was administered at 70 minutes after induction (routine practice).

- The tourniquet was inadvertently deflated. Clinical signs of lightening anesthetic depth including increased heart rate and nystagmus were noted.
  - This required administration of a bolus of xylazine and increased vaporizer setting.
  - The increase in heart rate and increased need for isoflurane indicate that the intravenous block had been providing analgesia.

11.7.2 A 5-Year-Old 500 Kg-Quarter Horse Stallion with a Luxated Hock

- The horse was scheduled for external reduction of the luxation and application of an external splint.
- TIVA was chosen for anesthesia with xylazine (1.1 mg/kg) and butorphanol (0.02 mg/kg) for premedication and induction of anesthesia with diazepam (0.05 mg/kg) and ketamine (2.2 mg/kg) IV.
- The horse was transported to the surgery room by hoist attached to the three sound limbs and positioned in lateral recumbency on the table with the injured limb uppermost.
- Before transportation, the trachea was intubated, and when the horse was on the table, the endotracheal tube was connected to an anesthesia machine and controlled ventilation with oxygen started.
- Anesthesia was maintained for approximately two hours by IV infusion of guaifenesin-ketamine-xylazine (650 mg xylazine and 1300 mg ketamine in 1 L of 5% guaifenesin) at 2 ml/kg/h.
- Routine monitoring included an ECG, invasive arterial pressure monitoring, and end-tidal capnography.
- Management specific to this patient included:
  - Induction of anesthesia was behind a swing door, but a rope was looped around the injured hind limb and held so that the limb was pulled forward as the horse subsided to the ground. The intention was to avoid buckling of the limb that might have induced further injury.
- A catheter was inserted into the epidural space at the first intercoccygeal junction and threaded approximately 20 cm cranially. The catheter was sutured where it exited the skin, a gauze pad sutured over that, and further protection sutured at that location to keep the catheter, filter, and injection port clean. Preservative-free morphine (0.05 mg/kg) was injected before the end of anesthesia and daily for two weeks when analgesia was needed.
- The horse was assisted in recovery by attachment of ropes to the halter and to the tail. The ropes were then passed through adjacent rings in the walls of the stall and then outside for traction by assistants. In this case, the horse was very quiet throughout recovery, remained in sternal position for longer than usual, and then stood at first attempt with no need for assistance despite the heavy cast.
- When walking the horse from the recovery room to the hospital stall, a rope was again looped around the cast so that the limb could be pulled forward whenever a forward step was taken. The intention was to avoid the horse tripping over the cast until he became accustomed to the required maneuvering.

FURTHER READING

Auckburally A, Nyman G (2017) Review of hypoxaemia in anaesthetized horses: Predisposing factors, consequences and management. *Vet Anaesth Analg* **44**:397–408.

Bohaychuk-Preuss KS, Carrozzo MV, Duke-Novakovski T (2017) Cardiopulmonary effects of pleural insufflation with CO_2 during two-lung ventilation in dorsally recumbent anesthetized horses. *Vet Anaesth Analg* **44**: 483–491.

Ccrasoli I, Cornillie P, Gasthuys F, Gielen I, Schauvliege S (2017) A novel approach for regional anaesthesia of the auricular region in horses: an anatomic and imaging study. *Vet Anaesth Analg* **44**:656–664.

de Linde Henriksen M, Brooks DE (2014) Standing ophthalmic surgeries in horses. *Vet Clin Equine* **30**:91–110.

Martin-Flores M (2013) Neuromuscular blocking agents and monitoring in the equine patient. *Vet Clin Equine* **29**:131–154.

Trim CM (2017) Anesthesia for horses with colic. In: *The Equine Acute Abdomen*, 3rd edn. (eds Blikslager A, White NA, Moore JN, Mair TS), Wiley-Blackwell, London, pp. 511–538.

CHAPTER 12

PAIN

Jarred Williams, Katie Seabaugh, Molly Shepard
and Dana Peroni

DOI: 10.1201/9780429190940-12

12.1 Physiology, Recognition, and Local Anesthetic Techniques

Jarred Williams

12.1.1 INTRODUCTION

Historically, pain management in large animal veterinary medicine has included non-steroidal anti-inflammatory drugs and local analgesia. In recent years, this practice has changed and advanced. This chapter discusses the principles of pain physiology and management in equine patients.

12.1.2 WHAT IS PAIN?

- Pain is an unpleasant or aversive sensation or feeling (a perception) that is associated with actual or potential tissue damage.
- Pain can be physiologic or pathologic.
  - Physiologic pain is short-lived, protective, and associated with minimal to no tissue injury.
  - Pathologic pain typically occurs following tissue injury, though it can also occur with no tissue injury (spontaneous pain), in response to an innocent stimulus (allodynia), or as an exaggerated response to a stimulus (hyperalgesia).
- Pain is the end product of a multistep process that begins with an injury or stimulus in the periphery (nociception), which is transmitted to the brain and results in conscious perception of the insult.

Nociception is the stimulation of peripheral nociceptors that initiate a signal via the spinal cord to the brain. There are 5 steps in this process: transduction, transmission, modulation, projection, and perception (**Figure 12.1**).

- Transduction: Initiation of a nerve impulse.
  - A noxious stimuli (chemical, electrical, mechanical, or thermal) occurs.
  - Peripheral afferent nerve endings (nociceptors) detect the stimuli and convert (transduce) the signal to electrical energy.
  - Types of nociceptors include mechanoreceptors, thermoreceptors, chemoreceptors, and visceral nociceptors (for visceral pain).
- Transmission: The transfer of the nerve impulse to the spinal cord.
  - Nociceptors have 2 distinct types of axons, A-delta and C fibers, that transmit the electrical energy or nerve signal to cells in the dorsal horn of the spinal cord.
  - A-delta fibers: these fibers are myelinated, so they transfer the energy very quickly, giving off the initial, fast, and sharp onset of pain detected following a stimulus.
  - C fibers: these are unmyelinated, so the conduction of the signal is much slower, giving off the more prolonged, less intense dull ache or burn sensation.
- Modulation: The impulse from the periphery is received at the spinal cord and modified to reflect amplification of the signal to the brain or suppression of the signal.
  - A-delta and C fibers send sensory input to the cell bodies of the dorsal root ganglion and on to the dorsal horn of the spinal cord, where neurotransmitters are released (i.e. glutamate) into the synapse between the primary and secondary neurons.

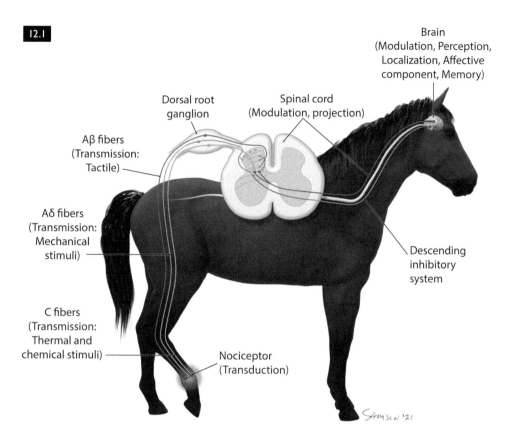

12.1

Brain
(Modulation, Perception, Localization, Affective component, Memory)

Dorsal root ganglion

Spinal cord
(Modulation, projection)

Aβ fibers
(Transmission: Tactile)

Aδ fibers
(Transmission: Mechanical stimuli)

Descending inhibitory system

C fibers
(Transmission: Thermal and chemical stimuli)

Nociceptor
(Transduction)

Figure 12.1 **Pain pathway (Illustrated by Joe Samson)**

- In the case of A-delta fibers the secondary neuron crosses, or decussates, the spinal cord and joins the spinothalamic tract.
- In the case of C fibers, there is a synapse on an interneuron prior to synapse onto the neuron that decussates and joins the spinothalamic tract.
- If there is a large or prolonged input along the C fibers, there can be a progressive "build up" of signal in the dorsal horn of the spinal cord from leakage of increased amounts of neurotransmitters out of the synapse and into supporting glial cells.
- Once activated, the glial cells can send neurotransmitters back into the synapse, propagating the nervous impulse without

the initial stimuli, or even after the initial injury has healed and no longer creates a signal.
- This process describes the "wind up" or increased sensitivity to pain.
- Projection: Transfer of the nerve impulse through the spinal cord to the brain.
  - The nervous impulse travels along fibers in the spinothalamic tract through the brainstem until synapsing on a third neuron in the thalamus.
  - The higher the frequency of this signal to the thalamus, the more intense the perception of pain.
  - The third neuron will project from the thalamus via the thalamocortical tract through the internal capsule and into

regions of the cortex, primarily the somatosensory cortex.

- In the case of C fibers, some fibers will branch off into the reticular and limbic systems, affecting sleep and emotions.
- Perception: Conscious awareness of the nerve impulse.
  - The magnitude of the pain is detected in the thalamus, but in the cortex, the origin or localization of the signal is determined and processed, and an efferent motor response can be initiated.

12.1.3 PRINCIPLES OF PAIN MANAGEMENT

- Once pain has been initiated and identified, management to minimize or eliminate its severity is vital.
- Pain management in veterinary medicine has been classified as acute, chronic, and cancerous. This chapter focuses on acute and chronic pain.
- Management of acute pain generally refers to pain encountered following an unplanned traumatic event, such as most accidents, or before, during, and after a planned traumatic event, such as surgery.
- Management of chronic pain has been described as treating pain that persists for greater than 3–6 months. Chronic pain is frequently acute pain that persists beyond the expected time frame, thus becoming chronic, and may be due to a "wind-up response".
- A wind-up response is when an initial injury leads to repeated peripheral and central sensitization, resulting in increased pain sensation over time.
- Adaptive vs maladaptive pain.
  - Adaptive pain is the appropriate and expected response to a painful event that is innate to a species for avoidance of further injury, healing, and survival. The goal of acute pain management is

to eliminate the painful stimulus for this response, which often involves stabilization of an injury, as well as management of the pain associated with the stabilization. If acute pain is not adequately eliminated, chronic or maladaptive pain may result.
  - Maladaptive pain is present following the healing of an injury and can become its own disease process due to abnormal sensory input and processing.

12.1.4 PAIN IDENTIFICATION, SCORING, AND MANAGEMENT

Recognition of pain is vital for its management. When an animal shows signs of discomfort, these have to be interpreted by a person. This can be subjective; however, when these signs are well-defined and obvious, the identification of pain is easy. When the signs are more subtle, pain recognition can be more difficult, as demonstrated by Dujardin and van Loon in 2011, who concluded that 40–60% of surveyed veterinarians classified their own ability to recognize pain in horses as moderate. Thus, many pain scoring systems have been developed to assess pain in experimental models and clinical cases.

12.1.4.1 Pain Scales
- Composite Pain Scale (CPS).
- Composite Measure Pain Scale (CMPS).
- Horse Grimace Scale (HGS).
- Equine Acute Abdominal Pain Scales 1 and 2 (EAAPS-1 and -2).
- Numerical Rating Scale (NRS).
- Post Abdominal Surgery Pain Assessment Scale (PASPAS).

- Each scale differs by their assignment of score or category to a variety of behaviors encountered. Regardless of which method is used, it is important to ensure that pain is ameliorated once identified.

- Pain negatively affects clinical outcomes.
  - Pain and inflammation can elicit systemic responses that have deleterious effects on organ systems (i.e. decreased gastrointestinal motility).
  - Horses undergoing exploratory celiotomy spend less time in locomotion and more time displaying painful behavior. They also have an increased NRS score, higher plasma cortisol, and higher heart rate as compared to control groups.
  - When CPS and NRS scores were used to assess survival after gastrointestinal surgery, animals without complications had significantly lower CPS and NRS scores compared to horses that were euthanized post-operatively or that had to undergo a repeat celiotomy.
  - Horses with prolonged discomfort in one limb can develop laminitis or deformities on the supporting limb.
- Many of the analgesic drugs administered in the pre-, intra-, and post-operative periods have side effects, particularly decreased gastrointestinal transit time and delayed mucosal healing.
- "The potential for ileus should not override the need to provide analgesia in a given case" (Sanchez and Robertson 2014).
- There are many methods of pain management. When considering medications, routes, and dosing regimens, it is important to understand where on the pain pathway the medication may alter the nerve impulse (i.e. peripheral vs central).

12.1.4.2 Classic Pain Management

- In equine veterinary medicine, the most common drugs used for pain management are NSAIDs, local anesthetics (i.e., lidocaine or mepivacaine) opioids, alpha-2 adrenergic agonists, and N-methyl-D-aspartate (NMDA) receptor antagonists (i.e., ketamine).

- NSAIDs and local blocks work peripherally by preventing transduction and transmission of nociceptive signals to the spinal cord.
- Alpha-2 adrenergic agonists and ketamine work centrally (at the level of the spinal cord to the brain) to alter modulation, projection, and perception of nociception.
- Opioids work centrally and peripherally to inhibit nociceptive input having an effect at transmission, modulation, projection, and perception.
- Clinicians can combine drugs to create a multimodal approach to pain management by altering the pain signal in multiple locations. Multimodal analgesia is the use of more than one analgesic class or technique for pain management.
- A variety of drugs have been used in conjunction and administered via constant rate infusion (**Table 12.1**).
  - Lidocaine and opioids (butorphanol or morphine).
  - Lidocaine and ketamine.
  - Lidocaine and alpha-2 agonists (xylazine, romifidine, or detomidine).
  - Opioids and alpha-2 agonists.
  - Ketamine and opioids.
  - Ketamine and alpha-2 agonists.
- Combinations can include up to 3 or 4 of these medications (i.e., morphine-lidocaine-ketamine and detomidine-ketamine-lidocaine).

12.1.4.3 Local Anesthetics and Techniques

- Regional anesthesia can be used preemptively or to manage pain after the tissue trauma has already occurred. Like systemic usage of pain medications, regional anesthesia must be repeatedly administered to remain effective.
- The areas of the body where anesthesia is most commonly applied include the distal

Table 12.1 **Example of doses (bolus and CRI) of some drug combinations used for pain management**

COMBINATIONS	BOLUS (IV)	CRI (IV)	COMMENTS
Xylazine + butorphanol	(X) 0.1–0.6 mg/kg + (B) 0.01–0.02 mg/kg	(X) 0.5–0.6 mg/kg/hour + (B) 0.01–0.02 mg/kg/hour	Can be used in standing or anesthetized horses.
Detomidine + butorphanol	(D) 2–5 µg/kg + (B) 0.01–0.02 mg/kg	(D) 0.1–0.3 µg/kg/min + (B) 0.01–0.02 mg/kg	Can be used in standing or anesthetized horses.
Detomidine + morphine	(D) 2–5 µg/kg + (M) 0.1 mg/kg (IM or IV slowly)	(D) 0.1–0.3 µg/kg/min + (M) 0.03 mg/kg/hour	Can be used in standing or anesthetized horses. If morphine bolus IV, administer slowly to avoid possible histamine release.
Xylazine + morphine	(X) 0.1–0.5 mg/kg + (M) 0.1 mg/kg (IM or IV slowly)	(X) 0.65 mg/kg/hour +/- (M) 0.03 mg/kg/hour	Can be used in standing or anesthetized horses. If morphine bolus IV, administer slowly to avoid possible histamine release.
Xylazine + ketamine	(X) 0.1–0.5 mg/kg (no ketamine loading dose)	(X) 0.5–0.6 mg/kg/hour + (K) 0.4–1.2 mg/kg/hour	Can be used in standing or anesthetized horses. In standing horses administer xylazine first and wait for signs of sedation before starting ketamine.
Xylazine + lidocaine	(X) 0.1–0.5 mg/kg + (L) 1.3–2 mg/kg	(X) 0.5–0.6 mg/kg/hour + (L) 3 mg/kg/hour	Can be used in standing or anesthetized horses.
Xylazine + lidocaine + ketamine	(X) 0.1–0.5 mg/kg + (L) 1.3–2 mg/kg (no ketamine loading dose)	(X) 0.5–0.6 mg/kg/hour + (L) 3 mg/kg/hour + (K) 0.4–1.2 mg/kg/hour	Can be used in standing or anesthetized horses. In standing horses administer xylazine first and wait for signs of sedation before starting ketamine.
Xylazine + lidocaine + ketamine	(X) 0.1–0.6 mg/kg + (L) 1.5–2 mg/kg + (K) 1–3 mg/kg	(X) 1 mg/kg/hour + (L) 3 mg/kg/hour + (K) 1–3 mg/kg/hour	In anesthetized horses. Decrease xylazine to 0.5 mg/kg/hour after first hour. Discontinue lidocaine 30 minutes prior to recovery. Decrease ketamine by 25% every hour.
Lidocaine + ketamine	(L) 1.5–2 mg/kg + (K) 1–3 mg/kg	(L) 3 mg/kg/hour + (K) 1–3 mg/kg/hour	In anesthetized horses. Discontinue lidocaine 30 minutes prior to recovery. Decrease ketamine by 25% every hour).

limb, head, epidural, intrathecal, and intra-articular space.
- When performing a nerve block, aseptic technique is recommended.
- Local anesthetic agents differ in onset and duration of effect (Table 12.2).

12.1.4.4 Nerve Blocks of the Limb

Palmar/Plantar Digital (Heel Block) (**Figure 12.2**).

- Location and method: A 25-gauge, 5/8-inch needle is inserted in a distal direction directly over the neurovascular bundle about 1 cm above the collateral cartilages on the foot.
- Desensitizes sole, navicular apparatus (bone, bursa, and supporting ligaments), heel bulb, digital cushion, coffin joint, deep digital flexor tendon (distal to the site of insertion), and distal sesamoidean ligaments.

Table 12.2 Dose, onset, and duration of commonly used local anesthetics

DRUG	DOSE (MG/KG)	ONSET OF ACTION (MINUTES)	DURATION OF ACTION (MINUTES)
Lidocaine	2–6	5–10	60–90
Bupivicaine	1–2	20–30	240–360
Mepivacaine	2–5	5–10	120–180

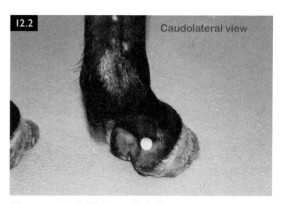

Figure 12.2 **Palmar digital**

- Proximal movement of local anesthetic solution can desensitize pastern joint and dorsal laminae.
- Volume: 1.5–3 ml of local anesthetic at each site.

Abaxial Sesamoid (**Figure 12.3**).
- Location and method: A 25-gauge, 5/8-inch needle is inserted in a distal direction directly over the neurovascular bundle along the abaxial border of the base of each proximal sesamoid bone.
- Desensitizes the entire foot, pastern joint, superficial and deep digital flexor tendons below the proximal sesamoids, the middle phalanx, mid-distal proximal phalanx, and distal sesamoidean ligaments.
- Proximal movement of local anesthetic solution can desensitize the fetlock joint.
- Volume: 1.5–3 ml of local anesthetic at each site.

Low Palmar/Plantar (Low 4 Point) (**Figure 12.4**).
- Location and method.
  - A 22-gauge, 1-inch needle is inserted beneath the distal end of the second and fourth metacarpal bones and directed towards the palmar aspect of the third metacarpal bone to anesthetize the medial and lateral palmar metacarpal nerves.

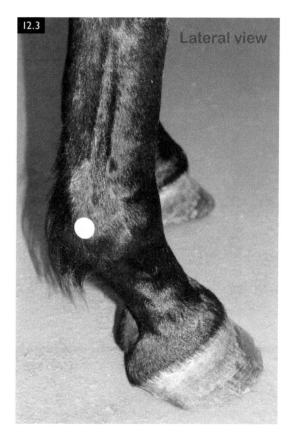

Figure 12.3 **Abaxial sesamoid**

  - Desensitizes the medial and lateral palmar nerves and the medial and lateral palmar metacarpal nerves.
  - A 25-gauge, 5/8-inch needle is inserted subcutaneously, along the dorsal aspect

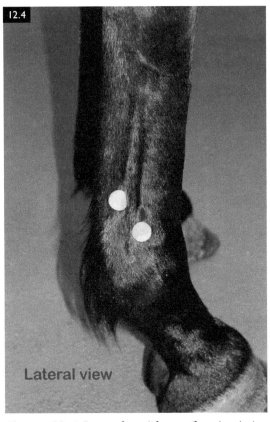

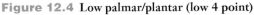

Figure 12.4 Low palmar/plantar (low 4 point)

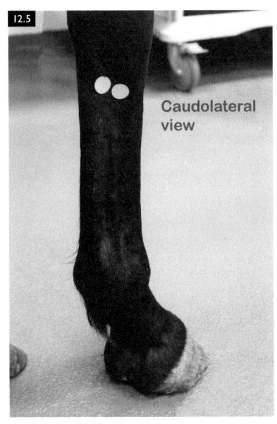

Figure 12.5 High palmar/plantar (high 4 point)

of the deep digital flexor tendon to anesthetize the medial and lateral palmar nerves.
  • Desensitizes the fetlock and structures distal to it.
• Volume: 1.5–3 ml of local anesthetic at each site.

High Palmar/Plantar (High 4 Point) (**Figure 12.5**).
• Location and method:
  • A 25-gauge, 5/8-inch needle is inserted below the level of the carpometacarpal joint adjacent to the dorsal surface of the deep digital flexor tendon to anesthetize medial and lateral palmar nerves.

• Desensitizes the medial and lateral palmar nerves and the medial and lateral palmar metacarpal nerves at the level of the carpometacarpal joint.
• A 20- to 22-gauge, 1.5-inch needle is inserted below the level of the carpometacarpal bone along the palmar aspect of the second and fourth metacarpal bones directed dorsally towards the palmar aspect of the third metacarpal bone to anesthetize the medial and lateral palmar metacarpal nerves.
  • Desensitizes the deep and superficial flexor tendons, second and fourth metacarpal bones, and the proximal aspect of the suspensory ligament.

- Proximal movement of local anesthetic solution can desensitize the carpometacarpal and middle carpal joints.
- Volume: 3–5 ml of local anesthetic at each site.

Other nerve blocks include the ulnar, median, cutaneous antebrachial, tibial, and peroneal; however, these are infrequently performed during anesthesia due to the potential for complication while attempting to stand during recovery.

12.1.4.5 Nerve Blocks of the Head
Maxillary (**Figure 12.6**).
- Location and method: A 20- to 22-gauge, 3.5-inch spinal needle is inserted ventral to the zygomatic process. The needle is directed rostrally and ventrally until the needle comes in contact with the

pterygopalatine fossa. The maxillary nerve is very close to this location, and the horse may abruptly move its head if it is contacted.
- Desensitizes the maxillary and premaxillary teeth, associated gingiva, as well as paranasal sinuses and nasal cavity.
- Volume: 15–20 ml of local anesthetic along the bone and as the needle is withdrawn.

Infraorbital.
- This block is not recommended due to possible nerve damage and potential for self-mutilation.

Mandibular (**Figure 12.7**).
- Location and method: A 20- to 22-gauge, 6-inch needle is inserted medially and

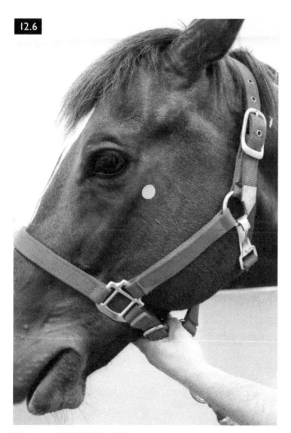

Figure 12.6 Maxillary nerve

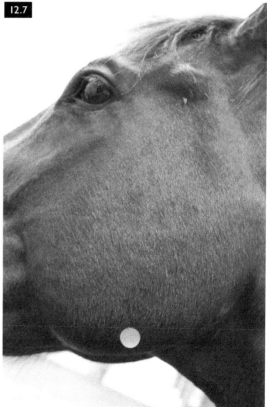

Figure 12.7 Mandibular nerve

dorsally along the ventral border of the mandible (the horizontal ramus) at the level of an imaginary line drawn from the lateral canthus to the spot of insertion on the mandible, just rostral to the angle of the mandible.

- Desensitizes the mandible and all of its dental structures.
- Volume: 15–20 ml of local anesthetic at the mandibular foramen.

Mental (**Figure 12.8**).

- Location and method: A 20- to 22-gauge, 1.5-inch needle is inserted through the mental foramen and into the mandibular canal. The foramen is palpated along the rostral aspect of the horizontal ramus of the mandible after elevating the tendon of the depressor labii inferioris dorsally.
- Desensitizes the lip, chin, mandibular incisors and canine, and associated gingiva.
- Volume: 5–10 ml of local anesthetic within the mandibular canal.

12.1.4.6 Sacro-Coccygeal Epidural Block

- Location and method (**Figure 12.9**): While flexing and extending the tail, the intervertebral space between coccygeal

vertebrae 1 and 2 or 2 and 3 is palpated. An 18- to 22-gauge, 1.5-inch needle is inserted perpendicular to the space through the skin and subcutaneous tissue.

- Desensitizes perineum, anus, vagina, and urethra with low volume (less 6 ml). With high volume (greater than 6 ml) it can provide analgesia to the bladder and hindlimbs.
- When administering high volume, use opioids only to avoid loss of motor to the hindlimbs.
- The hub of the needle is filled with sterile saline, and the needle is advanced until the saline is taken up into the needle.
- The disappearance of fluid indicates that the needle entered the epidural space. The drug can then be slowly injected. This is referred to as the "hanging drop" method.

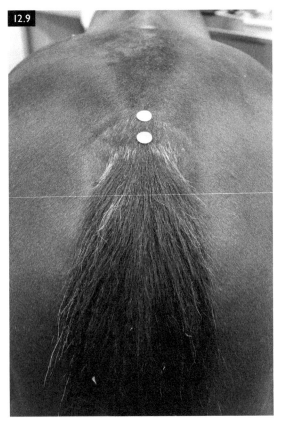

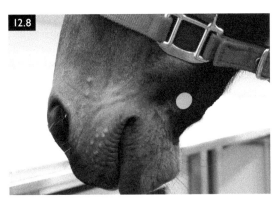

Figure 12.8 **Mental nerve**

Figure 12.9 **Sacro-coccygeal epidural**

- Alternatively, an 18- to 22-gauge, 3.5-inch needle is inserted caudal to either space at a 45° angle until it touches the caudal body of the cranially located coccygeal vertebra.
- The hub is again filled with sterile saline, and the angle of the needle is increased as the tip of the needle is "walked" off the vertebrae until the saline disappears, and the remainder of the volume is injected.
- Volume: For an average-sized adult, 2–3 ml of local anesthetic of choice is expanded with 2–3 ml of saline. This combination can have a very small amount of an alpha-2 agonist added (i.e. 30–50 mg xylazine) for enhanced effect.

12.1.4.7 Pudendal Block

- Location and method (**Figure 12.10**): A 20- to 22-gauge, 1.5-inch needle is inserted 1 inch lateral to the left and right of the anus, approximately 1 inch dorsal to the palpable aspect of the ischial arch. The needle is angled ventrally until it contacts the arch, and local anesthetic solution is injected.
- Desensitizes the penis and internal prepuce.
- Volume: 5 ml of local anesthetic at each site (left and right of anus).

12.1.4.8 Intra-Articular Blocks

- Intra-articular analgesia is most commonly performed following arthroscopy or

joint lavage. While any local anesthetic can be added to the joint for complete desensitization, morphine is more commonly added to provide analgesia without complete desensitization.
- Local anesthetics have been associated with chondrotoxicity. Mepivacaine is the local anesthetic least likely to cause chondrocyte damage. Therefore, if intra-articular local anesthetic is required, mepivacaine is preferred.
- This is a technique used to aid anesthetic recovery in the patient with a painful joint.

Distal interphalangeal (Coffin) (**Figure 12.11**).
- Location and method: A 20- to 22-gauge, 1.5-inch needle is inserted towards the midline, approximately 0.5 inches proximal

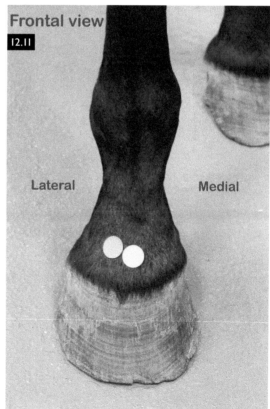

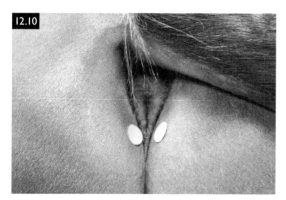

Figure 12.10 Pudendal

Figure 12.11 Distal interphalangeal (coffin)

to the coronary band and 0.75 inches lateral to midline. The needle is inserted perpendicular to the ground.

- Alternatively, the needle can be inserted parallel to the ground, approximately 0.5 inches proximal to the coronary band on midline.
- Volume: 4–6 ml of local anesthetic.

Proximal interphalangeal (Pastern) (**Figure 12.12**)
- Location and method: A 20-gauge, 1- to 1.5-inch needle is inserted towards the midline, approximately 0.5 inches distal to the lateral eminence of distal P1 and parallel to the ground surface.
- Volume: 8–10 ml of local anesthetic.

Metacarpo (-tarso) phalangeal (Fetlock) (**Figure 12.13**).

- Location and method: A 20-gauge, 1- to 1.5-inch needle is inserted into the palmar/plantar pouch just proximal to the proximal sesamoid bone, dorsal to the suspensory ligament, and palmar/plantar to the 3rd metacarpus/metatarsus in a lateral to medial direction.
  - Alternatively, the needle can be inserted dorsally, also in a lateral to medial direction, just palmar/plantar to the common digital extensor tendon.
- Volume: 8–12 ml of local anesthetic.

Carpus (Radiocarpal) (**Figure 12.14**).
- Location and method: With the forelimb lifted off the ground and flexed at the carpus, an 18- to 22-gauge, 1- to 1.5-inch needle is inserted in a dorsal to palmar/plantar direction medial or lateral to the

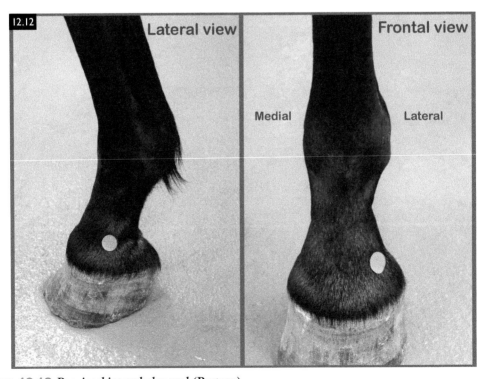

Figure 12.12 Proximal interphalangeal (Pastern)

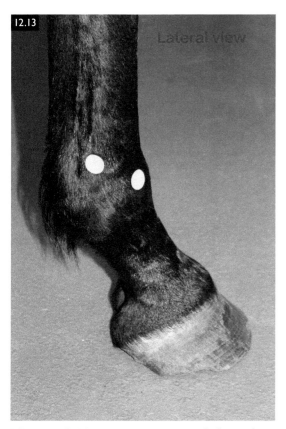

Figure 12.13 **Metacarpo (-tarso) phalangeal (Fetlock)**

extensor carpi radialis, distal to the distal end of the radius, and proximal to the proximal row of carpal bones.
- When flexed, there is an obvious indentation created within these borders.
- Volume: 7–10 ml of local anesthetic.

Carpus (Middle Carpal) (**Figure 12.15**).
- Location and method: With the forelimb lifted off the ground and flexed at the carpus, an 18- to 22-gauge, 1- to 1.5-inch needle is inserted in a dorsal to palmar/plantar direction medial or lateral to the extensor carpi radialis, distal to the distal

end of the proximal row of carpal bones, and proximal to the distal row of carpal bones.
- When flexed, there is an obvious indentation created within these borders.
- Volume: 7–10 ml of local anesthetic.

Tarsus (tarsocrural or tibiotarsal) (**Figure 12.16**).
- Location and method: An 18- to 20-gauge, 1.5-inch needle is inserted approximately 1–1.5 inches distal to the medial malleolus, medial or lateral to the saphenous vein.
- Volume: 10–20 ml of local anesthetic.

Tarsus (tarsometatarsal [**Figure 12.17**] and distal intertarsal [**Figure 12.18**]).
- The distal hock joints are 2 of the more commonly injected joints for purposes of routine anti-inflammation and lameness evaluation.
- They are infrequently injected for the purposes of analgesia and desensitization for anesthetic recovery.

Other articular blocks include the elbow, shoulder, stifle, and hip. While less risky than regional analgesia at sites more proximally located on the limb, these blocks are also less frequently performed during anesthesia due to the potential for complication while attempting to stand during the recovery process. When performed, they are more typically added to the joint following an arthroscopy.

12.1.4.9 Intrathecal Blocks
Navicular bursa (**Figure 12.19**).
- Location and method: With the foot on the ground, an 18- to 22-gauge, 3.5-inch spinal needle is inserted midway between the heel bulbs, just proximal to the coronary band, until it hits bone.

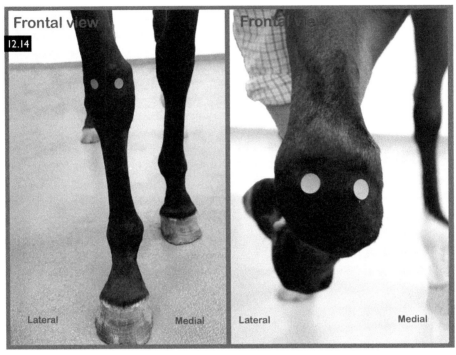

Figure 12.14 Carpus (radiocarpal)

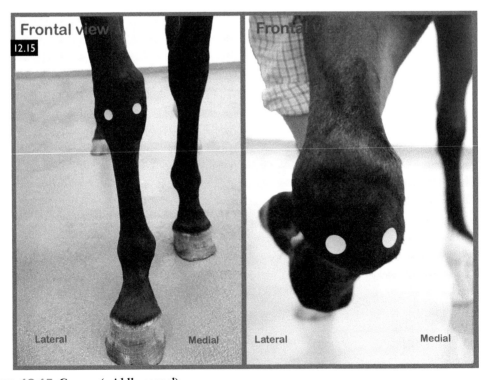

Figure 12.15 Carpus (middle carpal)

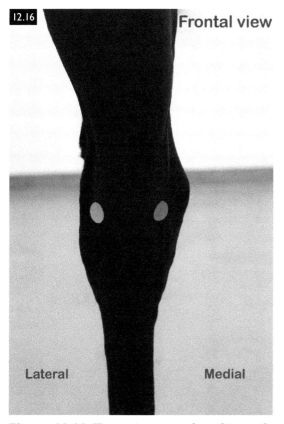

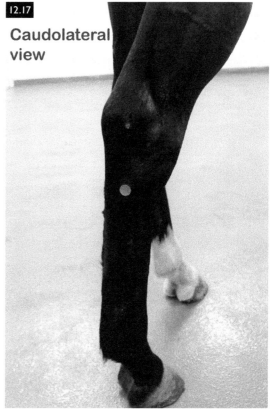

Figure 12.16 Tarsus (tarsocrural or tibiotarsal)   Figure 12.17 Tarsus (tarsometatarsal)

- This is frequently done with radiographic guidance.
- Volume: 2–4 ml of local anesthetic.

Digital tendon sheath (**Figure 12.20**).
- Location and method: An 18- to 22-gauge, 1- to 1.5-inch spinal needle is inserted into the sheath at numerous locations.
- The most reliable approach is palmar/plantar axial sesamoid approach. With the limb flexed, the needle is injected at the level of the midbody of the medial or lateral proximal sesamoid, just axial to either bone.
- The needle is inserted in a transverse plane and aimed towards midline to a depth of 0.5–0.75 inches.
- Volume: 8–12 ml of local anesthetic.

Other bursae that are infrequently injected, particularly during an anesthetic event, are the bicipital bursa, bursae of the calcaneus, and supraspinous bursa.

12.1.4.10 Local Anesthetic Catheters

Catheters (**Figure 12.21**) can be placed in some of the areas mentioned to provide constant analgesia without the need to continually stick the patient. The most common catheter sites are epidural, perineural, and intra-articular.

12.1.5 CASE EXAMPLES

- A 16-year-old Quarter Horse gelding, weighing 450 kg, presented for an acute non-weight-bearing lameness on the right

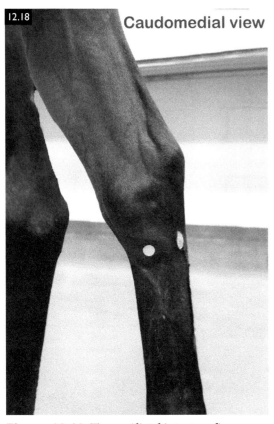

Caudomedial view

Figure 12.18 Tarsus (distal intertarsal)

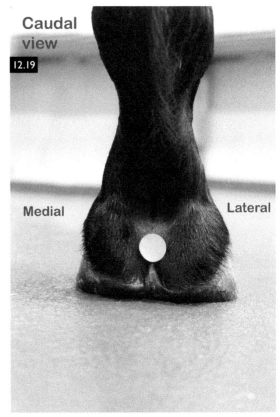

Caudal view

Medial   Lateral

Figure 12.19 Navicular bursa

hindlimb. The horse was sensitive across the solar surface when hoof testers were applied.
- A plantar digital (PD) nerve block was administered with 3 ml of 2% lidocaine medially and laterally.
  - Approximately 10 minutes later the lameness was gone, and the horse would readily stand without discomfort.
- Radiographs revealed a gas shadowing within the sole of the hoof, consistent with a subsolar hoof abscess.
- The foot was soaked in water and Epsom salts overnight. In anticipation of discomfort after the nerve block had worn off, the gelding received 2 grams of phenylbutazone orally.
- Approximately 5 hours after the block was performed, the gelding was again

non-weight-bearing on the right hindlimb, had a heart rate of 80 beats/minute, was sweating profusely, and had muscle fasciculations.
- The PD nerve block was repeated with 5 ml of mepivacaine, and 10 mg of butorphanol was administered intramuscularly.
  - The patient was weight-bearing with a heart rate of 40 beats/minute approximately 20 minutes later.
- The next morning, the patient was once again very painful and had the PD nerve block with mepivacaine. He also received 10 mg of butorphanol IM and 1 gram of phenylbutazone orally, while the foot soak was removed and the hoof sole debrided in an effort to identify and open the abscess.

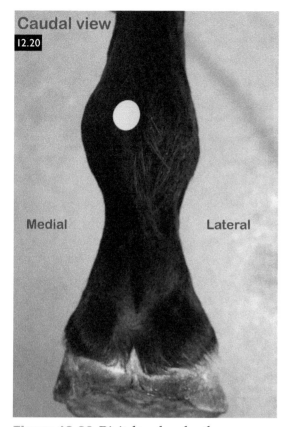

Caudal view

Medial   Lateral

Figure 12.20 **Digital tendon sheath**

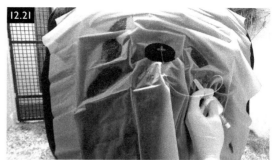

Figure 12.21 **Epidural catheter**

- Exploration was unsuccessful. A second soak was applied to the foot, and the patient had an epidural catheter placed without complications.
- Through the epidural catheter approximately 15 mg of preservative free morphine and 30 mg xylazine were administered every 6 hours.
- The IM butorphanol was discontinued, and the oral phenylbutazone was continued at a dose of 1 gram every 12 hours.
- After the PD nerve block wore off, the patient returned to his non-weight-bearing state, and his heart rate increased to 56 beats/minute.
- Approximately 24 hours later the soak was again removed, the foot was assessed,

and the abscess could not be identified or successfully drained.
- Due to the persistent tachycardia, most likely from pain, an intravenous catheter was placed, and the patient was started on a detomidine-ketamine-lidocaine constant rate infusion (D-K-L CRI). The epidural drugs were continued at 6-hour intervals, and the oral phenylbutazone was discontinued.
  - The patient remained non-weight-bearing for the next 24 hours; however, his heart rate never went above 36 beats/minute, and his appetite was great.
- The following morning the PD nerve block was once again performed, and the sole was assessed.
- Upon assessment, a small bruise was identified and opened with a hoof knife. Immediately after opening the sole, purulent material was evacuated, and a draining track to the abscess was encountered.
  - The draining track was opened and lavaged with a dilute betadine solution. The patient was maintained on the D-K-L CRI and epidural administration of morphine and xylazine every 6 hours.
  - Throughout the remainder of the day and overnight, the patient was weight-bearing with a heart rate of 36 beats/minute and a great appetite.

- The next morning the area of debridement on the sole was lavaged and deemed to be healing.
- The D-K-L CRI was discontinued, intravenous phenylbutazone at 1 gram every 12 hours was administered, and the epidural administration of medication was decreased to every 12 hours.
  - The patient remained comfortable for the next 24 hours, at which time the epidural catheter was removed and the intravenous phenylbutazone was continued at an amount of 1 gram every 12 hours.
  - The patient remained comfortable for the following 24 hours and the sole was reassessed the next morning, at which time it was determined the sole was healing nicely.
- The patient was kept on phenylbutazone, but the route was switched from intravenous to oral following removal of the IV catheter.
- The patient was maintained on oral phenylbutazone every 12 hours for 3 days before decreasing the amount to 1 gram orally for 5 days.
- The foot was assessed for healing daily and kept clean.
- Approximately 10 days later the foot was healed and the patient was comfortable without any medication.

12.2 Rehabilitation Techniques

Katie Seabaugh

12.2.1 INTRODUCTION

Musculoskeletal pain (MSP) in horses is common and can result in significant reduction in performance and financial loss for owners. Common treatments for MSP in horses involve targeted or systemic medications. Such treatments include, but are not limited to, intra-articular corticosteroid treatments or systemic non-steroidal anti-inflammatory drugs (NSAIDs). Repeated or continuous treatment with these drugs can have consequences.

12.2.2 MUSCULOSKELETAL REHABILITATION

- Musculoskeletal rehabilitation has been an increasing focus in the veterinary literature in the last decade.
- Rehabilitation from injury in horses is not a novel idea and has undergone many changes for as long as horses have been performing.
- Current theories regarding rehabilitation from injury are a fine balance between minimizing strain while not completely restricting exercise.
- As we learn more about rehabilitation from injury, as well as extrapolate information from the human and canine literature, rehabilitation programs are targeted at injury prevention and pain management.
- Human literature has found benefit in physiotherapy for pain reduction. People with chronic musculoskeletal pain showed improvements in pain and function following a 15-week multidisciplinary rehabilitation program.

- Evidence-based clinical practices recommended therapeutic exercises for chronic and subacute low back pain, knee osteoarthritis, and chronic neck pain.
- A more recent study in people found that a musculoskeletal rehabilitation program was associated with lower purchases of prescribed pain medications.
- Equine practitioners are beginning to extrapolate this success in humans to horses.
- The multidisciplinary rehabilitation program described for humans by Volker et al. (2016) utilized a team comprised of a rehabilitation physician, an occupational therapist, a social worker, a psychologist, and a physical therapist.
  - When dealing with horses, the veterinarian wears all these hats. They diagnose the injury (physician), understand the desired function of the patient (occupational therapist), predict the interaction between pasture-mates and owner (social worker), assess the demeanor of the horse (psychologist), and create a controlled exercise program (physical therapist).
  - Most commonly, veterinarians balance stall rest and paddock turnout, deciding between hand walking and tack walking and fine-tuning rehabilitation timelines. Intermixed within these programs is the encompassment of additional rehabilitation techniques.

12.2.2.1 Passive Range of Motion
- In the early stages following injury, a horse's activity level is restricted. During this time,

however, passive range of motion exercises can be utilized to regain or maintain normal joint function and neuromotor function.

- These exercises can easily be instituted during stall rest. Such exercises include maximum flexion and extension of target joints for a series of repetitions.
  - Example: Passive range of motion for the fetlock. The toe is pulled up for maximum flexion (**Figure 12.22**) and pushed away for maximum extension (**Figure 12.23**).
- During each grooming session the target joint should be manually flexed and extended maximally. This should be done for 10 repetitions and each position held for 5 seconds.

12.2.2.2 Dynamic Mobilization Exercises

- Rehabilitation techniques can be utilized for pain management by providing muscle strengthening and increased range of

motion. Stabilization of the back by preactivation of the multifidus muscle and transversus abdominus reduced low back pain in people.

- Dynamic mobilization exercises (DME) have been found to increase diameter of the multifidus muscle in horses.
  - Atrophy of this multifidus muscle occurs in horses with thoracolumbar pain, especially associated with spinous impingement and facet joint osteoarthritis.
  - A common DME is a baited stretch or "carrot stretch".
    - "Carrot stretch" can be performed by asking the horse to extend its neck (**Figure 12.24**), flex its neck ("chin between carpi," **Figure 12.25**), and bend laterally ("chin to girth," **Figure 12.26**, and "chin to flank," **Figure 12.27**).
- In the equine literature, DME are stretching exercises to increase the strength of the neck and back.

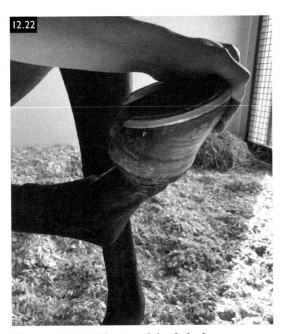

Figure 12.22 Flexion of the fetlock

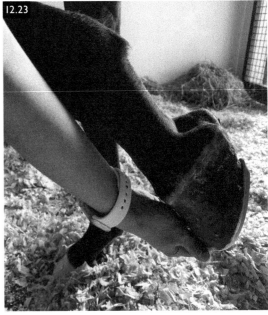

Figure 12.23 Extension of the fetlock

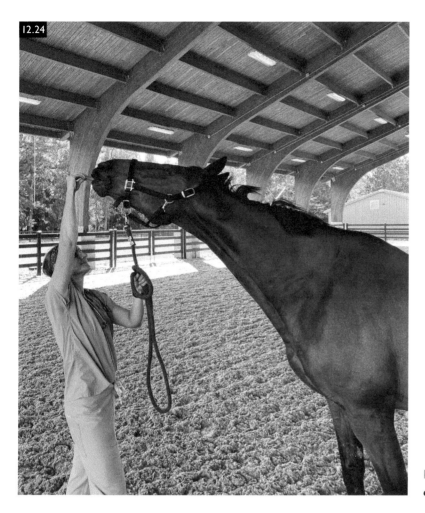

Figure 12.24 Extension of the neck

- Any form of active range of motion can be utilized in a rehabilitation program with the goal of decreasing pain. Walking on an underwater treadmill has been found to increase range of motion in various joints of horses.
- This modality can be incorporated into a rehabilitation program following arthroscopic surgery to regain range of motion and reduce pain.
- The use of weights and tactile stimulators has also been described to increase active range of motion.
- Stimulation devices placed on the hind pasterns of trotting horses resulted in an increased range of motion of the fetlock, tarsus, and stifle.
- Increasing the range of motion of the hind limb improves movement but also strengthens the muscles of the hind end, which will help return the horse to soundness following injury.

12.2.2.3 Gymnastic Training
- Gymnastic training is another option for exercise that can be performed while horses are in a rehabilitation program.
- In-hand gymnastics include walking over poles, backing, walking in tight circles, and pelvic tilting.

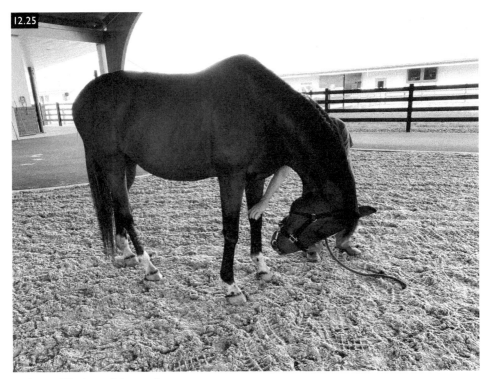

Figure 12.25 Flexion of the neck

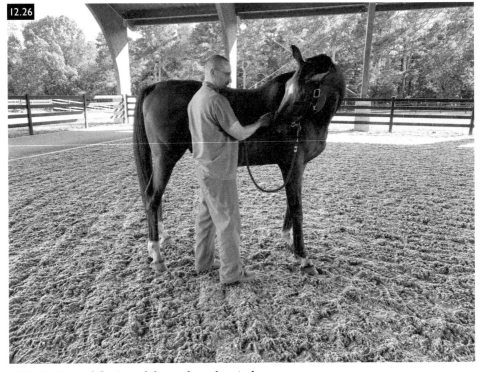

Figure 12.26 Lateral flexion of the neck to the girth

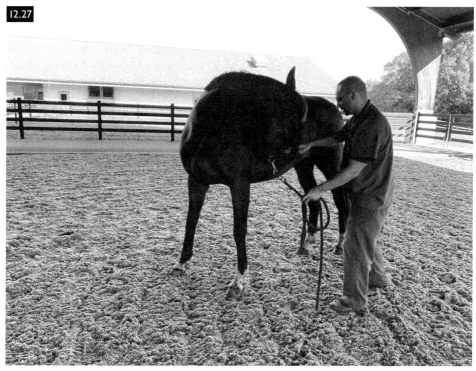

Figure 12.27 Lateral flexion of the neck to the flank

- de Oliveira et al. (2015) found that DME in combination with gymnastic training increased stride quality in healthy horses.

12.2.2.4 Aquatic Therapy
- The therapeutic effects of water immersion have been recognized for centuries.
- Pain may be relieved due to the effects of pressure and temperature on nerve endings as well as a result of muscle relaxation in people.
  - Patients suffering from rheumatoid arthritis showed significant improvement of joint tenderness and knee range of motion following treatment with hydrotherapy.
- Aquatic therapy has been widely used in rehabilitation programs for humans.
- There are five variables that are involved in aquatic therapy: temperature, osmolality, buoyancy, viscosity, and hydrostatic pressure.
  - Many of these parameters have not been subjected to controlled clinical studies in horses, but increased range of motion has been reported.
- Benefits that have been described in human and canine patients can be extrapolated to our equine patients.

12.2.3 SPECIFIC EXERCISES

12.2.3.1 Baited Stretches ("Carrot Stretches")
- Are an easy exercise that can be done to strengthen the muscles of the horse's core.
- This will help stabilize the back and abdomen, resulting in pain reduction.

- It may appear that the horse is only moving their neck, but you will see that they are flexing and extending their back as well.
- Baited stretches as described by Stubbs and Clayton (2008).
  - Flexion.
    - Chin to chest.
    - Chin between carpi.
    - Chin between fore fetlocks.
  - Extension.
    - Neck extended (chin as far forward as possible).
  - Lateral flexion (to each side).
    - Chin to girth.
    - Chin to flank.
    - Chin to tarsus.
  - These exercises should be performed approximately 3 times a week.
    - Each stretch should be performed for 5 repetitions.
    - The goal should be to get the horse to hold the stretch for 5 seconds.
    - Avoid a jerking motion to achieve the stretch. If the horse is unable to reach all the way to your target, start with a shorter distance.
    - Stop the exercises if the horse displays any signs of pain or discomfort.
      - In the early stages, it is helpful to place the horse with one side against a wall so that they cannot move away when you ask them to bend to each side.
    - After 1 month of exercises you may be able to increase the hold time to 10 seconds.

12.2.3.2 Gymnastic Training Exercises
- Walking over poles.
- Backing.
- Walking in tight circles.
- Pelvic tilting.

12.2.3.3 Hind-End Strengthening
- The specific exercises listed here are targeted to increase muscle strength in the hind end.
- We are specifically targeting the quadriceps, gluteal, biceps femoris, semimembranosus, and semitendinosus muscles.
- These muscles are important for lumbosacral and sacro-iliac joint extension, pelvic limb retraction, hip extension, and stifle flexion. They are also engaged during the weight-bearing portion of the stride.
- The following exercises should be performed 3 days a week. They do not *all* have to be done every session.
  - Hill work.
    - Walk up hills.
    - Make sure they don't shorten their stride.
    - Start with mild slopes and slowly increase the grade.
    - Don't walk straight down; zig-zag down.
  - Lateral tail pulls.
    - Weight shifting to engage the stabilizer muscles used during weight bearing.
    - Pull and hold (**Figure 12.28**).
    - Start with 2 sets of 5 seconds each direction and build on the length of time that you hold (up to 20 seconds).
    - It should take several weeks to build to 20 seconds.
  - Walk over ground poles.
    - Start with 4–6 single poles (**Figure 12.29**).
    - Walk over the poles for 10 minutes.
    - After two weeks elevate one of the poles to a height of 40 cm.

12.2.3.4 Pelvic Stabilizing
- These final series of exercises will help strengthen the abdominal muscles and pelvic stabilizing muscles.

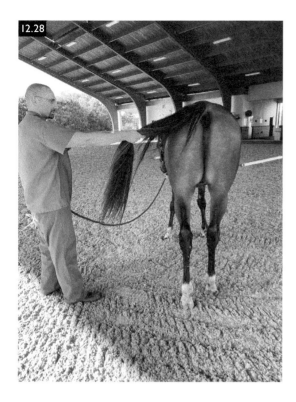

Figure 12.28 Tail pull and hold

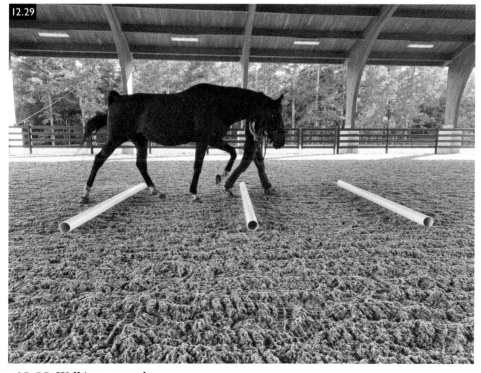

Figure 12.29 Walking over poles

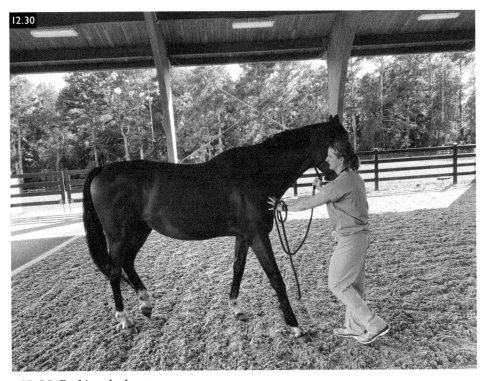

Figure 12.30 Backing the horse

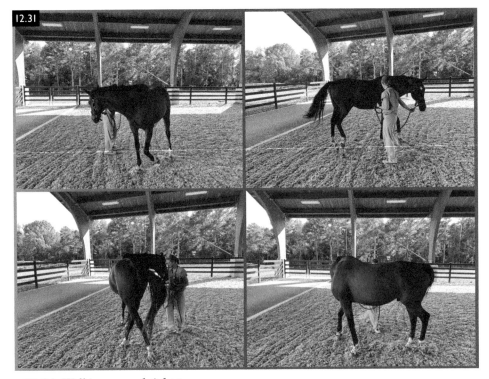

Figure 12.31 Walking around tight turns

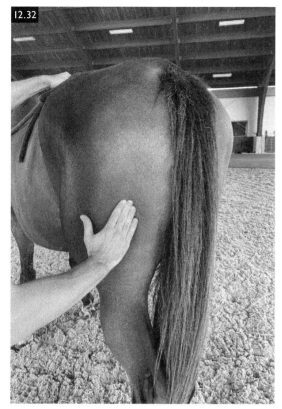

Figure 12.32 **Applying pressure to biceps femoris and semitendinosus**

- This too is aiming to strengthen the core.
  - Backing.
    - Straight lines on firm footing (**Figure 12.30**).
    - Progress to softer footing and then to backing up mild slopes.
    - Start with 10 strides.
  - Walking around tight turns (**Figure 12.31**).
    - Circle to the left for 5 turns.
    - Rest.
    - Circle to the right for 5 turns.
    - Figure eight for 5 repetitions.
    - Make sure there isn't just pivoting but walking forward in a small circle.
    - Walking around a barrel may be helpful.
  - Pelvic tilting.
    - Apply pressure to a point located between the biceps femoris muscle and semitendinosus muscle (**Figure 12.32**).
    - Hold the tilt for 5 seconds for 5 repetitions per session.

12.3   Equine Acupuncture

Molly Shepard

12.3.1   INTRODUCTION

Acupuncture is a medical technique first developed in China between 2,000 and 4,000 years ago. The term "acupuncture," meaning "needle puncture," was coined by a Danish physician, Willem Ten Rhyne, who visited Nagasaki, Japan, in the early 17th century, where he witnessed this technique in practice. Following that trip, he returned to Europe and shared his experiences with the Western world of medicine.

12.3.2   PHILOSOPHIES OF TEACHING

Any veterinarian interested in performing acupuncture is advised to complete one of several certification courses available at the time of this writing:

- Medical Acupuncture for Veterinarians (MAV, https://curacore.org/vet/courses/acupuncture/).
- Chi Institute (www.tcvm.com).
- International Veterinary Acupuncture Society (IVAS, www.ivas.org).
- These programs all provide a solid background for safe practice, despite their philosophical differences.

12.3.2.1   Traditional Chinese Medicine (TCM)

- This philosophy describes acupuncture as a means of changing the flow of "Qi" in the body and appeals to the balance of five properties believed to govern the balance of the universe as well as normal physiology and overall health, and predict an individual's response to acupuncture: Water, Wood, Fire, Earth, Metal.
- "Qi" is translated into the word "energy" by many Western practitioners but may, in fact, be a mistranslation due to the limitation of the English language to capture the original meaning.
- Chi Institute and IVAS follow this philosophy.

12.3.2.2   Western Medical Acupuncture

- This philosophy describes acupuncture as a means of stimulating the central and peripheral nervous system via local access to nerves and connective tissue surrounding nerves, thereby modulating release of neurotransmitters on a local and systemic level.
- MAV follows this philosophy.

12.3.3   PRESUMED MECHANISMS OF ACTION

12.3.3.1   Systemic

- Gate Control Theory.
  - Originally developed by Ronald Melzack and Patrick Wall, suggests that non-noxious stimuli (e.g. mechanical, thermal) serve to block the transmission of nociceptive stimuli (A-delta and C fibers) before they arrive at the brain, effectively overriding or suppressing the intensity of those nociceptive signals.
  - The nerves responsible for transmitting these non-noxious stimuli have a higher conduction velocity (30–120 meter/second) than A-delta (5–25 meter/second) and C fibers (0.7–1.3 meter/second),

thereby reaching the spinal cord more quickly and influencing the modulation process of those signals.

- Endogenous neuropeptide release.
  - Acupuncture has been shown to stimulate release of endogenous antinociceptive neuropeptides including opioids such as met-enkephalin, beta-endorphin, endomorphin, dynorphin-A, and serotonin.

12.3.3.2 Locoregional

- Blood flow augmentation.
  - Acupuncture needles stimulate blood flow to the skin and muscle around the needle, allowing the immune system to send inflammatory cells and compounds produced by the central nervous and immune systems to stimulate growth, healing, or pain relief.
  - In animals and people with light or thinly haired skin, this response can be seen as a wheal and flare around the needle within 5–10 minutes of needle placement.
- Fibroblast traction.
  - Electron microscopy studies have demonstrated that acupuncture needles inserted into the skin cause collagen fibers to adhere to the needle.
  - Rotation or agitation of the needle subsequently applies greater traction on these fibers and the surrounding fibroblasts, thereby stimulating local blood flow.
  - Myofascial mobilization is the application of acupuncture, massage, or static pressure to acupuncture points ("acupressure" or "shiatsu" massage) overlying tense areas of muscle known as myofascial trigger points (MTrPs).
  - Focal, sustained pressure (transient ischemia) and release or needle insertion at these sites allows restoration of blood flow, and relaxation of that muscle.

12.3.4 INDICATIONS

- Acupuncture has been documented to address conditions ranging from pain, nerve injury, nausea, ileus or gastrointestinal hypermotility, infertility, anxiety, depression, addiction, allergies, sinusitis, immune-mediated disease, endocrine disease, and dermatologic conditions.
- The focus of this chapter will be on its analgesic utility and usefulness for treatment of superficial wounds or nerve injury.
- Acupuncture is a valuable tool for pain management in horses but should always be considered an adjunctive treatment, in combination with other analgesic therapies.
- It should be considered a component of an "integrative" approach to pain management, not an alternative to Western medical approaches.
- Acupuncture frequently serves to reduce the dosage or frequency of drug therapy, thereby reducing the risk of drug-related side effects.
  - It may help restore normal gastrointestinal (GI) motility in colic horses, thereby reducing the pain of gas accumulation and ileus, or reducing the discomfort of borborygmi.
    - Acupuncture is not a substitute for surgery in cases of surgical colic but may provide symptomatic relief.
  - The success of this intervention may allow the practitioner to reduce requirement for other analgesics such as opioids, which may adversely affect GI motility.
- It may help restore lymphatic and venous drainage to edematous tissues, when used in combination with massage, heat therapy, and cryotherapy.

12.3.4.1   Clinical Significance of Acupuncture Point Locations

- TCM and medical acupuncture utilize many of the same point locations for needle placement and oftentimes reference these points as they fit into a "channel" or "meridian" scheme of orientation on the body.
- These point "channels" were determined hundreds of years ago for the human body and originally named according to the ancient Chinese understanding of organ function.
  - Anatomical and physiological knowledge has expanded, making the names of these channels essentially arbitrary today, with respect to the physiologic effects of acupuncture. For the sake of simplicity, these names have remained.
  - The channels are named as followed: Heart, Pericardium, Lung, Liver, Kidney, Spleen, Stomach, Large Intestine, Small Intestine, Gallbladder, Bladder, Triple Heater, Governor Vessel, Conception Vessel.

12.3.5   ACUPUNCTURE POINT LOCATIONS AND ANATOMICAL RELATIONSHIPS

- The points assigned to each "channel" typically share the same nerve supply or embryological germ layers, which give rise to dermatomes and myotomes through the course of fetal development.
- Dermatomes explain why during a heart attack, pain is often felt in the left arm.
  - The muscle of the heart shares a similar nerve supply with the muscles and nerves in the left arm.
- For the same reason, placing a needle at the tip of the finger or at the level of the wrist along the "heart channel" is believed to stimulate normal function in the heart. This is only one example of how acupuncture

points along a particular channel can provide a clinical effect in the associated but distant tissues (**Table 12.3**).

- Other acupuncture points do not fall in line with a "channel" but may overlie areas of a muscle commonly affected by focal tension or myofascial restriction, giving rise to myofascial trigger points (MTrPs).
  - MTrPs are localized, hyperirritable spots within a taut band of skeletal muscle fibers that are very sensitive to palpation.
  - These are bundles of muscle fibers that have become fixed in a contracted state as a result of stress, injury, repetitive use, or poor posture.
  - While humans frequently develop these trigger points in the trapezius, rhomboideus, and other muscle groups in the neck, upper back, and shoulder area, horses frequently develop trigger points in the strap muscles of the neck (e.g. cleidobrachialis, epaxial lumbar muscles, and triceps muscle group).
  - If allowed to persist, trigger points can restrict joint range of motion and stimulate referred pain in adjoining

Table 12.3 **Acupuncture channels and relationships with nerve anatomy**

CHANNEL	ASSOCIATED NERVE(S)	POINTS (EXAMPLES)
Heart	Ulnar nerve, median nerve	HT1, HT7, HT9
Pericardium	Median nerve, ulnar nerve	PC6, PC9
Liver	Radial nerve	LI6, LI7, LI10, LI11
Bladder	Spinal nerves; sciatic, tibial and fibular nerves	BL11—BL30; BL36, BL39, BL40, BL60, BL62, BL67
Gallbladder	Sciatic nerve, fibular nerve	GB30, GB34, GB39, GB44
Kidney	Tibial nerve	KI3, KI1

muscles or distant muscles which share a similar nerve supply, resulting in significant discomfort and reduced quality of life.

- Horses commonly develop MTrPs when compensating for an abnormal gait or posture, such as those recovering from an orthopedic or neurologic injury, e.g. forelimb lameness frequently precipitates compensatory neck pain.
- Horses with a poorly fitting saddle also may demonstrate sensitivity or trigger points in the muscles dorsal to the shoulder girdle, e.g. thoracic and cervical trapezius.
- Acupuncture is one of many manual therapies which effectively address MTrPs and compensatory muscle pain and should be considered alongside stretching, massage, heat, and cryotherapy for maximal patient benefit.

12.3.6 CLINICAL EFFECTS OF ACUPUNCTURE

12.3.6.1 Spinal Nerves

- The central location of these nerves gives rise to their role in providing innervation to much of the peripheral and visceral tissues, including voluntary and autonomic organ function.
- The points that are needled determine which spinal nerve is stimulated, and thereby have a clinical effect in the tissues receiving nerve supply from that segment of the spinal cord.
- One channel, the "bladder" channel, is particularly useful for stimulation of the spinal nerves, as its points follow either side of the dorsal midline, overlying the epaxial muscles (longimus dorsi m., iliocostalis m.) (**Figure 12.33**).
  - For example, stimulation of points near the thoracolumbar junction (e.g. BL21) may stimulate stomach motility.

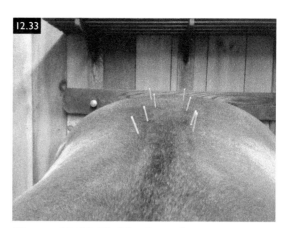

Figure 12.33 Bladder channel
Courtesy of Dr. Jenna Donaldson

- Another example is that acupuncture near the sacral spine (e.g. BL25, BL27, BL35) may stimulate normal urinary or colonic function, due to the fact that the colon and urinary bladder receive nerve supply from fibers that exit the sacral spinal canal.

12.3.6.2 Peripheral Nerves

- Many acupuncture points lie in close proximity to peripheral nerves.
- When nerves suffer injury (e.g. trauma, stroke, inflammation), their ability to heal depends on the severity of the injury, blood flow to the nerve, and time.
- If it has not been irreparably damaged, a nerve may still only grow 1–5 millimeter/day.
- In theory, acupuncture near the site of injury may help stimulate the injured nerve to secrete growth factors and accelerate healing. Anecdotally, acupuncture appears to increase the responsiveness of animals to the benefits of therapeutic exercise and other physical rehabilitation.

12.3.6.3 Neurovascular Bundles

- There are numerous locations in the body where large nerve fibers lie in close proximity to large veins and arteries. The nerve activity in these bundles influences vascular blood flow.

- There are acupuncture points overlying these locations to stimulate normal function, or homeostasis, in the nervous and vascular systems.
- In the case of very ill animals, these points are approached with caution, with the consideration that stimulation of these nerves may change systemic blood pressure.
  - Examples of this phenomenon in horses are the "Ting" points, found along the coronary band of each foot.

12.3.6.4 Trigger Points

- As described above, trigger points respond to acupuncture because acupuncture restores blood flow to these chronically hyperirritable bundles of muscle fibers.
- Once blood flow returns, delivery of energy substrates and oxygen is restored to the muscle, allowing it to relax.

12.3.6.5 Relaxation Points

- In addition to stimulating particular peripheral nerves, some acupuncture points reportedly relieve agitation (**Figure 12.34**), or provide a feeling of relaxation (**Table 12.4**).

12.3.6.6 Expected Patient Response

- The majority of horses undergoing acupuncture gain some benefit from it.
- Acupuncture reportedly has a cumulative effect, so it may be more likely to provide a clinical benefit (improved nerve function, alleviation of chronic pain) after 3–4 sessions than after the first session.
- An estimated 10% of individuals do not gain an apparent benefit from acupuncture, but this outcome cannot be predicted until several sessions have been attempted.

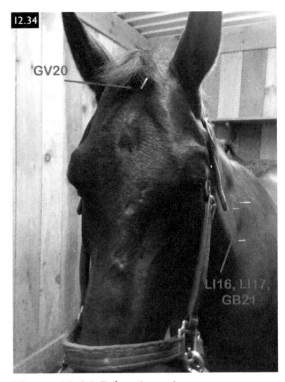

Figure 12.34 Relaxation points
Courtesy of Dr. Jenna Donaldson

- In the case of trigger point therapy with acupuncture, one session is likely to alleviate much of the pain caused by the trigger points.
- Acupuncture needles are *solid* and very small: 0.14–0.3 mm in diameter, so depending on the location of needle insertion, most patients do not notice when these needles are inserted.
- They do not typically produce an unpleasant sensation, as one would expect from a hypodermic needle, and often will create a sensation previously described as a non-localized, dull ache or heaviness.
- If the needles are inserted into a tense, painful muscle, they may cause mild discomfort at first, but the muscle-relaxing effects of the needle quickly alleviate this discomfort.

Table 12.4 **Acupuncture points useful for anxiolysis**

POINT	ASSOCIATED NERVE(S)	LOCATION
GV-20	Trigeminal nerve, cranial cervical nerves	Dorsal midline, highest point of the poll, rostral to nuchal crest
HT-7	Ulnar nerve	Caudolateral radius, proximal to insertion of flexor carpi ulnaris
PC-1	Cranial thoracic spinal nerves	Lateral thorax, caudal to tip of olecranon, in 5th intercostal space, ascending pectoral muscle
KI-27	Cervical/thoracic spinal nerves	1 cun* ventrolateral to manubrium, overlying ascending pectoral m.
Da Feng Men (GV-24 plus two auxiliary points)	Trigeminal nerve, facial nerve	GV24: Point where lateral ridges of external sagittal crest of the parietal bone meet on midline; other points—1 cun* ventrolateral to GV24
LI-16	Cervical/thoracic spinal nerves	Immediately cranial to scapula, between cranial margin of supraspinatus and dorsal margin of brachiocephalicus
Bai Hui	Lumbosacral spinal nerves	Dorsal midline, overlying lumbosacral junction
ST-45	Tibial nerve, fibular nerve, nervi vasorum of the coronary venous plexus	Cranial midline of the hind foot, proximal to coronary band

*cun = translation from Chinese is "body inch"; a unit of measurement used to describe point locations relative to a patient's body size; equal to the width of the patient's rib, usually ~3 cm in most adult equine patients.

- Many acupuncture needle types are coated with silicon, which makes their insertion more comfortable.
- Rarely, some animals do not tolerate acupuncture and are very sensitive to needle insertion.
- The majority of equine patients tolerate it very well, however, as long as they experience it in a quiet, calming, stress-free environment. Each patient is different.
- Horses are creatures of habit, so very frequently, they may not learn that they are safe and can relax in that new environment during acupuncture until their 3rd or 4th session.
- The handler's or clinician's state of mind can profoundly influence the horse's ability to relax, particularly in stressful environments. Any trepidation or stress on the part of the handler may cause the horse to be more restless than relaxed during his/her therapy.

- Release of catecholamines under conditions of stress may antagonize the relaxing effects of acupuncture.

12.3.7 RECOMMENDED PRACTICE TIPS: PRACTICAL AND LOGISTICAL CONSIDERATIONS

- Getting started: Prior to the initiation of any acupuncture program, the practitioner should perform a thorough physical exam, including the examination and palpation of large muscle groups (myofascial exam) (**Figure 12.35**) and a lameness evaluation, if applicable.
- A "holistic" perspective on the patient's health status will inform a more appropriate treatment plan or recommendations for further diagnostics (e.g. ultrasound, nerve blocks).

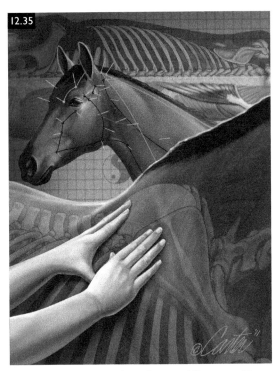

Figure 12.35 Myofascial exam (Illustrated by Kip Carter)

- The most thorough practitioners offer recommendations which may include pharmaceutical or surgical therapies as well as physical medicine modalities such as physical rehabilitation (e.g. therapeutic exercise, laser, shockwave), massage, and acupuncture.
- Clients presented with all the indicated treatment options can discuss them with their veterinarian and collaboratively determine the best course of action for their horse.
- Location of treatment: an ideal environment for acupuncture treatment is a calm, low-stress area free from excessive noise or other stimuli. The floor should be free from bedding or other debris that may prevent the practitioner from finding needles that prematurely fall out.
- Duration of treatment.

- For horses that have not experienced acupuncture before, it's customary to keep the first treatment brief, < 15 minutes, and to use fewer than 8–10 needles, in order not to overwhelm the central nervous system. The practitioner should instead focus on ensuring that animal's first session is a relaxing, calming experience.
- Once the patient has become accustomed to the experience of acupuncture, depending on the goals of therapy (stimulate nerve function vs chronic pain management), more needles may be used, or an extra stimulus may be applied to the needles (e.g. electroacupuncture) to increase the effect of the treatment.
- The longest period of time for needles to remain in place would be 50 minutes, and this would only be appropriate for horses that have gradually "worked up" to this level, appear to relax during the treatment, and do not develop excessive lethargy or interruptions in their normal routine for more than 12–24 hours after treatment.
- Patients exhibiting this exaggerated response may benefit from a reduction in the duration of treatment or the number or size of needles used. In addition, these animals should ideally not be asked to ride in a trailer for 2–3 hours after their treatments, in order to allow them time to maintain an alert state of mind for safe transport.

12.3.7.1 Needle Types and Technique
- Many varieties of needle widths, lengths, hubs, and added features exist. The least stimulating needles are of narrower width and are coated with silicon, which makes their insertion more comfortable for the patient.

- Each needle should be newly opened from packaging and sterile, in order to maintain patient safety.
- Practitioners aiming for a stronger stimulus may select larger, longer, or uncoated needles.
- Each practitioner must discover their own technique, but new acupuncturists may benefit from the use of needles individually packaged with a guide tube, designed to assist in accurate needle placement.
- Needles should never be inserted up the hub. This error may result in needle breakage.
- Needles should never be inserted into a wound or infected tissue.
- Once a needle is inserted, it may be gently, slowly twirled within the tissue bed until it appears to stick and resist further movement.
  - This event does not always occur on agitation of the needle but indicates that either fibroblasts and collagen in the tissue have engaged the needle or that muscle tissue has contracted around the needle.
  - The practitioner should leave the needle alone at that time; it is likely to loosen after blood flow improves to the tissue bed, or after the needle has caused the surrounding muscle to relax.
  - If an attempt is made to remove a needle and it will not easily slide out, the practitioner may place needles in a circle surrounding the "stuck" needle. After a few minutes, this technique typically serves to relax the tissue bed and release the needle in question.

12.3.7.2 Restraint

- Due to the unpredictable nature of patient response to acupuncture, horses undergoing treatment should not be restrained in the stocks.

- Ideally, patients should wear halters and be held on lead by an assistant that is prepared to respond to any sudden movements the patient could make during treatment, and guide them in a direction away from potential hazards.
- The use of cross ties should be approached with caution, and always consider the temperament, training level or previous response of the patient to acupuncture.

12.3.8 POTENTIAL NEGATIVE CONSEQUENCES OF ACUPUNCTURE

- Acupuncture is very noninvasive, and generally low-risk. Most states require that acupuncture on animals must be performed by a licensed veterinarian.
- The rare case in which acupuncture harms a patient is most likely to occur in the hands of an untrained person who has a poor understanding of equine anatomy.
  - An untrained person would not recognize, for example, that there are points overlying the abdomen, joint spaces, large vessels and the chest.
- When performed by knowledgeable, trained individuals, however, it is rare for acupuncture to carry any significant risk.
- A patient's immediate response to acupuncture is very individualized.
  - An estimated ~10% of patients will respond strongly, exhibiting lethargy and/or decreased appetite for 24–48 hours after the treatment session.
  - This response should not cause alarm, but may inform the selection of future needling technique, e.g. fewer or smaller needles, shorter duration of treatment.
  - The possibility of this outcome should be communicated to clients, so they are mindful of their animal's possible responses to therapy.

12.3.9 MODIFIERS OF ACUPUNCTURE

12.3.9.1 Aquapuncture

- The use of a hypodermic needle to inject fluids (e.g. saline, vitamin B12) into the tissue associated with an acupuncture point.
- Practitioners historically have used this technique for patients that will not remain standing or stationary for the duration of an acupuncture treatment.
- Practitioners should use caution with this technique, as hypodermic needles and subcutaneous injections present greater risks for bacterial introduction and abscess.

12.3.9.2 Moxibustion (Moxa)

- A Chinese medicine technique requiring the burning of the herb, mugwort (*Artemisia Vulgaris*), a species of chrysanthemum flower, directly over an inserted acupuncture needle, which serves to warm the needle.
- Practitioners should use caution with moxa, as the smoke created by this technique can be objectionable to some clients and patients.

12.3.9.3 Electroacupuncture (EA)

- A means of intensifying the acupuncture stimulus via application of a low intensity electrical current to the needle.
- EA requires the use of needles of at least 0.2mm width, with metal hubs that allow the electrical signal to conduct into the tissues.
- Silicon-coated needles should not be used for EA, lest it heats and melts the silicon into surrounding tissue.
- Low frequency (~2–10 Hz), continuous wave EA, has been shown to stimulate the CNS to release endogenous antinociceptive compounds such as endomorphin, met-enkephalin and beta-endorphin, as well

as inhibit release of stress hormones (e.g. corticosterone).

- This technique is most commonly used for control of chronic or neurogenic pain, for example, osteoarthritis or cancer pain.
- Another EA technique is a pattern of "mixed mode" or dense and disperse (DD) waveforms, alternating between high (~100 Hz) and low (2 Hz) frequency.
  - For example, the pulse generator connected to two acupoints would apply a square wave at 2 Hz for 3 seconds then immediately switch to 100 Hz for 3 seconds, and then back to low frequency, and so on.
  - This EA technique has been shown to stimulate more significant endogenous release of endomorphin (mu agonist) as well as dynorphin A, a neurotransmitter shown to reduce pain behavior in acute, neuropathic, and inflammatory models.
  - This technique has been shown to reduce postoperative opioid requirements in people, and improve pain scores in chronic human pain states such as diabetic neuropathy and lower back pain.

12.3.10 FREQUENCY OF TREATMENT

- Each patient's needs may be different.
- A general recommendation for patients with acutely painful conditions or acute neurologic injuries may be for acupuncture therapy twice to three times per week.
- Patients with chronic pain conditions or chronic neurologic deficits may receive treatments once per week, but may not exhibit a response for at least 4–5 weeks.
- Note: acupuncture should always be considered an adjunct treatment in addition to other medical therapies prescribed by the patient's primary clinician.

- Through the course of 5 treatments, practitioners are often able to gauge whether acupuncture is benefiting the patient, and whether the frequency of treatment or technique (e.g. electroacupuncture versus dry needling) should be changed.
- After an "induction" phase where treatments are given on a twice weekly or weekly basis for about 1 to 2 months, particularly in cases of chronic pain, the practitioner is usually able to decrease treatment frequency to every other week, then sometimes once per month.
- The patient's pain level should be serially evaluated by the owner and practitioner in order to optimize treatment frequency and technique, via a trial and error process.
- Some patients may need a treatment once every 10–14 days, while others may need a treatment once every other month in order to stay comfortable and active.
- Older or more debilitated patients tend to be more sensitive, so they may require less frequent treatments or just a lower-intensity treatment (e.g. no electroacupuncture).

12.3.11 TREATMENT RESPONSE: HOW TO IDENTIFY A POSITIVE RESPONSE

- For a patient receiving acupuncture for neurologic disease, a positive response may be defined as an improvement in neurologic function, for example, resolution of paralysis or paresis to an affected limb or tissue or a faster response to the physical therapy than previously expected.
- A positive response in chronic pain patients may be defined by more subtle observations, for example, a greater willingness to be active and interactive, more normal weight-bearing or posture, improved appetite or weight gain, or quicker transitions between recumbency and standing posture.
- Another sign that the patient is more comfortable includes a greater willingness to stretch their back ("down dog" or "cat" stretch) on a regular basis again. Animals with chronic pain have difficulty doing these daily, "normal" behaviors, and the return of normal behaviors are good indicators that therapy is working.

12.4   Chiropractic

Dana Peroni

12.4.1   INTRODUCTION

Chiropractic treatments have recently become more popular in management of equine musculoskeletal pain. The addition of chiropractic care to a multimodal pain management plan can be more beneficial for the patient compared to traditional treatments alone.

12.4.2   CHIROPRACTIC CARE

- Can be used as an alternative, drug-free therapy for pain relief in horses.
- Does not replace traditional veterinary medicine but works very well when used in conjunction with traditional medicine.
- Can enhance and improve a horse's overall health and comfort.
- Works to eliminate the cause of the problem rather than simply treating the symptoms.
- When a horse is being treated for lameness, chiropractic can help with compensatory issues.
  - For example, a horse may have sore hocks and need joint injections, but may also have a sore back secondary to hock pain.

12.4.2.1   What Is the Goal of Chiropractic?

- Help relieve pain and restore normal function.
- Restore proper motion of the affected joint.
- Decrease pain and muscle spasms in the area of the subluxated joint.
- Restore correct alignment of the axial skeleton.
- Help restore normal joint motion and normal physiology.
- Help slow the progression of degeneration.

12.4.2.2   Who Should Perform a Chiropractic Adjustment?

- Licensed veterinarian who is also certified by either the International Veterinary Chiropractic Association or the American Veterinary Chiropractic Association.
- Licensed chiropractor certified by one of the same associations.

12.4.3   BEFORE AN ADJUSTMENT IS PERFORMED

12.4.3.1   History

- Signalment, including breed, age, discipline, body condition score.
- History of illness, injury, surgery, or joint injections.
- What is the owner's complaint?
- Desired work level, intensity, and frequency.

12.4.3.2   Physical Exam

- Observation at the walk and trot.
- Analysis of posture and conformation.
- Evaluation of feet: Assessment for balance, toe length, sole depth, thrush or other infection, shod or barefoot?
- Static palpation: Evaluation of signs of pain, heat, or swelling.
- Motion palpation.
  - A joint with decreased range of motion indicates that an adjustment is needed.

12.4.4   THE CHIROPRACTIC ADJUSTMENT

- The chiropractor must have a thorough understanding of equine anatomy.
- Brute force is not necessary.
- Mallets and other tools are not necessary.

- High velocity, low force adjustments are used.
- Only one joint is adjusted at a time.
- Adjustment made within the normal range of motion of a joint.
- Some adjustments are so subtle that they may not be obvious to the owner.
- Adjustment must be done in the appropriate line of correction.
  - Line of correction is determined by the type and shape of the facet.
- The chiropractor may need to get above the horse's back in order to achieve the correct angle (**Figure 12.36**).
- Some joints require another person to stabilize the joint for an adjustment (such as the poll and the withers).

12.4.4.1 Common Symptoms that May Be Relieved by a Chiropractic Adjustment

- Abnormal posture or head carriage.
- Pain in the temporomandibular joint.
- Head tossing.
- Bucking.
- Neck, back, shoulder, or hip soreness.
- Poor performance.
- Snapping and pinning the ears.
- Behavior problems.
- Difficulty getting up and down.
- Hollowing the back.
- Swishing the tail.
- Refusing to jump.
- Resisting collection.
- Sensitivity to touch.
- Abnormal gait or lameness.
- Stiffness.
- Muscle wasting.
- Shortened stride.

12.4.5 AFTER THE CHIROPRACTIC ADJUSTMENT

- The horse often licks and chews; this is a sign of comfort.

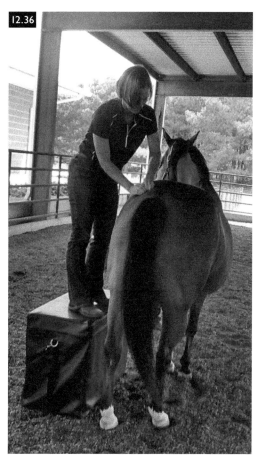

Figure 12.36 Chiropractor over the horse's back

- Horses should not be ridden for 12–24 hours.
- Normal turnout and feeding schedules.
- The number of chiropractic adjustments needed depends on the horse's specific problem.
- Performance horses and older horses benefit from regular adjustments done every 4 to 6 weeks.

12.4.6 OTHER CONSIDERATIONS WHEN PROVIDING CHIROPRACTIC CARE

- Saddle fit.
  - Poor saddle fit can lead to painful pressure points, muscle swelling after the

saddle is removed, abnormal sweating under the saddle pad, white hair growth, and atrophy of muscles along the withers.
- It is very important to have a saddle that fits the horse and is comfortable for both the horse and the rider.
- Hoof balance.
  - Affects the health and soundness of the horse.
  - Improper shoeing or trimming can lead to a change in gait.
  - Routine hoof care will help keep the foot balanced and keep the toe from getting too long.
  - If the foot is unbalanced, additional stresses are placed on the joints and soft tissue structures of the legs. These stresses can lead to long-term lameness issues.
- Dental care.
  - Routine dental care is important to reduce the presence of sharp enamel points, hooks, ramps, and waves.
  - By correcting these malocclusions, the horse will be able to chew more efficiently and pain free.
  - The bit seating will also be examined and teeth floated as needed.
  - A horse that is unable to chew comfortably will suffer from temporomandibular joint pain and be irritable when the bit is placed.

FURTHER READING

Physiology, Recognition, and Local Anesthesia Techniques

Doherty T, Valverde A (2006) Management of sedation and anesthesia. In: *A Manual of Equine Anesthesia & Analgesia* (eds Doherty T, Valverde A), Blackwell Publishing, Ames, pp. 206–259.

Gonzalo-Marcilla M, Gasthuys F, Schauvliege S. (2015) Partial intravenous anaesthesia in the horse: A review of intravenous agents used to supplement equine inhalation anaesthesia. Part 2: Opioids and alpha-2 adrenoceptor agonists. *Vet Anaesth Analg* **42**:1–16.

Moyer W, Schumacher J, Schumacher JR (2011) *Equine Joint Injection and Regional Anesthesia*, Academic Veterinary Solutions, Chadds Ford.

Sanchez LC, Robertson SA (2014) Pain control in horses: What do we really know? *Equine Vet J* **46**:517–523.

Yamashita K, Muir WW (2009) Intravenous anesthetic and analgesic adjuncts to inhalation anesthesia. In: *Equine Anesthesia Monitoring and Emergency Therapy*, 2nd edn. (eds Muir WW, Hubbell JAE), Saunders Elsevier, St. Louis, pp. 260–276.

Rehabilitation Techniques

Bender TS, Karagülle Z, Bálint GP et al (2004) Hydrotherapy, balneotherapy, and spa treatment in pain management. *Rheumatol Int* **25**:220–224.

Clayton HM, Lavagnino M, Kaiser LJ et al (2011) Evaluation of biomechanical effects of four stimulation devices placed on the hind feet of trotting horses. *Am J Vet Res* **72**:1489–1495.

de Oliveira K, Soutello RVG, da Fonseca R, Costa C, de L Meirelles PR, Fachiolli DF et al (2015) Gymnastic training and dynamic mobilization exercises improve stride quality and increase epaxial muscle size in therapy horses. *J Equine Vet Sci* **35**:888–893.

Hall J, Skevington SM, Maddison PJ et al (1996) A randomized and controlled trial of hydrotherapy in rheumatoid arthritis. *Arthritis Care Res* **9**:206–215.

Harris GR, Susman JL (2002) Managing musculoskeletal complaints with rehabilitation therapy: Summary of the Philadelphia panel evidence-based clinical practice guidelines on musculoskeletal rehabilitation interventions. *J Fam Pract* **51**:1042–1046.

Hides JA, Jull GA, Richardson CA (2001) Long-term effects of specific stabilizing exercises for first-episode low back pain. *Spine* **26**:E243–E248.

King MR, Haussler KK, Kawcak CE et al (2012) Mechanisms of aquatic therapy and its potential use in managing equine osteoarthritis. *Equine Vet Educ* **25**:204–209.

Mendez-Angulo JL, Firshman AM et al (2013) Effect of water depth on amount of flexion and extension of joints of the distal aspects of the limbs in healthy horses walking on an underwater treadmill. *Am J Vet Res* **74**: 557–566.

Saltychev M, Laimi K, Oksanen T et al (2014) Nine-year trajectory of purchases of prescribed pain medications before and after in-patient interdisciplinary rehabilitation for chronic musculoskeletal disorders: A prospective, cohort, register-based study of 4,365 subjects. *J Rehabil Med* **46**:283–286.

Stubbs NC, Clayton HM (2008) *Activate Your Horse's Core*, Sport Horse Publications, Mason.

Stubbs NC, Kaiser LJ, Hauptman J et al (2011) Dynamic mobilisation exercises increase cross sectional area of musculus multifidus. *Equine Vet J* **43**:522529.

Stubbs NC, Riggs CM, Hodges PW et al (2010) Osseous spinal pathology and epaxial muscle ultrasonography in Thoroughbred racehorses. *Equine Vet J* **42**:654–661.

Volker G, van Vree F, Wolterbeek R et al (2016) Long-term outcomes of multidisciplinary rehabilitation for chronic musculoskeletal pain. *Musculoskelet Care* **15**:59–68.

Equine Acupuncture

Habacher G, Pittler MH, Ernst E (2006) Effectiveness of acupuncture in veterinary medicine: Systematic review. *J Vet Intern Med* **20**:480–488.

Joaquim JGF, Luna SPL, Brondani JT, Torelli SR, Rahal SC, Freitas FP (2010) Comparison of decompressive surgery, electroacupuncture, and decompressive surgery followed by electroacupuncture for the treatment of dogs with intervertebral disk disease with long-standing severe neurologic deficits. *J Am Vet Med Assoc* **236**:1225–1229.

Kim MS, Xie H (2009) Use of electroacupuncture to treat laryngeal hemiplegia in horses. *Vet Rec* **165**:602–603.

Langevin HM, Bouffard NA, Badger GJ et al (2005) Dynamic fibroblast response to subcutaneous tissue stretch ex vivo and in vivo. *Am J Physiol Cell Physiol* **288**:C747–C756.

Langevin HM, Bouffard NA, Badger GJ et al (2006) Subcutaneous tissue fibroblast cytoskeletal remodeling induced by acupuncture: Evidence for a mechanotransduction-based mechanism. *J Cellular Physiol* **207**(3):767–774.

Langevin HM, Konofagou EE, Badger GJ et al (2004) Tissue displacements during acupuncture using ultrasound elastography techniques. *Ultrasound Med Biol* **30**:1173–1183.

Macgregor J, Graf von Schweinitz D (2006) Needle electromyographic activity of myofascial trigger points and control sites in equine cleidobrachialis muscle—an observational study. *Acupunct Med* **24**:61–70.

Merritt AM, Xie H, Lester GD et al (2002) Evaluation of a method to experimentally induce colic in horses and the effects of acupuncture applied at the Guan-yuan-shu (similar to BL-21) acupoint. *Am J Vet Res* **63**:1006–1011.

Noguchi E (2010) Acupuncture regulates gut motility and secretion via nerve reflexes. *Autonom Neurosci* **156**:15–18.

Skarda RT, Muir WW (2003) Comparison of electroacupuncture and butorphanol on respiratory and cardiovascular effects and rectal pain threshold after controlled rectal distention in mares. *Am J Vet Res* **64**:137–144.

Skarda RT, Tejwani GA, Muir WW (2002) Cutaneous analgesia, hemodynamic and respiratory effects, and beta-endorphin concentration in spinal fluid and plasma of horses after acupuncture and electroacupuncture. *Am J Vet Res* **63**:1435–1442.

Steiss JE, White NA, Bowen JM (1989) Electroacupuncture in the treatment of chronic lameness in horses and ponies: A controlled clinical trial. *Can J Vet Res* **53**:239–243.

Trinh K, Graham N, Irnich D et al (2014) Acupuncture for neck disorders. *Cochrane Database Syst Rev.* doi:10.1002/14651858. CD004870.pub4.

Wilson DV, Lankenau C, Berney CE et al (2004) The effects of a single acupuncture treatment in horses with severe recurrent airway obstruction. *Equine Vet J* **36**:489–494.

Xie H, Colahan P, Ott EA (2005) Evaluation of electroacupuncture treatment of horses with signs of chronic thoracolumbar pain. *J Am Vet Med Assoc* **227**:281–286.

Chiropractic

Boldt E Jr (2002) Use of complementary veterinary medicine in the geriatric horse. *Vet Clin North Am Equine Pract* **18**:631–636.

Gaumer G, Koren A, Gemmen E (2002) Barriers to expanding primary care for chiropractors: The role of chiropractic as primary care gate keeper. *J Manipulative Physiol Ther* **25**:427–449.

Haussler KK (1999) Back problems: Chiropractic evaluation and management. *Vet Clin North Am Equine Pract* **15**:195–209.

Haussler KK (2010) The role of manual therapies in equine pain management. *Vet Clin North Am Equine Pract* **26**:579–601.

Haussler KK (2018) Spinal manual therapies in sport horse practice. *Vet Clin North Am Equine Pract* **34**:375–389.

Sullivan KA, Hill AE, Haussler KK (2008) The effects of chiropractic, massage and phenylbutazone on spinal mechanical nociceptive thresholds in horses without clinical signs. *Equine Vet J* **40**:14–30.

Willoughby S (1998) Chiropractic care. In: *Alternative and Complementary Veterinary Medicine: Principles and Practices* (eds Schoen AM, Wynn SG) Mosby, St. Louis, pp. 185–200.

CHAPTER 13

ANESTHESIA AND ANALGESIA FOR DONKEYS, MULES AND FOALS

Tomas Williams and Michele Barletta

13.1 INTRODUCTION

Despite similarities, donkeys and mules present several behavioral, anatomical and physiological differences from horses. Neonates and pediatric patients are at higher anesthetic risk and the anesthetist should focus on anatomical and physiological differences compared to adults.

13.2 DONKEYS AND MULES

13.2.1 Behavioral Differences

- Patience when handling a donkey is of paramount importance, since they usually become unwilling to move when confronted, especially if in an unfamiliar environment (**Figure 13.1**). It may take a long time to get them to perform a task (walking into a stock or into the induction stall etc.).
- Nose twitches (**Figure 13.2**) are usually ineffective in restraining donkeys (the twitch is hard to place on their noses and slides off easily).
- Mules may be considered more dangerous than donkeys due to their larger size. Both mules and donkeys can kick without warning.
- Pain is not as easy to assess in donkeys and mules as it is in horses. They are stoic, which makes the behavioral assessment of illness and pain very challenging. It is possible that they are much sicker and more painful than they look.
- Failure to judge pain or degree of cardiovascular compromise before

anesthesia and surgery may lead to cardiovascular decompensation after induction of anesthesia.

13.2.2 Anatomical Differences

- When placing a jugular catheter it is important to remember that even though the veins are located in the same position as in horses, the skin is much thicker. The cutaneous colli muscle extends over the jugular groove and can make it difficult to see the distention of the vein. It is recommended to block the skin using a local anesthetic and make a small incision at the site of insertion prior to catheter placement. The catheter should be angled slightly more perpendicular to the skin than when placed in a horse. Use of long catheters, 9 cm (3.5 inch), is recommended.
- Endotracheal intubation can be more difficult in donkeys than in horses. The pharynx opens into the larynx with a greater angle, which tilts caudally. The pharyngeal recess is more developed than in horses. Full extension of the neck should help guide the endotracheal tube into the trachea (**Figure 13.3**).
- The presence of excess pharyngeal mucosa and long paired laryngeal saccules makes intubation more difficult.
- In donkeys nasal intubation can be challenging since they have narrow nasal passages. The ventral meatus is smaller than in horses of similar size and a smaller tube should be used.

DOI: 10.1201/9780429190940-13

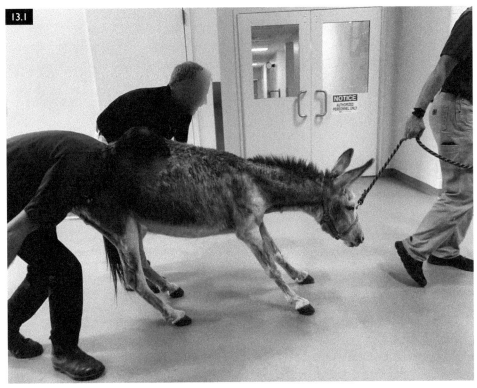

Figure 13.1 Donkey, unwilling to move

- The facial artery can present several branches, making the placement of an arterial catheter difficult. Usually the facial, transverse facial and auricular arteries are preferred to monitor invasive blood pressure. Similarly to jugular catheter placement, it is advised to make a small skin incision at the site of catheter insertion, due to their thick skin.

13.2.3 Physiological Differences

- Increases in hematocrit only occur when donkeys are at least 30% dehydrated. Assessing mild to moderate dehydration by hemoconcentration is difficult and inaccurate. Clinical signs and laboratory values should be considered before general anesthesia.
- Hyperlipidemia is frequently noticed during anorexia, stress, and illness in donkeys.

Triglyceride levels should be checked in these animals.
- Donkeys (especially miniature donkeys) metabolize some drugs (i.e. some NSAIDs and ketamine) much faster than horses, resulting in the use of higher doses and/or shorter dosing intervals.

13.2.4 Normal Values

- Heart rate is similar to horses and it is a good indicator of stress and pain.
- Resting respiratory rate is higher than in horses and averages around 20–30 breaths/ minute.
- Their body temperature can increase more after exercise compared to horses.
- ACTH and triglycerides are higher, insulin levels are lower, and cortisol values are similar compared to horses.

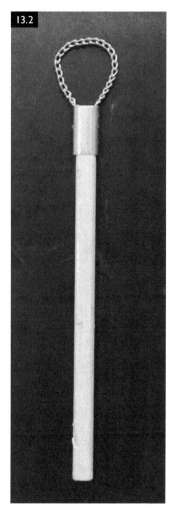

Figure 13.2 Nose twitch

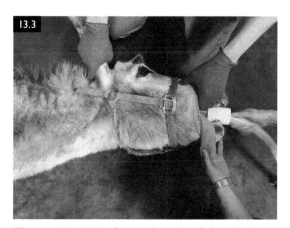

Figure 13.3 Donkey, induced with head and neck extended for endotracheal intubation

13.2.5 Premedication

- In donkeys detomidine at 5–10 ug/kg IV provides adequate sedation and analgesia. Higher doses (20–40 ug/kg IV) provide better analgesia but similar sedation.
- Mules require approximately 50% higher doses of xylazine compared to horses. Usually a dose of 1.6 mg/kg is needed to adequately sedate mules. It has been reported that higher doses of romifidine might be required in untamed mules. These higher doses of alpha-2 agonists are usually not required in donkeys.
- It has been shown that detomidine oral gel (**Figure 13.4**) provides sedation and analgesia in donkeys and mules. The label dose for horses can be used for these species (approximately 40 ug/kg). Approximately 30–40 minutes should be allowed to appreciate the clinical effects.
- After sedation, donkeys might lie down in sternal if they feel unstable. Anesthesia can be induced with the animal in sternal recumbency.

13.2.6 Induction and Maintenance with Injectable Drugs

- After adequate sedation, induction of anesthesia can be achieved with xylazine and ketamine in donkeys and mules. Ketamine at 2.2–2.5 mg/kg IV can also be combined with either diazepam or midazolam at 0.02–0.08 mg/kg for induction.
- After sedation, induction can also be achieved with IV midazolam at 0.05 mg/kg followed by IV alfaxalone at 1 mg/kg. Time to standing may be longer and the quality of recovery a bit lower when compared to ketamine.
- Anesthesia can be maintained with intermittent boluses of xylazine/ketamine. These boluses may need to be administered more frequently than in horses

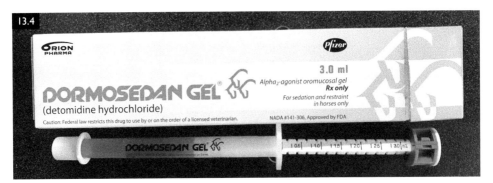

Figure 13.4 Detomidine gel

(approximately every 10 minutes) based on the patient's anesthetic depth.

- "Triple drip" of "GKX" (1 liter of guaifenesin 5% + ketamine 2000 mg + xylazine 500 mg) has been safely used for induction and maintenance of anesthesia in donkeys after sedation with xylazine. Induction is achieved by rapid administration of the mixture. Maintenance of general anesthesia is accomplished by administration to-effect (approximately 1–2 ml/kg/hour).
  - Notice that in this GKX combination the ketamine dose is doubled compared to standard GKX used in horses: 1) donkeys metabolize ketamine faster; 2) guaifenesin causes more respiratory depression than is observed in horses.
- Thiopental alone or in combination with guaifenesin can be used for induction at 7–8 mg/kg IV, but recovery is generally slow.
- In miniature donkeys the use of tiletamine/zolazepam (Telazol) at 1 mg/kg IV is recommended for induction after sedation, since they metabolize ketamine faster than horses.
  - Alternatively, propofol 2 mg/kg IV can be used for induction followed by 0.2 mg/kg/minute for maintenance. Use an endotracheal tube and oxygen supplementation since apnea can occur.

13.2.7 Maintenance with Inhalant Anesthetics, Support and Monitoring

- Recommended for procedures longer than 60–75 minutes.
- Isoflurane and sevoflurane can be used: minimum alveolar concentrations and side effects are similar to horses.
- Induction via face mask has been used in tame adult donkeys. If the animal is calm and accustomed to handling, mask induction can be performed after sedation without difficulty or danger.
- As mentioned above, endotracheal intubation can be more challenging than in horses. This is especially evident in dwarf-like miniature donkeys (**Figure 13.5**), that can have hypoplastic trachea.
- If the donkey is not intubated (injectable anesthesia) monitor for normal airflow with no excessive respiratory noise and efforts. If this occurs, straighten the head and neck and administer oxygen flow by.
- Basic monitoring is similar to the anesthetized horse. Heart rate, respiratory rate, blood pressure, mucous membrane color, capillary refill time, eye signs (palpebral reflex, presence/absence of nystagmus) and degree of muscle relaxation should all be monitored.
- Respiratory rate can be higher in anesthetized donkeys than in horses. Breath

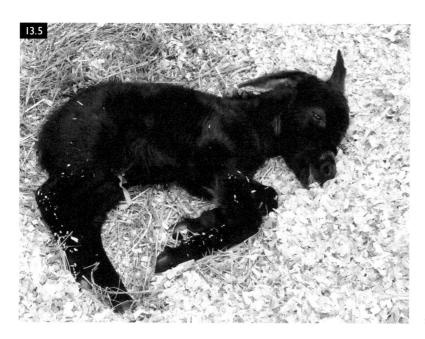

Figure 13.5 Dwarf-like mini donkey

holding instead of increased frequency can be seen during light plane of anesthesia.
- Nystagmus and palpebral reflex are similar to horses, but not as reliable.
- Arterial blood pressure (either direct or indirect) is more reliable than eye signs when assessing the depth of anesthesia.
- During inhalational anesthesia, administration of intravenous fluids (Lactated Ringer's Solution) is recommended at a rate of 5–10 mg/kg/hour.
- Myositis is less of a concern in donkeys than in horses, due to lower muscle mass, however preventative measures are still recommended. Myopathies can be more frequent in draft mules. Appropriate positioning to protect radial and peroneal nerve and padding are recommended.

13.2.8 Recovery
- Due to their calmer demeanor, donkeys experience a calmer recovery without excitement compared to horses. For this reason, hand-recovery is generally not necessary.

- Most donkeys lie quietly in sternal until they are ready to stand (**Figure 13.6**). If they are uncoordinated during their first attempt, they may lie down back in sternal until they are more stable.
- They usually stand by extending their hind legs first, like a cow, but some may stand like horses do.
- Mules can act more like horses in recovery. If the mule is not tame or manifests more horse-like behavior before anesthesia, the animal should be treated as a horse in recovery.

13.2.9 Standing Surgery in Donkeys
- Proper sedation is necessary for standing surgical procedures.
- Similar protocols used for horses can be used in donkeys and mules. Constant rate infusions of alpha-2 agonists +/- opioids can be used. Local anesthetic techniques should be added when appropriate.
- Detomidine at 10 µg/kg IV with buprenorphine at 6 µg/kg followed by

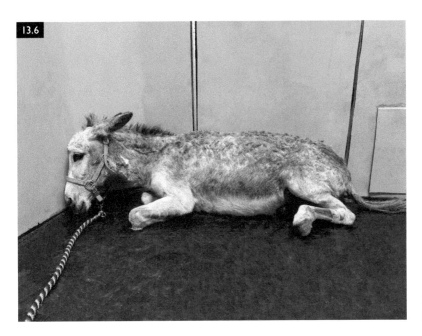

13.6

Figure 13.6 Donkey
lying quietly in sternal

detomidine CRI at 0.16 µg/kg/min can
produce adequate sedation.
- Morphine epidural at 0.1 mg/kg can help
reduce systemic drugs required and provides
analgesia for the patient.
- Caudal epidural injection is usually
performed between the second and third
coccygeal vertebra. This space is preferred
because the first intercoccygeal space is
narrower in donkeys compared to horses.
The spinal processes at this level are easy
to palpate. The epidural needle should be
directed at a 30° angle from the horizontal
plane.

13.3   FOALS

13.3.1 Anatomy and Physiology
- Pulmonary changes occur in their first
hours after birth and changes of the
cardiovascular system take place during
their first 72 hours of life.
- Respiratory rate and minute ventilation are
higher than in adults.

- They have decreased pulmonary functional
reserve, compliant lungs and chest wall
and high oxygen consumption rate which
increase the risk of hypoxia and hypoxemia.
- Partial pressure of oxygen in arterial
blood is lower (40–75 mmHg) for several
hours after birth and becomes normal
approximately at day 7.
- Anatomical shunts (foramen ovale and
ductus arteriosus) completely close 2–4
weeks after birth and they can reopen if
acidemia, hypoxemia or hypercarbia is
present.
- Their cardiac output is heart rate
dependent, due to less contractile tissue.
They have minimal cardiac reserve,
increased cardiac index and immature
sympathetic system.
- Neonates have lower mean arterial blood
pressure (40–60 mmHg).
- At birth the blood-brain barrier can be
more permeable to drugs and neonates may
require lower doses to achieve the desired
sedation/plane of anesthesia.

- Nociception occurs in very young animals and it can lead to chronic pain conditions even later in life. Pre-emptive analgesia should always be provided if nociception is expected.
- Their thermoregulation is less efficient, due to immature thermoregulatory center, high surface area to body mass ratio and low body fat. They are prone to hypothermia under general anesthesia.

13.3.2 Preparation and Sedation

- Physical restraint can be accomplished by standing on the side of the foal, wrapping one arm around the neck and grabbing the ear and holding the tail with the other hand (**Figure 13.7**). Holding both ears and extending the neck can be useful to restrain for jugular catheter placement (**Figure 13.8**).
- When working with foals, it is important to sedate and control the mare. After sedation,

foal and mare can be led together to the induction stall and after induction of the foal, the mare can be brought back to the stall. Foals can be recovered in front of the mare's stall. This allows the mare to see the foal and still provides a physical barrier between the two until the foal has recovered.

- Suckling neonatal foals should not be fasted prior to anesthesia. Bottle fed foals should be fasted for approximately 2 hours prior to anesthesia due to slower gastric emptying. Withhold food in older foals for approximately 4–6 hours.
- Neonates may require lower doses of injectable drugs due to immature nervous system, more permeable blood-brain barrier, decrease in plasma protein binding and increased volume of distribution.
- Young foals might become recumbent when sedated. This can facilitate

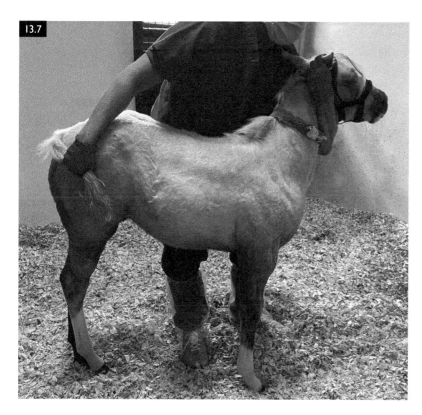

13.7

Figure 13.7 Restraint of foal—wrapping one arm around the neck and grabbing the ear and holding the tail with the other hand

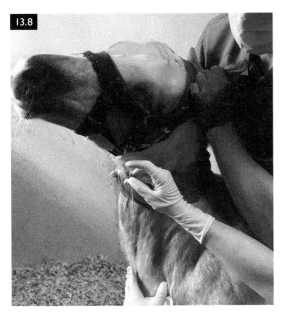

Figure 13.8 Holding both ears and extending the neck may be helpful for catheter placement

nonpainful procedures; nonetheless, oxygen supplementation should be provided.

- Although benzodiazepines should be avoided for sedation in adult horses, midazolam and diazepam can be administered at 0.05–0.1 mg/kg in neonatal foals.
- Opioids should be used if pain is expected.
- Alpha-2 agonists should be used with caution in very young patients. They cause cardiovascular depression by increasing afterload and decreasing heart rate, which can be detrimental in neonates. Bradycardia, respiratory depression and severe ataxia can be noticed. In older foals xylazine 0.5–1 mg/kg can be used if necessary.

13.3.3   General Anesthesia: Management and Monitoring

- Induction of general anesthesia can be achieved by the use of IV injectable agents, such as ketamine/diazepam (1–3 mg/kg and 0.05–0.1 mg/kg, respectively) and propofol (2 mg/kg to effect), or inhalant anesthetics.

Isoflurane or sevoflurane can be delivered via face mask or nasotracheal tube (which can be placed without sedative drugs or with minimal sedation if necessary).

- Although smaller in size, positioning, padding and protection of bony prominences under general anesthesia is important to avoid post-operative complications.
- Cardiovascular support should be provided when necessary. Mean arterial pressure can be lower than in adults, but the heart rate should be higher than 50 beats per minute.
- Controlled ventilation should be initiated if $ETCO_2$ is above 50–60 mmHg. This scenario is very common under general anesthesia, regardless of the technique used (injectable vs inhalant). Foals tend to hypoventilate and become hypoxemic if ventilatory support and oxygen supplementation are not provided.
- Body temperature should be monitored and every effort should be made to minimize heat loss.
- Blood glucose should be monitored for long procedures and for sick foals. If hypoglycemia is present, supplement intravenous fluids with 2–5% dextrose.
- During recovery, the foal should be kept warm. Assisted recovery is recommended for neonates and pediatric patients.

FURTHER READING

Bidwell LA (2010) How to anesthetize donkeys for surgical procedures in the field. *Proceedings of the 56th Annual Convention of the American Association of Equine Practitioners*, Baltimore, pp. 38–40.

Doherty T, Valverde A (2006) *Manual of Equine Anesthesia and Analgesia*, Blackwell Publishing, Ames.

Matthews NS (2009) Anesthesia and analgesia for donkeys and mules. In: *Equine Anesthesia Monitoring and Emergency Therapy*, 2nd edn. (eds Muir WW, Hubbell JAE), Saunders Elsevier, St. Louis, pp. 353–357.

Matthews NS, Peck KE, Mealey KL et al (1997) Pharmacokinetics and cardiopulmonary effects of guaifenesin in donkeys. *J Vet Pharmacol Ther* **20**:442–446.

Matthews NS, Taylor TS (2002) Anesthesia of donkeys and mules: How they differ from horses. *Proceedings of the 48th Annual Convention of the American Association of Equine Practitioners*, Orlando, pp. 110–112.

Matthews NS, van Loon JPAM (2013) Anaesthesia and analgesia of the donkey and the mule. *Equine Vet Educ* **25**:47–51.

Taylor EV, DVM, Baetge CL, Matthews NS et al (2008) Guaifenesin-ketamine-xylazine infusions to provide anesthesia in donkeys. *J Equine Vet Sci* **28**:295–300.

14.1 INTRODUCTION

Complications that arise during recovery from general anesthesia are a major contributor to perioperative equine fatalities. The recovery period is associated with the greatest risks.

- Recovery quality scoring systems (RQSSs) have been used to evaluate equine recoveries. There are 3 common forms of RQSSs:
  - A numerical rating.
  - Composite measure.
  - Visual analogue scale (VAS).
- A reliable, reproducible, and repeatable scoring system for recovery quality is a prerequisite to identifying factors contributing to poor quality and potentially fatal recoveries after general anesthesia. As of now there is no universally accepted RQSS.
- Perioperative fatality is reported to occur in 0.24 to 1.8% of horses with no systemic illness undergoing general anesthesia. Twenty-five to fifty percent of fatalities (euthanasia) occur as a direct result of injury sustained during recovery.
- In 2016, anesthesia/recovery related mortality was 1.1% for all cases, 0.9% for elective cases, 1.6% for colics and 0% for non-colic emergencies. Fractures and dislocations accounted for the majority (71.4%) of deaths.
- Risk factors for mortality include:
  - Increasing age.
  - ASA status.

- Fracture repair.
- After hours surgery.
- Absence of any premedication.
- Age of less than 1 month (neonates).
- Stress may also be a potential risk factor for death associated with anesthesia.
- Fractures remain responsible for the largest proportion of recovery-associated deaths.
- The use of acepromazine and intravenous anesthetic agent maintenance of anesthesia is associated with reduced risk.
- Recovery quality is associated with:
  - Body mass.
  - ASA status 3 and 4.
  - Duration of anesthesia.
  - Horse temperament.
  - After hours anesthesia.
  - Non-fatal complications in the immediate recovery period include postanesthetic myopathy/neuropathy and postanesthetic respiratory obstruction.

14.2 CATASTROPHIC INJURY

- In adult horses those aged 14 years or higher were at increased risk for death. Very old horses may develop osteoporosis increasing the risk of fracture, which is one of the most common causes of anesthetic-related death. Broodmares may be more prone to osteoporosis.
- Fracture repair was the surgery with the highest risk.
  - This may be related to the long duration of surgery which increases the risk. Other features of fracture cases may

DOI: 10.1201/9780429190940-14

include pain, previous hard exercise leading to stress, excitement, exhaustion, and dehydration. These conditions are less than ideal to handle the insult of surgery and anesthesia.
- Some fractures may be as a consequence of myopathy-induced pain or weakness.
- Fractures have been described as responsible for 26 to 64% of all anesthesia-related fatalities. A study in which dislocations were included increased the number to 71%.
- Long duration of anesthesia and surgery time contribute by causing:
  - Inadequate perfusion, hypoxia, and acid-base abnormalities.
  - Supporting blood pressure to maintain a MAP of > 70 mmHg may result in fewer deaths and reduce the severity of post-anesthetic myopathy.
- For horses undergoing colic surgery intra-operative mortality was positively associated with heart rate and packed cell volume (PCV) at admission, and inversely related to the severity of pain.
  - Post-operative mortality increased with increasing age and PCV at admission.
  - Draft horses, Thoroughbreds, and Thoroughbred-cross horses carried a significantly worse prognosis.
  - Cardiovascular compromise, level of pain, age, and breed are all associated with the risk of mortality in equine surgical colic cases. There is an increased likelihood of intra-operative mortality in horses that showed less severe signs of abdominal pain on admission to the hospital. This may reflect the extent of devitalization of bowel (pain reduces as ischemia becomes more advanced) and thus the severity and/or duration of vascular compromise and endotoxemia.
  - An alternative explanation is that horses showing moderate or severe pain generally undergo immediate surgery.

Surgery may be delayed in horses showing less obvious signs of pain.
- Reduced long-term prognosis is associated with increasing age, larger breeds of horse, and elevated PCV on admission to the hospital.

14.3   CARDIOPULMONARY ARREST

- Cardiac arrest in the anesthetized horse is responsible for approximately 30% of mortalities. Factors that may predispose to arrest are an excessively deep anesthetic plane leading to cardiovascular collapse and hypotension. Signs of impending arrest include:
  - Loss of palpebral and corneal reflexes, pupillary dilation.
  - Loss of anal pinch reflex.
  - Hypoventilation, < 4 breaths/min to apnea.
  - Tachypnea > 20 breaths/min.
  - Dyspnea or abnormal breathing pattern and agonal gasps.
  - Cyanosis, injected or gray to white mucous membranes, prolonged CRT of > 2.5 seconds.
  - Weak or irregular peripheral pulses, hypotension, MAP < 70 mmHg.
  - Rapid > 60 beats/min or slow < 25 beats/min heart rate, muffled or absent heart sounds.
  - Abnormal ECG, asystole.

14.4   CARDIOPULMONARY RESUSCITATION (CPR)

- A trained prepared team is needed along with appropriate supplies for successful resuscitation. Everything that is needed for resuscitation should be easily accessible. A well-organized crash cart should always be available and kept in the same place in the hospital, so it is easily found when needed.

- Prognosis for a successful outcome is poor in the adult due to the difficulty of performing effective CPR. The prognosis may be better for foals if they are not compromised by systemic illness.
- If the arrest occurs during anesthesia, discontinue anesthetic administration and consider reversal of anesthetic agents. If possible, corrections of major acid-base and electrolyte disturbances are advisable.

14.4.1 Basic Life Support

- Consists of intubation, ventilation, and chest compressions. This is the immediate response to cardiopulmonary arrest (CPA).
- Recognize the need for CPR and rapidly institute treatment.
- Intubate and start ventilation at a rate of 6 to 10 breaths/min. It is a common mistake to ventilate too frequently. Ventilatory rates higher than 10 to 12 breaths/min should be avoided as time spent without cardiac compressions in single-rescuer scenarios should be minimized and increased time with positive intrathoracic pressure will have a negative effect on hemodynamics.

- Start chest compressions at a rate of at least 100 per minute in foals, 80 in adult equines.
  - Compressions are best performed with the patient in lateral recumbency.
  - In the case of an adult horse, the compressor stands on the ventral aspect of the patient, facing the heart. Thoracic compressions are done by delivering a blow to the chest wall immediately posterior to the left elbow with the knee as a person drops from a standing or crouched position (**Figure 14.1**).
- In foals, chest compressions are performed much like for a large dog, applying compressions by hand over the thorax (see below).
- Change the person doing the chest compressions every 2 minutes, if possible, to maintain effective compressions. Knee drop compressions performed by adults is an exhausting endeavor.
- In adult horses compression rates of 80 per minute produced significantly greater blood flows and mean arterial blood pressures than did slower rates. The blood flows produced by 80 thoracic

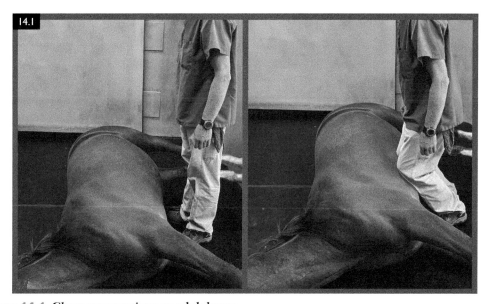

Figure 14.1 Chest compressions on adult horse

compressions/min were approximately 50% of those reported for deeply anaesthetized horses and while not sufficient to sustain life might be used to prolong life in order to facilitate distribution of resuscitative drugs to vital tissues.

- The lack of an applicable and practical electrical defibrillator for large animals dooms horses with ventricular fibrillation. If thoracic compressions are effective in producing blood flow to allow the distribution of cardiovascular stimulants to the myocardium and other vascular tissues, then short-term thoracic compressions would be of benefit, particularly in hypotensive and bradycardic horses and those in shock.

- The goal of cardiopulmonary resuscitation is to restore normal cardiopulmonary function, to provide time for resuscitative drug and fluid administration, and to distribute drugs to target tissues.

- Normal cardiac output in the resting conscious adult horse is 30–40 L/min. Cardiac output falls to 15–20 L/min in anesthetized horses. Increases in intrathoracic pressure, rather than direct compression of the heart are responsible for the blood flow.

- On a practical basis, the duration of application of thoracic compressions is limited by the endurance of the operator. Rising and dropping at a rate of 80 compressions/min is exhausting. In the absence of unlimited numbers of personnel, compressions can be applied for short periods only. Compressions during CPR is valuable in the adult horse, if only for facilitating the delivery of drugs to vital organs, most notably the heart.

- CPR is almost always a failure in adults once blood pressure becomes undetectable.

14.4.2 Advanced Life Support

- Consists of monitoring, emergency drugs, and defibrillation.
  - Monitoring.
    - The time to verify an absent pulse should be brief to avoid delaying the onset of CPR.
    - ECG analysis of an unresponsive patient may be used to identify arrhythmias requiring specific treatment.
      - The use of ECG to diagnose CPA must be done with caution as pulseless electrical activity can be mistaken for a perfusing rhythm. ECG analysis does enable the identification of rhythms that can be treated with defibrillation (i.e. ventricular fibrillation). Pauses in chest compressions to evaluate the ECG should be minimized to avoid the loss of intrathoracic pressure and blood flow.
      - End-tidal carbon dioxide ($EtCO_2$) monitoring is useful to identify return of spontaneous circulation (ROSC) and may be prognostic. $EtCO_2$ and $PaCO_2$ are indicative of pulmonary blood flow and cardiac output and therefore are prognostic indicators of effective CPR.
    - Monitoring after successful CPR should be tailored to each patient.
  - Drugs used for resuscitation.
    - Epinephrine: 0.01 mg/kg IV every 3 to 5 minutes.
    - No studies on the use of vasopressin have been done in the equine.
    - There is no evidence to support the use of atropine.
    - Drugs that could be given via intratracheal (IT) administration include epinephrine, vasopressin, and atropine. The absorption of these drugs has been shown to be effective during

anesthesia but the absorption during CPA is unknown. If given IT, the use of epinephrine should be increased 10-fold to 0.1 mg/kg. These drugs should be diluted in sterile water or saline and delivered via a catheter to at least the level of carina and ideally further down in the tracheal tree (**Figure 14.2**), followed by a manually delivered breath to help disperse the drug.

- Calcium gluconate, 10 to 20 mg/kg IV, can be used to counteract hyperkalemia, and hyperkalemia induced dysrhythmias, and to support blood pressure.
- Lidocaine, 1 to 2 mg/kg IV, is used to treat ventricular arrhythmias.
- Sodium bicarbonate, 0.5 mEq/kg IV, may considered for prolonged resuscitations.
- Defibrillation.
  - Rapid defibrillation is warranted in animals with observed progression to ventricular tachycardia (VT)

or ventricular fibrillation (V-fib). Defibrillation can be done in the foal but is not commonly attempted in the adult due to their large size and lack of adequate defibrillator effectiveness.

14.5   FOALS

- The first thing to do is to evaluate if the foal is suitable for CPR. Not all foals are suitable candidates for resuscitation due to severe congenital malformation, disease, or injury.
- In neonates, respiratory arrest usually precedes cardiac arrest. Hospitalized foals require resuscitation if the heart rate is less than 50 beats/min and falling or there is apnea. Decreases in venous oxygen saturation, $EtCO_2$, and muscle tone may be early signs of arrest.
- Cardiac arrest in neonatal foals is usually secondary to other systemic conditions, such as septic shock or respiratory failure, and not caused by primary cardiac failure.

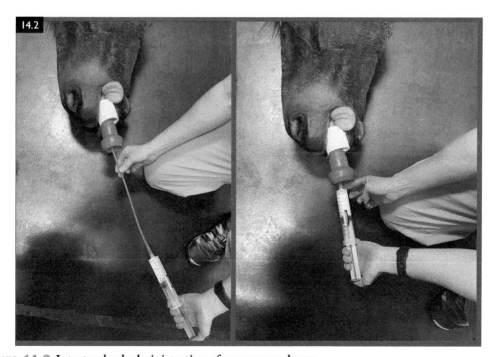

Figure 14.2 Intratracheal administration of emergency drugs

This explains why V-fib is not a common presenting arrhythmia. In the rare occasions where CPA is cardiac in origin, it is usually secondary to hypoxic-ischemic or cytokine-mediated myocardial damage, congenital cardiac defects, myocarditis, endocarditis with coronary artery embolism, or cardiac tamponade.

- If resuscitation is begun before a non-perfusing cardiac rhythm develops, the likelihood of revival is good (survival rate as high as 50%). If resuscitation efforts are delayed until after development of asystole, however, a less than 10% survival rate is to be expected.

- Place the foal in lateral recumbency on a hard, flat surface.

- The best way to ensure an adequate airway is to endotracheally intubate the foal. Intubation via the nose in the non-anesthetized foal is preferred to intubation via the mouth to prevent the foal chewing the tube if consciousness is regained. However, time is of the essence so only 2 quick attempts should be used for nasotracheal intubation after which the oral route should be used. A 55-cm long, cuffed endotracheal tube is recommended. The diameter of the tube should be matched with the size of the foal and be as large as possible to decrease the resistance to flow. As a rough rule, a 9 to 10 mm tube fits most newborn thoroughbred foals, whereas large Warmbloods may need tubes as large as 10 to 12 mm. Arabian and pony foals may need smaller tubes.

  - When an endotracheal tube is not immediately available, ventilation with a mask (**Figure 14.3**) or mouth-to-nose ventilation can be effective. The fact that foals are obligate nasal breathers makes these methods relatively effective. For both methods, the head and neck should be maximally extended to reduce the risk of aerophagia, which fills the stomach

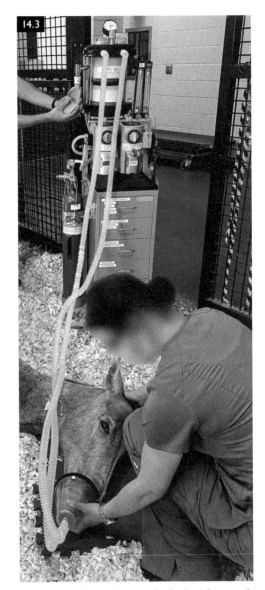

Figure 14.3 Ventilation of a foal with a mask

with gas and can prevent the lungs from fully expanding. For mouth-to-nose resuscitation, the opposite nostril should be held closed. While blowing into the nostril or squeezing the re-breathing bag one should observe the chest rising, ensuring that the air is reaching the lungs and that the tidal volume is adequate.

- Inspiratory time should be 1 second with a longer expiratory time, and a rate of 10 breaths per minute.
- The goal is to achieve normocapnia while avoiding arterial hypoxemia. Tidal volume is 10 ml/kg. Increased thoracic pressure induced by positive-pressure ventilation can interfere significantly with cardiac return and decreases coronary and cerebral perfusion. The peak inspiratory pressure should be between 10 and 20 cmH$_2$O to avoid increased intrathoracic pressure.
- The foal should be reassessed 30 seconds after starting the ventilation.
- Thoracic compressions should be started if the heartbeat is absent or less than 50 beats per minute.
  - The person performing the thoracic compressions should kneel parallel to the foal's spine and place his or her hands on top of each other, just caudal to the foal's triceps, at the highest point of the thorax (**Figure 14.4**).

- The shoulders should be directly above the hands, enabling use of the body weight to help compress the thorax. This helps to deliver enough force and also to reduce resuscitator fatigue (**Figure 14.5**).
- Defibrillation in the foal is similar to the technique done in large dogs. Defibrillator paste is applied to the paddles. Paddles are placed firmly on opposite sides of the thorax at the level of the costochondral junction. In foals in lateral recumbency, a posterior paddle is placed on the down side and the hand paddle on the up side.
  - Once the machine is set, the person using the defibrillator announces an audible "clear" and visually ensures all personnel including the one providing the shock are not in contact with the table or the patient.
  - One single shock is provided after which chest compressions and ventilation should immediately resume. ECG should only be evaluated after one cardiac compression cycle (2 minutes)

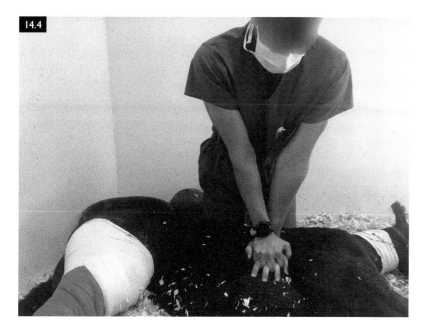

Figure 14.4 Kneeling next to foal for thoracic compressions
Courtesy of Dr. Jessica Bramski

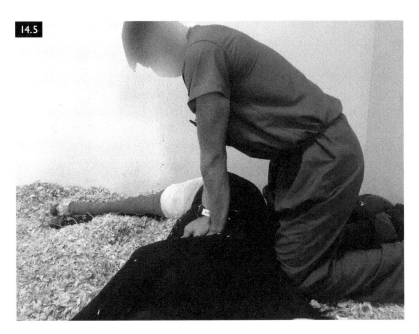

Figure 14.5 Shoulders directly over hands for chest compressions
Courtesy of Dr. Jessica Bramski

is complete and then determine if a second defibrillation is necessary. The dose is 2 to 4 J/kg (100–200 J/50 kg foal), increasing the energy by 50% with each defibrillation attempt.

- Ventilation should be stopped when the heart rate is greater than 60 beats/min in the foal, and spontaneous breathing is well established. This can be tested by stopping ventilation and disconnecting the bag for 30 seconds. The first few breaths may be gasping but after these the foal should have a respiratory rate greater than 16 breaths/min, a regular respiratory pattern, and normal respiratory effort.
- Chest compressions should be continued until a regular heartbeat of more than 60 beats/min has been established. There should be no lag period between the stopping of support and the onset of a spontaneous heartbeat.
  - When testing for adequacy of heartbeat, CPR should not be stopped for longer than 10 seconds at a time. Clinical experience suggests that if spontaneous

circulation and respiration are not present after 10 minutes, then survival is unlikely.

14.6   POST-CARDIAC ARREST CARE

- Organ perfusion should be optimized with fluid therapy and possibly inotropes and vasopressors. Dobutamine, 0.5 to 5 µg/kg/min IV, is the most commonly used inotrope in equine medicine. This drug also has chronotropic effects. Dobutamine is used to help maintain cardiac output and arterial blood pressure.
- Aim for normoxemia, not hyperoxemia.
- Mild hypothermia may be beneficial in the early post-resuscitation period.
- Myocardial stunning, a reversible phenomenon that happens early after global myocardial ischemia in which left and right ventricular ejection fractions decrease and end diastolic pressure increases, may contribute to the hemodynamic dysfunction. Patients suffering from this generally respond to inotropic therapy.

- The goal of post-cardiac arrest care is to avoid hypotension and maintain adequate perfusion to the tissues.
  - Perfusion depends on blood flow not blood pressure alone.
  - It is advisable to not only monitor blood pressure but also to measure global perfusion metrics such as central venous oxygen saturation ($ScvO_2$) and blood lactate.

FURTHER READING

Doherty T, Valverde A (2006) Complications and emergencies. In: *Manual of Equine Anesthesia & Analgesia* (eds Doherty T, Valverde A), Blackwell Publishing, Ames, IA, pp. 305–337.

Dugdale AHA, Obbrai J, Cripps PJ (2016) Twenty years later: a single-centre, repeat retrospective analysis of equine perioperative mortality and investigation of recovery quality. *Vet Anaesth Analg* **41**:171–178.

Dugdale AHA, Taylor PM (2016) Equine anaesthesia-associated mortality: Where are we now? *Vet Anaesth Analg* **43**:242–255.

Farmer E, Chase-Topping M, Lawson H, Clutton RE (2014) Factors affecting the perception of recovery quality of horses after anesthesia. *Equine Vet J* **46**:328–332.

Hubbell JAE, Muir WW, Gaynor JS (1993) Cardiovascular effects of thoracic compression in horses subjected to euthanasia. *Equine Vet J* **25**:282–284.

Johnston GM, Eastment JK, Wood JLN, Taylor PM (2002) The confidential enquiry into perioperative equine fatalities (CEPEF): mortality results of Phases 1 and 2. *Vet Anaesth Analg* **29**:159–170.

Jokisalo JM, Corley KTT (2014) CPR in the neonatal foal, has RECOVER changed our approach? *Vet Clin North Am Equine Pract* **30**:301–316.

Proudman CJ, Dugdale AHA, Senior JM et al (2006) Pre-operative and anaesthesia-related risk factors for mortality in equine colic cases. *Vet J* **171**:89–97.

Suthers JM, Christley RM, Clutton RE (2011) Quantitative and qualitative comparison of three scoring systems for assessing recovery quality after general anesthesia in horses. *Vet Anaesth Analg* **38**:352–362.

15.1 INTRODUCTION

Respectful and humane treatment at the end of life is just as important as during the course of it. Veterinarians provide leadership in most aspects of the prevention and relief of animal suffering, and this extends to the matter of humane taking of animal life. The American Veterinary Medical Association (AVMA) has convened a Panel on Euthanasia (POE) since 1963 to evaluate methods and create guidelines for veterinarians who carry out or oversee the euthanasia of animals. Although it initially focused on dogs, cats, and small mammals, since 1993 the POE has included recommendations for horses as well. The following summary is based on the most recent (2020) edition of the AVMA POE guidelines for equids.

15.2 GENERAL CONSIDERATIONS

- Personnel safety
  - Unpredictable falling or thrashing is a risk in euthanizing any equid. There may also be exaggerated muscle movements after the fall, which may pose significant danger. All personnel should be vigilant during the euthanasia process, and care must be taken to avoid undue risk of exposure.
- Disposition of remains
  - The veterinarian is advised to consult federal, state, and local regulations regarding disposal of remains. As a general guideline, when pentobarbital is used, disposal must be prompt

to avoid poisoning of wildlife and domestic animals with barbiturate residues. On-farm burial, incineration/cremation, commercial rendering, direct haul to a solid waste landfill, and biodigestion are all acceptable disposal methods.

15.3 ACCEPTABLE METHODS OF EUTHANASIA

- Barbiturates or barbituric acid derivatives
  - Pentobarbital 100 mg/kg IV alone or in combination with other agents is the euthanasia method of choice. Due to the large volume required, administration through an intravenous (IV) catheter placed in the jugular vein is recommended. The use of acepromazine, $\alpha2$ adrenergic receptor agonists and/or opioids may facilitate restraint in fractious patients, but may also prolong the time to loss of consciousness due to effects on cardiac output.

15.4 ACCEPTABLE METHODS OF EUTHANASIA WITH CONDITIONS

- Penetrating captive bolt and gunshot
  - These methods are only to be used by well-trained personnel with well-maintained firearms. The animal must be adequately restrained and personnel protected from the ricochet from free bullets. The site of entry should be centered at the intersection of two

DOI: 10.1201/9780429190940-15

diagonal lines each running from the outer corner of the eye to the base of the opposite ear (**Figure 15.1**).

15.5   ADJUNCTIVE METHODS

- Adjunctive methods of euthanasia can be used after the horse has been anesthetized. Use of these methods in an awake patient is unacceptable. Following induction of anesthesia using traditionally used injectable agents (e.g., xylazine, ketamine) euthanasia is completed by one of the following:

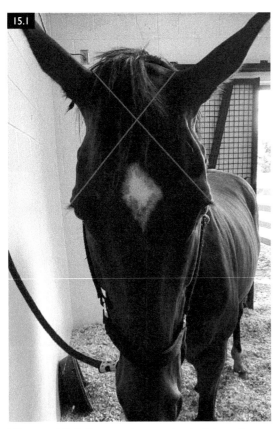

Figure 15.1 **Penetrating captive bolt/gunshot target—the site of entry should be centered at the intersection of two diagonal lines each running from the outer corner of the eye to the base of the opposite ear**

- Potassium Chloride at 75–150 mg/kg IV or intracardiac injection with rapid administration.
- Magnesium sulfate (supersaturated solution) at 1–2 ml/kg IV.
- Lidocaine 2% at 4 mg/kg intrathecal injection, over 30 seconds.

15.6   EXCEPTIONS IN CASE OF EMERGENCY

- Neuromuscular blocking agents (NMBAs)
  - Serious injury at a racetrack or other event may necessitate immediate euthanasia of a horse that is too difficult and dangerous to obtain IV access in. Sedation may have a prolonged onset, and the horse may injure itself or others before it takes effect. Under these circumstances, intramuscular or IV injection of an NMBA such as succinylcholine may be used to control the horse, immediately followed by an appropriate euthanasia method. NMBAs alone are not acceptable methods.

15.7   AVOIDING EUTHANASIA PITFALLS

Not only is euthanasia a part of equine practice, it also is a very difficult and emotional procedure for horse owners to experience. The following is a checklist for veterinarians to use in order to ensure that it goes as quickly, smoothly, and safely as possible.

- Use a large-sized needle (14 gauge) or intravenous catheter with an extension set when a horse is being euthanized.
  - An average sized adult horse (450 kg or 1000 lb) requires 120 ml of euthanasia solution to be euthanized, and it is important that this volume be administered quickly.

- To facilitate this process, two 60 ml syringes should be used because they are easy for the veterinarian to handle and exchange.
- The large-sized needle and extension set allow the veterinarian to increase the speed of administration of the euthanasia solution.
- If the solution is given too slowly, the horse may collapse before the entire amount is given, requiring the veterinarian to administer the rest of the solution while the horse is down. Under such circumstances, the horse may continue to move, which will make the jugular vein difficult to access. As a result, the entire procedure will become more dangerous than necessary.
- Sedate the horse before administering the euthanasia solution.
  - It is ideal for the horse to be relaxed before the large needle is placed in the jugular vein for administration of the euthanasia solution. To achieve this level of sedation, 0.5–0.8 mg/kg of xylazine should be given IV. Heavier sedation with a larger volume of xylazine or with detomidine should be avoided because the subsequent reduction in cardiac output will make it take longer for the euthanasia solution to have its full effect.
- Always have an extra bottle of euthanasia solution, extra needles, and syringes on hand when you euthanize a horse.
  - If extra solution or supplies are needed during the euthanasia procedure, they should be immediately available, not in your truck.
- It is essential to have the assistance of an experienced horse handler while the euthanasia solution is being administered by the veterinarian.
  - The horse handler needs to be comfortable around horses and capable

of safely holding a horse's halter and lead rope during the procedure.
- A veterinarian should not attempt to euthanize a horse when alone. This is not safe for the veterinarian and the potential for something to go wrong increases greatly.
- The horse handler should hold the horse's head in its normal position (**Figure 15.2**) and help keep the horse still while the sedative and the euthanasia solution are being administered. Holding the horse's head too high or too low will hinder a smooth injection into the jugular vein.
- Once the entire amount of euthanasia solution is injected, there is typically enough time for the horse handler to safely move away and the veterinarian to hold the horse's halter and lead rope when the horse falls.
- Give the entire amount of euthanasia solution intravenously.
  - If any of the euthanasia solution becomes visible subcutaneously during the injection, the needle should immediately be removed and placed in the opposite jugular vein.
  - Euthanasia solution given extravascularly can be very irritating to the horse.
  - It is also important that the entire amount of solution be given IV so the veterinarian knows how much solution the horse has received and can better predict the outcome of the procedure.
- If the horse has a cardiac murmur, additional euthanasia solution may be needed.
  - An additional 60 ml of euthanasia solution should be drawn up and ready to administer when a horse with a heart murmur is being euthanized.
  - It is also common for horses with heart issues to have a rougher euthanasia

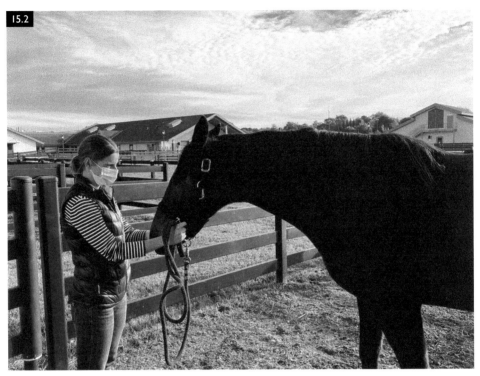

Figure 15.2 Horse head held in normal position

(falling over backwards, longer time to pass away after the solution is given, etc.). If the client wishes to stay during the euthanasia procedure it is best to warn them of this possibility.

- Never remove the halter and lead rope until after the horse is deceased.
  - This would seem to be common sense, but there have been numerous occasions when a handler or owner has removed the halter and lead rope while the euthanasia solution is being given. While they are trying to be helpful, this is very dangerous. The owner and handler should be gently told that the halter and lead rope will be removed after the horse has died. It is important to have a way of restraining the horse in a safe position until the animal falls to the ground and is determined to be deceased.

- When a horse is on the ground, never auscultate the heart when standing near the horse's legs.
  - A horse can make sudden movements or violent jerks after the euthanasia solution has been given which may result in the veterinarian being kicked. Therefore, it is important to always auscultate the chest while leaning across the horse's back rather than standing between the horse's legs.
- Avoid having extra people or animals in the immediate area where the horse is being euthanized.
  - It is the veterinarian's responsibility to keep any observers or other animals at a safe distance during the euthanasia procedure, as horses may take several steps in any direction or may lunge forward or backward quickly.
  - Similarly, other animals, such as dogs and cats, must be kept away both during

the euthanasia process (so they are not accidentally stepped on) and after the horse is deceased. There is a concern that other pets may lick the horse's neck where the euthanasia solution was injected, which potentially could be fatal to a dog or cat.

- The horse should be covered with a tarp or sheet until the horse is either buried or hauled away for disposal.

- Do not euthanize a horse directly next to the hole that has been dug for the horse to be buried.
  - It is often unpredictable where the horse will fall once euthanized. Consequently, it is possible for the horse to accidentally step into the hole before all of the euthanasia solution has been administered, which would be harmful to itself and others. If the burial hole has been dug before the horse is euthanized, a spot several yards away should be selected for the euthanasia procedure. The horse can then be moved to the hole using a tractor or backhoe.
  - Ideally, if the horse is to be buried, it is best to euthanize the horse first, and then have the burial hole dug next to the horse.

- Use extra caution when euthanizing a horse on a trailer.
  - Whenever possible, avoid euthanizing a horse on a trailer as this can be very dangerous for the veterinarian and the handler.
  - If this is unavoidable, make sure there is an escape door on the trailer for the horse handler and the veterinarian to use in case the horse rears or falls sideways.
  - Plan to use adequate sedation to ensure that the horse is as calm and relaxed as possible. It is advisable to premedicate the horse with a sedative given IM and IV, as mentioned previously.

- If you do not have an adequate amount of euthanasia solution with you, do not attempt to euthanize the horse.
  - Call another veterinarian to help or pick up more euthanasia solution from your office or from another veterinarian's office. If the euthanasia procedure can be rescheduled to ensure that sufficient euthanasia solution is on hand, plan to do this.
  - Do not be tempted to use other medications or solutions to euthanize a horse. It is very important that the euthanasia procedure be as painless and smooth as possible.

- The veterinarian should not leave the farm until the horse's heartbeat can no longer be auscultated and there is an absence of a corneal reflex.
  - If 120 ml of euthanasia solution has been given and a heartbeat is still audible 5–10 minutes later, the veterinarian should administer another 60 ml of euthanasia solution intravenously. This can be repeated if necessary.

15.8   EUTHANASIA COUNSELING

- It is often necessary for veterinarians in equine practice to counsel clients about euthanizing a horse. A typical scenario the equine veterinarian may face is that of a geriatric horse that has gradually deteriorated with age. Most owners find it very difficult to make the choice for a planned euthanasia in such situations on their own, and many look to their veterinarian for guidance.
  - If possible, a geriatric horse should be euthanized as a scheduled appointment and not as an emergency situation. The concept of a planned euthanasia is difficult for many owners to appreciate. However, if the benefits of a planned euthanasia are explained, many owners will decide

that this is their preferred route for their beloved equine companion.

- Many chronic health conditions in a geriatric horse justify recommending a planned euthanasia. These include significant weight loss, chronic diarrhea, difficulty walking or getting up, metabolic disease, neurologic disease or other debilitating, painful conditions such as uveitis, laminitis, or severe degenerative joint disease.
  - Many horse owners naturally humanize these situations and feel guilty about considering euthanasia even though they recognize the severity of their horse's condition. This can be an excellent opportunity for veterinarians to help horse owners realize that their decision needs to be based on what is best for their animal and not based on what is less painful or easier for them to manage.
  - Sometimes these chronic conditions are not treatable, or are difficult and expensive to treat. A planned euthanasia can also avoid an emergency situation, such as a painful colic episode or a recumbent horse that cannot get to its feet, both of which would require an emergency euthanasia.
- Veterinarians should suggest that owners make a few important considerations before euthanizing their horse:
  - Does the owner want to be present during the euthanasia procedure?
    - The author's recommendation would be for the owner to stay with the horse until the horse is sedated, then leave before the euthanasia solution is given. When a horse falls after the solution is given, this is very upsetting to the owner and it is best for them not to be present.
    - It is also unpredictable how smoothly the horse will go down. Sometimes horses lunge forward or backward, which can be very disturbing for an owner to witness. It is usually explained

to the owner that this is not a memory they want to have, and recommended that they leave the rest of the euthanasia process to the veterinarian.

- Will the horse be buried on the property? Or will the horse be picked up and disposed of by a rendering company?
  - Ideally, the veterinarian should be able to share with the owner contact information for businesses that own and operate the equipment used to dig a hole large enough to bury a horse.
  - It should be the horse owner's responsibility to call one of these companies to schedule the equipment to arrive about one hour after the horse is scheduled to be euthanized. This will allow the hole to be dug in proximity to where the horse has been euthanized, and the owner doesn't need to see the horse after it is deceased.
  - If owners have pre-arranged plans for either disposal or burial of their horse, this makes the process much smoother and they will also be prepared for the cost associated with these services.
- When dealing with younger healthy horses, it may still be important for the farm veterinarian to discuss with owners the circumstances of euthanasia. The main goal of this discussion is to establish the best process to pursue in case of an emergency situation which may require referral to a hospital facility or possibly euthanasia.
  - This discussion should occur during a stress-free, routine farm appointment and should focus on determining whether the horse owner would consider referring the horse to a hospital for an emergency procedure (such as colic surgery).
  - This degree of preparation will also prevent wasting precious time and avoiding the need to make a hard decision, such as euthanasia, during a high stress moment.

- As a veterinarian, it's always best to leave the ultimate decision to the horse owner, while playing an advisory role if they ask for it. The veterinarian should not assume what a client would or wouldn't do in an emergency situation. Furthermore, it is very important to be supportive, regardless of the decision made.

FURTHER READING

Aleman M, Davis E, Williams DC, Madigan JE, Smith F, Guedes A (2015) Electrophysiologic study of a method of euthanasia using intrathecal lidocaine hydrochloride administered during intravenous anesthesia in horses. *J Vet Intern Med* **29**:1676–1682.

American Veterinary Medical Association (2020) *AVMA Guidelines for the Euthanasia of Animals*, AVMA, Schaumburg, IL.

CHEMISTRY

Fibrinogen	100–400 mg/dl
Urea nitrogen	9–27 mg/dl
Total protein	5.1–8.2 g/dl
Albumin	2.0–3.7 g/dl
Glucose	55–123 mg/dl
Globulin	2.62–4.04 g/dL
Serum amyloid A	0–2.0 mg/dL
Total bilirubin	0.10–3.50 mg/dl
Bilirubin direct	0.0–0.4 mg/dL
Bilirubin indirect	0.2–2.0 mg/dL
Bile acids	0.0–15.0 µmol/L
GGT	3–54 U/L
SDH	1.0–8.0 U/L
AST	153–409 U/L
ALP	84–395 U/L
SGOT	157–253 U/L
Lactic dehydrogenase	100–412 U/L
Sorbitol dehydrongenase	3.3–15.5 U/L
Alanaine amino transferase	5–13 U/L
Amylase	1–5 U/L
Anion Gap	10–24
Triglycerides	10–61 mg/dl
Cholesterol	59–189 mg/dl
Creatine kinase	92–548 U/L
Fructosamine (non-diabetic animals)	227–347 µmol/L
Betahydroxybutyrate	1.2–4.4 mg/dL
Bicarbonate	21–33 mmol/L
Bile Acids, post-prandial or non-fasting	1.2–4.4 µmol/L
Globulin	2.3–5.3 g/dL
Haptoglobin	0.01–0.17 mg/dL
Insulin	0.5–10.0 uU/ml
Lactate	0.60–7.97 mmol/L
Lipase	10–32 U/L
Total T4	0.5–3.1 µg/dL
Uric acid	0.1–0.6 mg/dL

CBC

WBC	4.1–14.3 × 10^3/µl
RBC	5.63–12.09 × 10^6/µl
HGB	9.8–17.2 g/dl
HCT	26.3–47.5%
MCV	33.5–55.8 fl
MCH	12.2–19.3 pg
MCHC	32.4–43.1 g/dl
RDW	20.6–29.0 %
Platelets	95–385 × 10^3/µl
MPV	5.0–7.5 fl
Segmented neutrophils	1.700–10.400 × 10^3/µl
Band neutrophils	0.000–0.100 × 10^3/µl
Lymphocytes	0.600–6.700 × 10^3/µl
Monocytes	0.000–0.900 × 10^3/µl
Eosinophils	0.000–0.780 × 10^3/µl
Basophils	0.000–0.300 × 10^3/µl
Nucleated RBC	0–5/100 WBC
PCV Hot-blooded horse	32–53%
PCV Cold-blooded horse	24–44%

ELECTROLYTES AND BLOOD GAS

Sodium	130–146 mmol/L
Potassium	2.2–5.5 mmol/L
Chloride	93–109 mmol/L
Bicarbonate	20–28 mmol/L
Anion gap	6–15 mEq/L
Creatinine	0.3–1.8 mg/dl
Calcium	10.3–13.6 mg/dl
Iron	73–213 µg/dL

DOI: 10.1201/9780429190940-16

Magnesium	1.5–2.8 mg/dL
Phosphorus	1.4–5.9 mg/dL
Osmolality	270–300 mOsm/kg
pH	7.32–7.44
PCO$_2$	38–46 mmHg
TCO$_2$	24–32 mEq/L

COAGULATION

Antithrombin III	10–1000 %
APTT	33.0–55.0 seconds
Fibrinogen (quantitative)	100–400 mg/dL
Fibrinogen (semi-quantitative)	100–400 mg/dL
PT	9.1–12.6 seconds

REFERENCES

Smith BP (2015) *Large Animal Internal Medicine*, 5th edn., Elsevier, Amsterdam.

Muir E, Hubbell J (2009) *Equine Anesthesia*, 2nd edn, Elsevier, Amsterdam.

Plumb's Veterinary Drug Handbook (2018) Wiley-Blackwell. https://www.wiley.com/en-us/Plumb%27s+Veterinary+Drug+Handbook%3A+Desk%2C+9th+Edition-p-9781119344452.

UGA College of Veterinary Medicine Clinical Laboratory (2018) https://vet.uga.edu/diagnostic-service-labs/veterinary-diagnostic-laboratory/.

STANDING RESTRAINT/SEDATION

Drug	Dose mg/kg IV	Doses mg/kg IM
Xylazine	0.3–1.0	0.2–1.1 sedation outlasts analgesia
Detomidine	0.005–0.02	0.005–0.04
Romifidine	0.03–0.1	
Xylaxzine	0.4–1.0	
Butorphanol	0.02–0.05	0.04–0.1
Romifidine	0.04–0.1	
± Butorphanol	0.02–0.05	
Detomidine	0.025–0.02	
Butorphanol	0.02–0.03	
Detomidine	0.004	
Xylazine	given 3 to 5 minutes after detomidine 0.5–0.8	
Acepromazine	0.02–0.04	0.02–0.05
Butorphanol	0.02–0.03	
Xylazine	0.2–0.6	
Xylazine	0.5–1.0	
Morphine	0.15–0.7 maximum total dose 300 mg, give slowly	0.25 co-administration with sedatives can minimize excitement, especially at higher doses
Xylazine	0.6–1.1	
Pentazocine	0.3–0.5 for sedation in foals	
Acepromazine	0.04	
Meperidine	0.6 maximum total dose 300 mg, give slowly	1–2
Acepromazine	0.04	
Methadone	0.1	0.1
Acepromazine	0.04	
Hydromorphone	0.02	0.02–0.04
Acepromazine	0.04	
Butorphanol	0.02	

DOI: 10.1201/9780429190940-17

Drug	Dose mg/kg IV	Doses mg/kg IM
Xylazine	0.6	
Buprenorphine	0.01	
Acepromazine	0.02	
Xylazine	0.5	
Acepromazine	0.02	
Xlyazine	0.6	
Pentazocine	0.3	
Detomidine	0.0025–0.004	
Buprenorphine	0.01	
Detomidine	0.0025–0.005	
Morphine	0.15–0.6 maximum dose 300 mg, give slowly	
Acepromazine	0.02	
Detomidine	0.0025–0.005	
Acepromazine	0.02	
Detomidine	0.0025–0.005	
Butorphanol	0.02–0.05	
Diazepam/midazolam	0.05–0.1 for sedation of neonatal foals	

INDUCTION FOR GENERAL ANESTHESIA FOLLOWING PREMEDICATION/SEDATION

Drug	Dose mg/kg IV
Thiopental	5–8
Ketamine	2.2
Guaifenesin	25–100 perivascular necrosis if not IV
Ketamine	1.7
Ketamine	2.2
Diazepam/midazolam	0.02–0.1
Propofol	0.4
Ketamine	2.2 following propofol
Tiletamine/zolazepam	0.5–2.0

TOTAL INTRAVENOUS ANESTHESIA (TIVA): FOLLOWING STANDARD INDUCTION

Drugs	Doses mg/kg IV	Comments
Xylazine	0.35	
Ketamine	0.7	Give both 8–12 minutes after the initial ketamine induction, repeat every 10–12 minutes for 2 to 3 times.

Guaifenesin/ketamine/xylazine constant rate infusion (CRI) or "triple drip". Add 650 mg xylazine and 1300 mg of ketamine to 1 liter of 5% guaifenesin. Infusion rate 2 ml/kg/hr IV, increase or decrease based on effect. Start immediately after induction of anesthesia. Jugular catheter is required when using guaifenesin.
Guaifenesin/ketamine/romifidine CRI, add 25 mg romifidine and 1000 mg ketamine to 1 L of 5% guaifenesin. Infusion rate 2 ml/kg/hr IV, increase or decrease to effect. Start immediately after induction of anesthesia. Jugular catheter is required when using guaifenesin.
Midazolam, 0.002 mg/kg/min plus ketamine 0.03 mg/kg/min plus xylazine 0.016 mg/kg/min has been use for TIVA.

ADJUNCTIVE DRUGS TO DECREASE THE LEVEL OF INHALANT, PARTIAL INTRAVENOUS ANESTHESIA (PIVA)

Drug	Dose IV
Xylazine	0.5–1.0 mg/kg/hr
Dexmedetomidine	0.0005–0.001 mg/kg/hr for 2 hours, may develop colic signs and decreased GI motility, may give prophylactic oral oil.
Ketamine	0.5–3.0 mg/kg/hr, can be used in the awake horse to provide analgesia at 0.4–1.2 mg/kg/hr
Lidocaine	1–2 mg/kg loading dose followed by 3–6 mg/kg/hr. Discontinue CRI 30 minutes before recovery to minimize possible ataxia.

Lidocaine, ketamine, and xylazine CRI's can be used simultaneously in the same horse for increased reduction in the inhalant levels.

POST-OPERATIVE DRUGS TO ASSIST IN SEDATION FOR RECOVERY

Drug	Dose mg/kg IV	Comments
Xylazine	0.1–0.2	Give 5–10 minutes after cessation of general anesthesia
Romifidine	0.01–0.02	Give 5–10 minutes after cessation of general anesthesia. May provide less ataxia than xylazine or detomidine in recovery.
Acepromazine	2–3 mg total dose	May be given in addition to an alpha 2 agonist

REVERSAL DRUGS

Drug	Dose mg/kg	Comments
Opioid Antagonists and agonist-antagonists		
Naloxone	0.01 IM, IV, intratracheal	Reverses all effects of opioids Limited data available. Titrate to effect
Butorphanol	0.02 IM, IV	Partial reversal of pure mu opioids Titrate to effect
Alpha 2 antagonists		
Tolazoline	2–4 mg/kg slow IV	
Yohimbine	0.12–0.25 IM, slow IV	
Atipamezole	0.15 or same volume as dexmedetomidine, IM preferred route, if IV give slowly	Titrate to effect

NON-STEROIDAL ANTI-INFLAMMATORY DRUGS

Flunixin	0.5–1.1 IV, can also be given orally, interval 12–24 hours. Not to be given IM	
Phenylbutazone	2.2–4.4 IV, can also be given orally, interval 12–24 hours	
Firocoxib	0.1 IV, can also be given orally, interval 24 hours	
Meloxicam	0.6 orally, interval 24 hours	

DRUGS USED FOR CAUDAL EPIDURAL ANALGESIA

Single drugs		
Lidocaine	0.2 mg/kg, duration 0.5–1.5 hrs, volume is 5–8 ml, not exceed 10 ml per 500 kg horse to avoid rostral spread and adverse effects	
Ropivacaine	0.8 mg/kg, duration 3 hrs, volume not to exceed 10 ml per 500 kg horse to avoid rostral spread and adverse effects	
Bupivacaine	0.04–0.06 mg/kg, duration 3.5–5 hrs, volume 5–8 ml, 0.25% concentration preferred	
Xylazine	0.03–0.35 mg/kg, duration 1–2 hrs	
Detomidine	0.01–0.06 mg/kg, duration 2–4 hrs	
Morphine	0.05–0.2 mg/kg, duration 3–8 hrs, dilute with preservative-free normal saline to 20–30 mls maximum volume in 450 kg horse, may cause pruritus	
Methadone	0.1 mg/kg, duration 5 hrs, dilute with preservative-free normal saline to 20–30 mls maximum volume in a 450 kg horse	
Combinations		
Lidocaine	0.22 mg/kg	
Xylazine	0.17 mg/kg, duration 4–6 hrs	

Lidocaine	2%, 5–8 mls
Morphine	0.1–0.2 mg/kg, duration 6–12 hrs
Xylazine	0.1–0.2 mg/kg
Morphine	0.1–0.2 mg/kg, duration 12–18 hrs
Detomidine	0.01–0.03 mg/kg
Morphine	0.1–0.2 mg/kg, duration 24–48 hrs

REFERENCES

Doherty T, Valverde A. (2006) *Manual of Equine Anesthesia & Analgesia*, Blackwell Publishing, Ames.

Muir E, Hubbell J (2009) *Equine Anesthesia*, 2nd edn, Elsevier, Amsterdam.

Sanchez LC, Robertson SA (2014) Pain control in horses: What do we really know? *Equi Vet J* **46**(4):517–523.

Page numbers in *italics* indicate a figure and page numbers in **bold** indicate a table on the corresponding page.

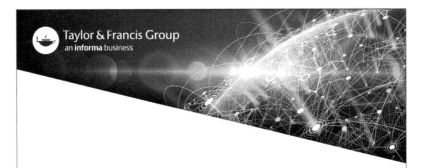